Laboratory Tests
and
Diagnostic Procedures
in Medicine

John H. Dirckx, M.D.

D0126597

Health Professions Institute

Modesto, California

2004

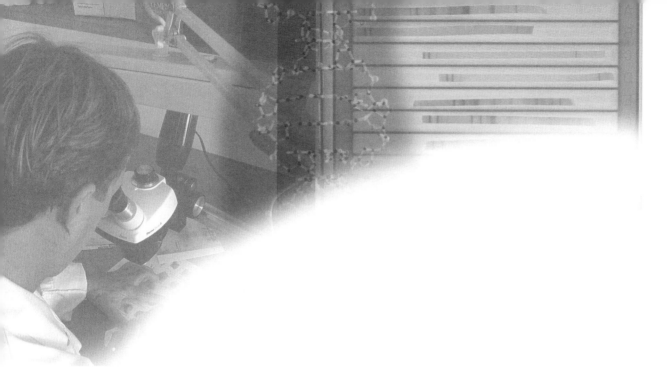

Laboratory Tests and Diagnostic Procedures in Medicine

by John H. Dirckx, M.D.

Cover design by Harrison Aquino E.

Published by
Health Professions Institute
P. O. Box 801
Modesto, CA 95353
Phone 209-551-2112
Fax 209-551-0404
Web site: http://www.hpisum.com
E-mail: hpi@hpisum.com
Sally Crenshaw Pitman, Editor & Publisher

Printed by
Parks Printing & Lithograph
Modesto, California

ISBN: 0-934385-49-1

Last digit is the print number: 9 8 7 6 5 4 3

For my daughter Janet,

with love

Contents

Preface

The purpose of this book is to bring together, in a single reference work, useful information on the broad range of special diagnostic examinations and laboratory tests that form an integral part of modern medicine. The book is designed for the use of medical transcriptionists and other professional handlers of health-care records and data, including legal and insurance personnel, technical writers and editors, and journalists.

Material is included here on six principal types of diagnostic procedure: physical measurements, electrodiagnostics, endoscopy, medical imaging, anatomic pathology, and clinical pathology. For each test or procedure, sufficient information is provided about methodology, indications or purposes, and range of results to enable the reader to recognize pertinent terminology and to grasp the general sense of a report. Because the book is intended for persons who are charged neither with performing diagnostic procedures nor with interpreting their results, details and technicalities that are irrelevant for that audience have been rigorously excluded. Normal ranges and other interpretive data are given solely for purposes of orientation or clarification and should not be applied to actual test results.

The style of presentation presupposes some basic knowledge of medicine, including particularly human anatomy, physiology, and pathology, as well as some familiarity with the terminology of those fields. Procedures have been grouped or classified principally by method or technical basis, and only secondarily by body system or type of disease.

The organization of material follows a logical developmental sequence so as to render the work suitable for use as a textbook. The workbook format is intended to augment and enhance the student's learning experience, whether the book is used for independent study or as an adjunct in a formal academic course. Because each division (sections, chapters, and discussions of individual tests) is more or less self-contained, the book can also be used strictly as a reference work. Cross-references between chapters have been kept to a minimum. The resulting occasional repetition of material already presented in a previous section provides an automatic review and reinforcement of learning when the book is read as a text.

It is a pleasure to acknowledge Sally Pitman's encouragement and technical support at every stage of the preparation of this book and to thank Ellen Drake for making valuable suggestions and for preparing the exercises and answer keys. Special thanks to Linda Campbell for compiling the table of normal lab values and helping the artist select appropriate medical images for graphic design.

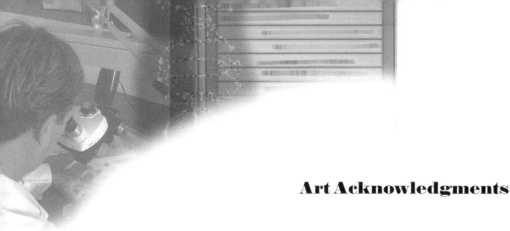

Art Acknowledgments

Illustrations of anatomy of the heart, conducting system of the heart, sample electrocardiogram with intervals, respiratory system, fiberoptic bronchoscopy, digestive system, gastroscope, cystoscope, cerebral circulation, coronary circulation, and karyotype are reprinted with permission from ***Melloni's Illustrated Medical Dictionary***, 4th ed. (London: The Parthenon Publishing Group, 2002).

Other figures from various educational and manufacturer Web sites were used with permission and are noted with each illustration. We appreciate their generosity. Additional images are available at each site for educational purposes.

MF Atletic Company, **http://www.performbetter.com**

Scott Moses, M.D., **http://www.fpnotebook.com**

**Mitek and Stryker. **.

Brian Mullan, M.D., Univ. of Iowa's *Currents Magazine*, and Virtual Hospital, **http://www.vh.org**

Greggory R. DeVore, M.D, **http://www.fetalecho.com**

J. Hornak, **http://www.cis.rit.edu**

Imaginis Corporation: **http://imaginis.com/cancer/cancer_medicalimaging.asp**

P. Gregory, Biology Laboratory Specialist at Tyler Junior College, **http://science.tjc.edu/images/histology/epithelium.htm**; tubular glands from Betsy Ott, Tyler Junior College, Tyler, TX, at the same site.

Clinical Chemistry and Hematology Laboratory, Wadsworth Center, NY State Dept. of Health; **http://www.wadsworth.org/chemheme**

http://mcdb.colorado.edu/courses/3280/lectures/class08.html

Finally, the cover and artistic graphic designs throughout the book were provided by Parks Printing, Modesto, CA.

List of Figures

General Introduction

1

LEARNING OBJECTIVES

Upon completion of this chapter, the student should be able to

- Describe the process of medical diagnosis and explain the role of laboratory tests and diagnostic procedures;

- Explain units and standards of measurement;

- Explain some ways by which the concept of *normal* is defined;

- Distinguish diagnostic from screening tests and sensitivity from specificity.

The Diagnostic Process

Medical diagnosis is the process by which a physician seeks to learn the nature, cause, and extent of an illness, injury, or congenital or developmental disorder. Obviously at least some tentative or general notion of what is wrong must precede any rational effort to treat it.

The diagnostic process begins with the medical history, an orderly narrative or chronology, established by careful inquiry, of the patient's symptoms, along with relevant surrounding events or experiences. The next step is the physical examination, a systematic assessment, general or focused, of parts of the patient's body that are accessible for inspection, palpation (feeling), manipulation, or auscultation (listening). For these diagnostic procedures the examiner uses eyes, ears, hands, and a few simple, handheld instruments (flashlight, reflex hammer, stethoscope).

The data gathered by history and physical examination often suffice to establish a precise diagnosis. Sometimes, however, more information is needed to determine whether disease is actually present, to distinguish among several disorders with similar features, to measure the severity or extent of the illness, to pinpoint the exact cause of the trouble, to guide the selection of treatment, or, later, to assess the response to treatment or to detect a relapse or recurrence of disease. For these and other purposes, the physician may perform, or arrange for the performance of, supplemental diagnostic tests that lie outside the scope of the physical examination.

A formidable number and variety of supplemental diagnostic procedures are currently available. These range from simple measurements performed with a scale or tape measure to the generation of computed three-dimensional images of internal structures by elaborate devices costing millions of dollars. This book surveys standard diagnostic procedures in each of six categories: physical measurements, electrodiagnostics, endoscopy, medical imaging, anatomic pathology, and clinical pathology.

Some of these tests, such as the measurement of blood pressure, are performed routinely as part of a general health evaluation, while others, such as DNA testing for a particular genetic abnormality, have application only in unusual circumstances. Procedures such as cardiac catheterization are performed directly on the patient, while others, such as a complete blood count, involve laboratory testing of specimens removed from the patient. Some tests can be carried out in a primary care physician's office or clinic, while others require the patient to go to a special laboratory, facility, or hospital department, or to be admitted to a hospital. A procedure may be within the competence of any nurse or physician, or it may require the special training and skills of a medical technologist, a radiologist, or a surgeon.

Not all diagnostic procedures are undertaken to clarify a disease or abnormal state. A **screening** examination or test is one that is performed on a person who is thought to be well or in whom this particular test has a low statistical probability of proving abnormal. Screening tests are done to identify common and potentially serious medical problems before they produce symptoms and perhaps cause irreparable damage. Screening may also be performed on certain classes of person for social, legal, or occupational reasons. For example, airline pilots undergo periodic testing to detect unsuspected cardiovascular disease and workers in asbestos are screened regularly for signs of lung damage.

There can be no sharp distinction between diagnostic tests and screening tests. The difference is largely one of clinical suspicion and statistical probability. A complete blood count done to assess the degree of blood loss in a patient who has had a hemorrhage would be a diagnostic test. The same set of examinations performed on an apparently healthy military recruit would be a screening test.

A third purpose for which laboratory testing may be performed is biomedical research, including clinical trials of new medicines or devices and research to develop new tests or refine existing ones.

Units and Standards of Measurement

The collection of scientific data is usually quantitative, that is, it involves measurements or numbers. Many basic diagnostic procedures consist in measuring something—height, weight, temperature, blood pressure, lung volume. Virtually all tests performed on blood and other specimens in a hematology or clinical chemistry laboratory yield quantitative results—for example, the number of red blood cells per cubic millimeter of whole blood or the concentration of glucose in cerebrospinal fluid.

The notion of measurement implies three fundamental elements or concepts: (1) a unit of measure, such as the centimeter or the Fahrenheit degree; (2) a standard or yardstick by which to gauge the dimension of the subject under study; and (3) a basis of interpretation, usually comparison to a norm.

When we count objects, we use the numbers 1, 2, 3, and so forth, naming the numbers according

---

Units and Standards of Measurement

The first units were probably adopted by primitive peoples for use in apportioning land and in measuring grain and other commodities for purposes of barter. The standardization of weights and measures has traditionally been one of the functions of government. In the 12th century King David I of Scotland officially defined the inch as the width of a man's thumb, measured across the base of the nail. In the 14th century King Edward II of England redefined it as "three grains of barley, dry and round, placed end to end lengthwise."

The metric system, based on the meter for length, the gram for weight, and the second for time, and with decimal multiples and submultiples, was adopted in France late in the 18th century by the government that came into power after the Revolution. By the early 20th century it was standard throughout Europe. Although the metric system gradually replaced the so-called English system (based on the foot and the pound) in England, the United States clung stubbornly to the English system. (In 1959 the inch was officially redefined as 2.54 centimeters.)

In 1937 the International Committee of Weights and Measures added three new units to the metric system: the newton for force, the joule for energy, and the watt for power. A revision of the metric system, called the International System of Units (in French, *Système International d'Unités*, abbreviated SI), was adopted in 1960. To the meter, kilogram, and second of the metric system, SI added the ampere (a unit of electrical current), the candela (a unit of luminous intensity), the kelvin (a unit of temperature), and the mole (a unit of amount of matter).

SI is a fully coherent system and its units are defined with the greatest possible precision. For example, the meter is defined as the distance traveled by light in a vacuum in 1/200,792,458 of a second, and the second is defined as the duration of 9,192,631,770 cycles of radiation from a cesium atom. In the United States the metric system never gained acceptance outside the scientific community, and SI has met with similar resistance from the building, manufacturing, and commercial world. Biology and medicine, however, have gradually changed over to SI units during the past decade. Inches, pounds, and Fahrenheit degrees are nonetheless still widely used in American medicine.

SI units and abbreviations are set forth in Appendix I.

to our own language and grouping or subdividing them, as needed, by ten and its multiples according to the decimal system that has been standard in the Western world for thousands of years. For types of measurement other than simple counting—length, volume, weight, time, force—we must use units.

A **unit** is a specific quantity or magnitude that we have agreed, by convention, to use for purposes of measurement or discussion. Virtually all units of measure in modern use are arbitrary. The inch was first defined as the breadth of the thumb, the foot as the length of a human foot (*see box on p. 3*). Since thumbs and feet vary substantially from person to person, it eventually became necessary to establish more rigorous standards.

Two or more units may be combined for more complex measurements. For example, velocity is the rate at which something moves, expressed as units of distance (e.g., miles) per unit of time (e.g., hour). Concentration is the mass or amount (e.g., milligrams or moles) per unit of volume (e.g., liter). Acceleration is the rate of change of velocity per unit of time, for example, feet per second per second.

Two measurements may be combined in such a way as to yield a fraction, percent, or ratio. For example, the hematocrit is that percent of a specimen of whole blood that consists of red blood cells, as determined by centrifugation (spinning a tube of blood at high speed to make the cells settle quickly). The heights of the entire column of blood and of the column of cells that settled to the bottom of the tube could both be measured and reported in millimeters, but in the computation of percent, the units "cancel out." Thus,

$$\frac{45 \text{ mm of red blood cells}}{100 \text{ mm of whole blood}} \times 100 = 45\%$$

For this reason, fractions (1/8), ratios (1:8), percents (12.5%), and similar expressions of comparison between two figures may be called dimensionless measurements.

In order to measure something, we need a yardstick—a **standard** that has been calibrated with known dimensions, perhaps an actual yardstick, by which to gauge the dimension of what is being measured. Yardsticks in regular use include rulers and calipers for measuring linear dimensions, scales for measuring weight, thermometers for measuring temperature, graduated vessels for measuring volume, and manometers for measuring pressure (*see box*). The validity and usefulness of any measurement depend on the reliability of the yardstick used to obtain it and the care and skill with which the yardstick is applied. Accuracy, in

Derivative Units

Sometimes the yardstick chosen influences the nature of the units used to make the measurement. Pressure (such as that of oxygen in a tank or of blood in an artery) can be expressed as units of weight (e.g., pounds) per unit of surface (e.g., square inch). But instead of measuring atmospheric pressure in pounds per square inch, we measure it in millimeters of mercury.

This is because the earliest form of barometer consisted of a column of mercury in a glass tube with a vacuum above it. Atmospheric pressure was measured as the height of the mercury column that was just balanced by the pressure of the atmosphere. Even though most modern-day sphygmomanometers (devices for measuring blood pressure) and barometers are of the aneroid type and contain no mercury, blood pressure is still recorded in millimeters of mercury (mmHg).

The unit of pressure corresponding to 1 mmHg is also called the torr in honor of Evangelista Torricelli (1608-1647), inventor of the mercury barometer. Neither the mmHg nor the torr is recognized as an SI unit.

this context, refers to the rightness or truth of the yardstick, while precision refers to the exactness or diligence with which the measurement process is carried out.

The collection of numerical data would be futile if it did not lead to some kind of conclusion or decision regarding what has been measured. After determining a person's pulse and blood pressure, a physician compares these data to known ranges of expected or normal pulse and blood pressure, and also perhaps to readings obtained on the same patient on previous occasions. These two forms of comparison illustrate the two basic ways in which numerical data are interpreted in medical diagnosis.

Concept of *Normal*

The concept of what is **normal** or expected depends on the collection and analysis of data from a sufficiently large population of subjects to provide a meaningful basis for comparison. Collecting, summarizing, analyzing, and interpreting numerical data are the province of the science of statistics. Statisticians apply complex mathematical methods to reduce masses of raw numbers to rule and order. Biostatistics, the branch of statistics that deals with numbers from biological and medical research, finds application particularly in the processing of data from clinical trials (rigorously designed and conducted experiments to determine the efficacy and safety of newly developed medicines, diets, medical devices, surgical procedures, and other treatment methods).

The orderly and diligent collection of data typically results in a spread of numbers that, when graphed, yield a so-called bell-shaped curve. That is, a majority of the numbers cluster around a middle figure, and the further one moves away from that middle figure, the fewer examples one finds.

Statisticians use various ways to define the central tendency of a sample or set of values. The **median** is the middle value in a distribution; the **mode** is the value occurring most frequently. The more familiar **average** (or **arithmetic mean**) is the sum of all the values divided by the number of values.

The **standard deviation** is a way of expressing how far a given value varies from the average or expected value. In any distribution of values, one standard deviation (SD, also symbolized by Σ, the Greek letter *sigma*) is defined as the square root of the average (arithmetic mean) of the squares of the deviations from the average. Although the definition may seem abstruse, the actual figure is easily determined from the raw data by a computer in a fraction of a second. In most distributions, 75% of the values are found to lie within one standard deviation above or below the mean, and 95% are found to lie within two standard deviations above or below the mean. Hence a normal range is often defined as being within two standard deviations above or below the mean.

Another way of comparing or relating a given value to all the other values in a distribution is by percentiles. A **percentile** is 1/100 of the total range of values. A value falling on the 50th percentile is thus halfway between the highest and the lowest number in the distribution. Percentile scores are widely used in comparing the heights and weights of children to those of other children of the same gender and age.

These statistical ways of handling data help to define what is normal in medical measurements. Established and published normal values for various measurements and test results are never absolute numbers. Rather, they express a spread of values, known as a reference range or range of normal. Reference ranges may be set forth as tables, graphs, nomograms (*see box on p. 6*), percentile charts, or equations. These ranges may vary substantially depending on the population studied and the methods used to obtain the figures.

In reporting the results of a quantitative test, a clinical laboratory also quotes its reference range for that test to facilitate interpretation and to prevent errors resulting from differences in method. Reference ranges may vary for the two sexes, or with the age of the subject. Requisition forms for

What Is a Nomogram?

A nomogram is a graphic representation of three interdependent quantities or values on three scales. These are so arranged that if two values are known, the third can be found simply by placing a straightedge across the scales. A straight line intersecting the two known values will intersect the third scale at the corresponding unknown value.

An example of a nomogram for determining body surface area when height and weight are known is given on page 21. Note that this nomogram does not set forth normal or ideal values or ranges, but only represents the mathematical relationship among three quantities. Moreover, the inset scale giving body surface area for children, based on weight alone, assumes normal height for weight.

laboratory tests therefore include spaces to enter the patient's sex and birth date. In computer-generated laboratory reports, any abnormal result (that is, a result outside the reference range for the test in question) is typically printed in a separate column to draw attention to it.

For some tests, action levels or panic levels may be established, above or below which a situation may exist that requires immediate treatment or further assessment. Examples of tests for which very low levels demand prompt attention are blood levels of calcium and glucose. It is standard procedure for the laboratory to inform the physician at once of results in the action or panic range.

As mentioned, diagnostic measurements are compared not only to established normal ranges but also to previous readings or determinations for the same patient, to note progression or remission of a disorder or assess the effectiveness of treatment.

An abnormal test result does not necessarily indicate abnormality in the patient. The result must be interpreted in the light of the patient's history and physical findings and of the results of other tests, or perhaps of the same test performed on different occasions. In some instances, the results of prior tests in a given patient may be the most useful indicator of what later results are to be considered normal for that patient.

Not all laboratory tests are of equal validity or reliability. Numerous factors can prevent the obtaining of a correct result, that is, a result reflecting the subject's true state of health or disease. Among these factors may be mentioned improper securing or preservation of the specimen, contamination of the specimen or of testing reagents or devices with extraneous substances or microorganisms, malfunction or improper calibration of equipment, mistakes in reading or recording results, and faulty identification of the source of the specimen.

In practice, all avoidable errors are assumed to have been excluded. It is nonetheless recognized that in any procedure performed by human beings there is a certain margin of error. In addition, because absolute control of test conditions and absolute precision of measurement are never possible, some variance in test results is a built-in feature of the test itself. Hence the reference range for a test allows not only for variations from one healthy subject to another but also for limitations of accuracy inherent in the test.

An abnormal or positive test result in a subject who is healthy or free from the condition tested for is called a **false positive**. A test result that is normal or negative despite the presence in the subject of a disease or condition that would be expected to produce an abnormal or positive test result is called a **false negative**.

Measures of Validity

Several measures of the reliability or validity of test procedures are applied by statisticians. The **accuracy** of a test, as mentioned earlier, is its correctness, that is, its ability to yield a result that truly measures or reflects the condition under investigation. The concept of accuracy implies that there is some independent means of checking on the correctness of the test. Sometimes no such check is possible. In that case, the best indication of the accuracy of a test may be its **reproducibility**. The reproducibility of a test is its ability to yield the same result time after time when performed on the same specimen or material.

The **sensitivity** of a test is its ability to yield abnormal results consistently when performed on abnormal material. Sensitivity is usually expressed as a percent. If the sensitivity of a given test is 90%, that means that when performed on 100 abnormal specimens it would yield 90 abnormal or positive results and 10 false negative results.

The **specificity** of a test refers to its ability to reflect only a specific abnormality, and not to be influenced by other factors. If the specificity of a given test is 84%, that means that when performed on 100 normal specimens it would yield 84 normal or negative results and 16 false positive results.

The terms defined in the preceding two paragraphs are often used incorrectly or carelessly interchanged. The term **precision** is somewhat ambiguous in that statisticians consider it synonymous with reproducibility, while physicists, chemists, and engineers use it to refer to the fineness of units (or to the number of significant figures) in a measurement.

CPT

The nomenclature of both diagnostic and therapeutic procedures has been standardized in *Physicians' Current Procedural Terminology* (CPT), published by the American Medical Association

What Is CLIA?

The Clinical Laboratory Improvement Amendments (CLIA) were passed by Congress in 1988 to establish uniform standards of quality for all clinical laboratories in the United States, as well as registration, surveillance, and enforcement procedures. For the purposes of this federal legislation, a clinical laboratory is defined as any facility where materials derived from the human body are examined for the purpose of providing information for the diagnosis, prevention, or treatment of disease or the assessment of health.

Standards applied under CLIA to laboratory personnel and procedures are based on the complexity of tests performed as well as the potential harm to the patient from improperly performed tests. Each laboratory must participate in a continuing program of proficiency testing whereby an independent laboratory periodically submits specimens of known composition for testing.

and revised annually. This system assigns a unique five-digit code number to each type of service rendered to a patient by a health care provider. For example, an appendectomy is coded as 44950 and determination of total serum cholesterol as 70123.

The ultimate purpose of CPT is to establish each service as a discrete, standardized entity to which a dollar value can be assigned for health insurance claim processing. CPT codes are required on all insurance and Medicare claims. In addition, they may be used to identify tests on laboratory or radiology requisitions and for recording and statistical purposes.

Exercises

Fill in the Blanks

1. In addition to the history and physical, _____ may be needed to determine whether disease is actually present, to distinguish among several disorders with similar features, to measure the severity or extent of the illness, to pinpoint the exact cause of the trouble, to guide the selection of treatment, or, later, to assess the response to treatment or to detect a relapse or recurrence of disease.

2. A _____ is performed on a person who is thought to be well or in whom this particular test has a low statistical probability of proving abnormal.

3. Three reasons for performing laboratory or other diagnostic tests include _____, _____, and _____.

4. _____ data usually involves measurements or numbers.

5. The notion of measurement implies three fundamental elements or concepts: (1) _____, such as the centimeter or the Fahrenheit degree; (2) a _____ by which to gauge the dimension of the subject under study; and (3) _____, usually comparison to a norm.

6. The _____ and _____ of any measurement depend on the reliability of the yardstick used to obtain it and the care and skill with which the yardstick is applied.

7. Comparisons between two figures of measurement, such as fractions, ratios, and percentages, may be called _____.

8. _____ refers to the rightness or truth of the yardstick, while _____ refers to the exactness or diligence with which the measurement process is carried out.

9. The two basic ways in which numerical data are interpreted in medical diagnosis are _____ and _____.

10. Statisticians use various ways to define the central tendency of a sample or set of values. The _____ is the middle value in a distribution; the mode is the value occurring most frequently. The more familiar _____ (or arithmetic _____) is the sum of all the values divided by the number of values.

Exercises

Multiple Choice: Circle the letter of the best answer from the choices given.

1. Screening tests are performed in order
   A. to identify common and potentially serious medical problems before they produce symptoms and perhaps cause irreparable damage.
   B. to measure the severity or extent of the illness.
   C. to contribute to biomedical research, including research on new drugs, devices, and diagnostic tests.
   D. to distinguish among several disorders with similar features.
   E. to assess the effectiveness of treatment.

2. The textbook discusses all of the following reasons for diagnostic studies except
   A. to provide a broader analysis of a disease or condition.
   B. to guide treatment or assess response to treatment.
   C. to screen apparently well patients for hidden problems.
   D. to evaluate the effectiveness of new drugs, devices, and diagnostic tests.
   E. to reassure the patient that there is really nothing wrong.

3. The middle value in a distribution of measurements is the
   A. ratio.
   B. bell curve.
   C. median.
   D. average.
   E. mean.

4. A normal range is often defined as
   A. being within two standard deviations above or below the mean.
   B. the square root of the average (arithmetic mean) of the squares of the deviations from the average.
   C. a so-called bell-shaped curve.
   D. a percentile of the total range of values.
   E. the average value in a list of values.

5. A graphic representation of three interdependent quantities or values on three scales that does not set forth normal or ideal values or ranges, but only represents the mathematical relationship among three quantities is called
   A. the median.
   B. the normal range.
   C. arithmetic mean.
   D. a percentile.
   E. a nomogram.

Exercises

6. Reference ranges may vary due to all of the following reasons except
   A. Different labs may have different reference ranges.
   B. Sex of patient.
   C. Age of patient.
   D. Testing method.
   E. Race of patient.

7. Factors contributing to incorrect results in laboratory tests include all of the following except
   A. Improper securing or preservation of the specimen.
   B. Patient's consumption of food just before specimen was taken.
   C. Malfunction or improper calibration of equipment.
   D. Mistakes in reading or recording results.
   E. Faulty identification of the source of the specimen.

8. The ability of a test to yield the same result time after time when performed on the same specimen or material is known as
   A. Sensitivity.
   B. Reliability.
   C. Reproducibility.
   D. Accuracy.
   E. Specificity.

9. The ability to yield abnormal results consistently when performed on abnormal material is known as
   A. Sensitivity.
   B. Reliability.
   C. Reproducibility.
   D. Accuracy.
   E. Specificity.

10. The ability to reflect only a specific abnormality, and not to be influenced by other factors is known as
    A. Specificity.
    B. Reliability.
    C. Reproducibility.
    D. Accuracy.
    E. Sensitivity.

Exercises

Short Answers

1. Define or explain:

   a. action level _____

   _____

   b. CLIA _____

   _____

   c. CPT _____

   _____

   d. percentile _____

   _____

   e. screening test _____

   _____

   f. SI _____

   _____

   g. torr _____

   _____

2. Give three examples of tests performed directly on the patient:

   a. _____

   b. _____

   c. _____

3. Give three examples of tests performed on specimens obtained from the patient:

   a. _____

   b. _____

   c. _____

4. How is the range of normal results established for a test?

   _____

   _____

   _____

   _____

Exercises

5. Distinguish the sensitivity and the specificity of a test.

    _____

    _____

    _____

    _____

    _____

    _____

6. List four possible reasons for a false negative test result.

    a. _____

        _____

    b. _____

        _____

    c. _____

        _____

    d. _____

        _____

7. Which of these could also cause a false positive test result?

    _____

    _____

    _____

    _____

Exercises

Activities for Application and Further Study

1. Research the history of the metric and SI systems of measurement in America. You may want to consult such documents as "A Metric America: A Decision Whose Time Has Come," and "Metric Conversion Act of 1975." Summarize your findings and discuss why America has been slow to adopt the systems of measurement used in the rest of the world.

2. Request from your private physician copies of reports of laboratory and other diagnostic studies performed on you and/or your immediate family members. Do the reports reflect the CPT codes for the tests performed? Are abnormal values in a separate column? Do the reports give reference ranges for normal values? Hold these reports to use later in the course.

3. Which is the more important measure of the validity of the test, sensitivity or specificity? Explain your answer.

Physical Measurements

This section discusses diagnostic tests that are essentially physical measurements, whether performed with such simple yardsticks as a tape measure or with sophisticated devices in which electronic sensors gather data that must be analyzed by a computer. Some of these measurements, such as determination of body weight or pulse rate, are purely objective, in that they do not depend on sensations, experiences, or interpretations of the patient and can theoretically be verified by any qualified observer. Other measurements, such as the determination of the acuity of vision and hearing, depend mostly or entirely on input from the patient.

Anthropometry, Musculoskeletal Measurements, and Clinical Pelvimetry

2

LEARNING OBJECTIVES

Upon completion of this chapter, the student should be able to

- Discuss the importance of body weight in health and disease;

- Describe various ways of measuring excess body fat;

- Explain the use of goniometry and quantitative strength testing in the diagnosis of musculoskeletal disease;

- Define clinical pelvimetry and explain its significance in obstetrics.

Anthropometry

Basic body measurements such as height, weight, girth, and arm span, and more complex values derived from them such as body mass index or waist-hip ratio, pertain to the science of anthropometry. Such measurements are of importance in assessing the growth and development of children and the nutritional status of persons of all ages. They may also help in identifying hereditary or acquired deformities and in coordinating physical capacities of workers with ergonomic measurements of job requirements.

The determination of **weight** is a routine part of well-baby care, as a means of comparing early childhood development with established norms of height and weight for chronologic age in months (*see Fig. 2.1, Fig. 2.2*). Low birth weight and failure to thrive (failure to gain weight at a normal rate) are nonspecific findings that may indicate a significant, even life-threatening disorder. Excessive birth weight and excessive weight gain may also signify serious abnormalities.

Appropriate dosages of medicines are usually expressed in milligrams per kilogram of body weight per day. Precise calculation of dosages is crucial for infants and small children to achieve therapeutic levels of medicine while avoiding toxic levels. Dosages for adults are not usually computed from body weight, except for medicines with narrow therapeutic ranges or for patients with renal failure or other disorders affecting their ability to metabolize and excrete foreign chemicals.

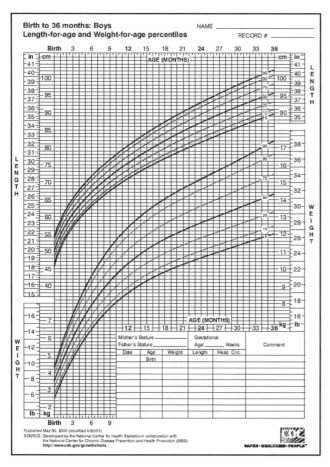

Fig. 2.1. Length-for-age and weight-for-age percentiles: boys, birth to 36 months. CDC Growth Charts: United States

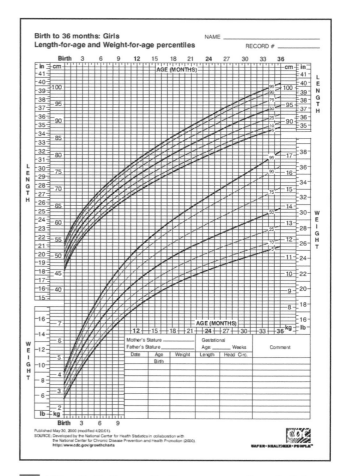

Fig. 2.2. Length-for-age and weight-for-age percentiles: girls, birth to 36 months. CDC Growth Charts: United States

Weight loss in adults is a symptom whose possible causes range from ill-fitting dentures to terminal cancer. In our culture, overweight is a more prevalent and more ominous departure from normal. Body weight is ideally measured by a balance type clinical scale that has been accurately calibrated. Spring type scales ("bathroom scales") and coin-operated scales in public places are notoriously unreliable. In outpatient medical practice, patients are usually weighed in indoor clothing, with or without shoes. Weighing without clothing may be necessary to ensure that patients with anorexia nervosa and other psychiatric disorders do not conceal heavy articles on their persons to increase scale readings. Body weight is recorded in either pounds (lb) or kilograms (kg).

$$1 \text{ lb} = 0.45 \text{ kg} \qquad 1 \text{ kg} = 2.2 \text{ lb}$$

Body weight in adults is often compared to actuarial tables of normal or "ideal" weights. These tables, giving appropriate weights for height, age, and gender, and sometimes further subdivided according to large, medium, or small frame, are based on comparison of mortality statistics with the height and weight measurements recorded during life insurance examinations.

One way of comparing a given body weight to these norms is to determine relative weight (RW) by dividing the subject's weight by the median desirable weight for a person of the same height and medium frame. Other measures of weight in proportion to height are the body mass index (BMI), determined by dividing the weight in kilograms by the square of the height in meters (kg/m^2), and the ponderal index, determined by dividing the weight in kilograms by the cube of the height in meters (kg/m^3).

If obesity is defined as body weight that is 20% or more in excess of ideal weight-for-height, then one-third of adults in the U.S. are obese. The National Institutes of Health has defined obesity as a BMI of 30 kg/m^2 or more, and over-weight as a BMI between 25 and 30 kg/m^2. By these criteria, two-thirds of adults are either overweight or obese.

The essence of obesity is an excess of subcutaneous fat in proportion to lean body mass. An objection to the use of actuarial tables and body mass index is that these measures do not differentiate between excess subcutaneous fat and increased lean body mass. The proportion of subcutaneous fat to total body mass differs in the two sexes. In men fat normally makes up 5-10% of total body weight, whereas in women the normal range is 10-15%.

Methods of assessing the percentage of body fat such as skinfold measurement and underwater weighing are considered more valid means of diagnosing and quantifying obesity. The thickness of a fold of skin lifted up between the thumb and index finger depends largely on the thickness of the subcutaneous fat layer. Measurement of skinfold thickness with a caliper designed and calibrated for that purpose provides data for determination of body fat composition according to various formulas. Skinfold calipers are spring-loaded to provide constant tension, and yield mechanical or digital (electronic) readings of skinfold thickness. Standard measurement sites differ for men and women. In men the measurements are taken on the chest, abdomen, and thigh; in women, over the triceps (back of the arm), iliac crest, and abdomen.

Underwater weighing is another means of assessing lean body mass. Whereas bones, muscles, and internal organs are heavier (have a higher specific gravity) than water, fat is lighter. A comparison of body weight, as determined in the usual way, with the weight determined while the subject is completely immersed in water permits calculation of the percent of fat in the body. The subject must expel as much air as possible from the lungs before immersion, and the calculation makes allowance for the buoyancy caused by the residual volume (RV), the small amount of air that cannot be expelled.

The health risks associated with excessive subcutaneous fat depend in part on the distribution of fat. Measurement of the circumference around the waist and around the hips permits determination of the waist-to-hip ratio (WHR). A high waist-to-hip ratio, indicating a relative excess of fat in the abdomen as contrasted with the hips and buttocks, betokens a more serious risk of cardiovascular disease and type 2 diabetes mellitus. WHR depends to some extent on race and body type. In addition, because of differences in the width of the pelvis, women normally have a lower WHR than men. A ratio of 0.95 or higher in men and a ratio of 0.80 or higher in women indicate significant health risks.

Estimates of health status and risk based on body weight for a given height imply the postulate that **height** is a fixed or constant figure, or at least one that is not subject to up-and-down variation or to control by change of lifestyle. The height of an individual depends largely on genetics—racial stock and, more particularly, parentage. The gain in height normally seen during childhood and adolescence can be curtailed by nutritional or metabolic disorders. Excessive gain in height is sometimes due to endocrine factors (functioning pituitary tumor producing growth hormone; delayed puberty). Height decreases slightly after middle age, mainly as a result of erosion of intervertebral disks. Marked reduction in height with aging suggests severe reduction in bone density (osteoporosis), possibly with compression fractures of vertebrae.

Height (length, in infants) may be measured in either English units (inches or feet and inches) or SI units (centimeters or meters and centimeters).

1 in = 2.54 cm	1 cm = 0.39 in
1 ft = 30.48 cm	1 m = 39.37 in

Measurement of the extremities (long bone length, arm span) and other body segments permits calculation of body **proportions** and identification of various congenital disorders. In achondroplastic dwarfism the extremities are shorter than normal in proportion to total height. In Marfan syndrome, the extremities are longer than normal in proportion to height. Measurement of head circumference is routine in well-baby care to detect hydrocephalus (increase in the pressure and volume of cerebrospinal fluid, causing enlargement of the head and compression of the brain). The circumference of the adult chest is increased in emphysema, while chest expansion (the increase in circumference from full expiration to full inspiration) is reduced.

Body surface area (BSA), as computed by various formulas from the height and weight, is sometimes preferred to simple weight as a means of computing the ideal dosages of certain drugs, as well as for determining fluid, electrolyte, and caloric needs of infants and small children. According to the Mosteller formula, the body surface area in square meters can be found by multiplying the height in centimeters by the weight in kilograms, dividing the product by 3600, and finding the square root of the quotient. The West nomogram (*see Fig.2.3*) is widely used to calculate BSA. The body surface area that is usually taken as standard or ideal for an adult male is 1.73 m^3.

Musculoskeletal Measurements

Methods for assessing joint mobility and muscle strength can provide important information about orthopedic and neuromuscular disorders of developmental, traumatic, or degenerative origin.

Goniometry is a standardized testing procedure to determine the mobility of a joint, irrespective of the strength of the surrounding muscles, their nerve supply, or the subject's coordination and ability to follow directions. It is an important adjunct in the diagnosis, treatment, and rehabilitation of injuries or diseases that affect joints and the structures around them. It is also useful in establishing job restrictions for disabled workers, in planning physical therapy and assessing its

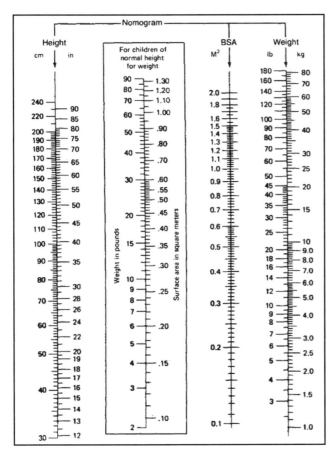

Fig. 2.3. Nomogram

laxity or damage of ligaments and other supporting structures.

A goniometer is a simple device of metal or plastic consisting of a round disk or body and two arms, one of them attached rigidly to the body (or forming a single piece with it) and the other capable of rotating around a pivot or fulcrum on the body (*see Fig. 2.4*). The body is calibrated to show degrees of rotation around the pivot, with gradations of 1° to 10°. Goniometers come in various sizes for various joints.

In performing goniometry, the examiner first places the joint to be examined in a neutral position (usually the standard anatomic position). The range of rotation, in a joint capable of rotatory motion (such as the shoulder), is measured with the limb half-way between flexion and extension. If the joint cannot be placed in the anatomic position, the examiner records the angle between the actual position of rest and the ideal anatomic position. Because joints differ widely in their structure (hinge vs. ball-and-socket, weightbearing vs. non-weightbearing), testing positions and procedures vary somewhat from joint to joint.

effects, and in designing braces and adaptive equipment.

Goniometry measures the passive range of motion—that is, the extent to which an examiner can move a joint in various standard directions, the limit of motion being the point at which the examiner feels resistance to further movement. (The active range of motion of a joint—the full extent to which the subject can move it voluntarily—provides information about muscle strength, coordination, and overall function, but is not assessed in goniometry.)

The passive range of motion depends in part on the anatomic structure of the joint and the type of motion tested, and it also varies with the gender and age of the subject. The range of motion may be reduced by swelling, inflammation, scarring, calcification, and other effects of disease or injury in and around the joint, and it may be increased by

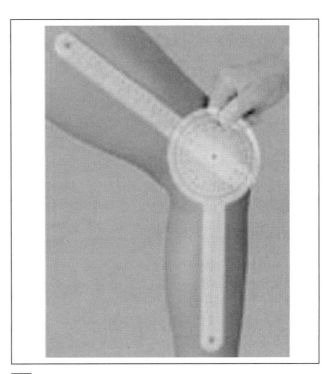

Fig. 2.4. Goniometer. Image used with permission from MF Athletic Company, http://www.performbetter.com

The stationary arm of the goniometer is aligned with the longitudinal axis of the body part that is proximal to the joint—that is, nearer to the center of the body. For example, to test the knee joint the stationary arm is aligned with the thigh. In addition, the pivot point of the instrument is aligned with the axis of movement of the joint, as noted by anatomic landmarks.

While stabilizing the stationary body part, the examiner determines the passive range of motion of the joint by moving the body part that is distal to it. Flexion (bending the joint to a sharper angle), extension (stretching the joint so that the two bones form a straight line), adduction (moving the part beyond the joint away from the midline of the body), and abduction (moving it closer to the midline) are tested in succession, with the mobile arm of the goniometer aligned with the moving, distal member of the joint. The angle formed by the distal member of the joint with the proximal member when the end of passive motion is reached is measured in degrees on the goniometer.

Local or general muscle weakness can be a sign of injury or disease affecting muscles, peripheral nerves, or the central nervous system, or can result from systemic, toxic, or metabolic disorders. **Quantitative muscle strength testing** (QMST) is an important step in the diagnosis of these disorders. It can also be used to measure disability and to select treatment and monitor its effects.

Estimates of muscle strength based on having the subject squeeze the examiner's hand or attempt to resist forces applied by the examiner are highly subjective and of limited diagnostic value. Quantitative muscle strength testing is an objective, standardized method of testing the strength of various muscles and muscle groups and of comparing the results with predicted or normal values based on age, gender, and body mass index. The testing method is isometric. That is, the subject exerts full force against a resistance that does not move appreciably, and the force is converted by a strain gauge (pressure transducer) into a measurable electronic signal. (In contrast, isotonic testing measures the distance through which the subject can move a weight or resistance of known force.)

The subject sits or lies at rest within a framework equipped with straps or bars attached to strain gauges. About 20 muscle groups are tested, one at a time. For each muscle group tested, the patient is appropriately stabilized to ensure that accessory or auxiliary muscles are not used to make up for deficient strength in the muscles under test. The results of the test are stored and analyzed by a computer. Interpretation of the data includes comparison of right and left sides and of proximal and distal muscle groups.

Clinical Pelvimetry

Dystocia (difficult or protracted labor) is one of the most common complications of childbirth and the principal reason for the performance of cesarean deliveries. Among the many possible causes for dystocia is cephalopelvic disproportion—a birth passage that is too small to allow passage of the fetal head. The normal fetal head measures about 11.5 cm from brow to occiput (occipitofrontal diameter) and about 9.5 cm in width (biparietal diameter). Although the fetal skull bones can shift and override slightly to conform to the birth passage, there is a limit beyond which such accommodation cannot occur and the progress of delivery is arrested.

Pelvimetry refers to any procedure for the determination of certain critical dimensions of the maternal pelvis in order to ensure an adequate passage for normal childbirth. X-ray pelvimetry, once widely practiced, has fallen into disuse, partly because of concerns about fetal damage early in pregnancy and partly because accurate determination of critical pelvic measurements from two-dimensional x-ray pictures demands both impeccable radiographic technique and skillful interpretation.

In clinical pelvimetry, measurements of the maternal pelvis are performed directly. For obstetrical purposes the bony pelvis is divided, from above downward, into three segments or levels: inlet, the midpelvis, and outlet.

The inlet, or brim of the true pelvis, is the bony passage into which the fetal head first enters as the birth process begins. The critical dimension here is the obstetric conjugate, or anteroposterior diameter as defined by the symphysis pubis anteriorly and the promontory of the sacrum posteriorly. The standard technique for estimating the adequacy of the pelvic inlet is to determine the diagonal conjugate. The index and middle fingers of the examiner are placed in the vagina and pressed firmly against the sacrum, and the point between the examiner's index finger and thumb that corresponds to the position of the pubic symphysis is noted (*see Fig.2.5*). The distance from this point to the end of the middle finger is the diagonal conjugate. Subtracting 1.5 cm from this dimension gives a good estimate of the true conjugate.

The critical dimension in the midpelvis is the interspinous diameter, the distance between the ischial spines, normally about 10 cm. Although direct clinical measurement of this diameter is not feasible, palpation of the ischial spines on vaginal or rectal examination gives the obstetrician a reliable estimate of the adequacy of this part of the birth passage.

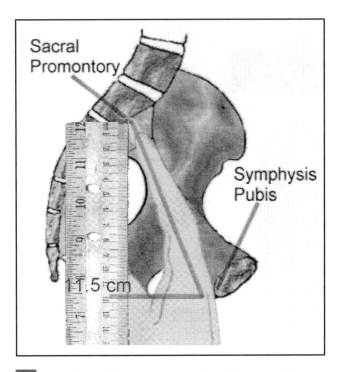

Fig. 2.5. Measurement of Diagonal Conjugate. Image used with permission from Scott Moses, M.D., http://www.fpnotebook.com

The narrowest dimension of the pelvic outlet is the intertuberous diameter, the distance between the ischial tuberosities, which is normally about 11 cm. This diameter can be directly measured, since the tuberosities are palpable through the soft tissues of the buttocks.

Exercises

Fill in the Blanks

1. _____ and _____, or failure to gain weight at a normal rate, are nonspecific findings that may indicate a significant, even life-threatening disorder in babies.

2. In adults, _____ is an independent risk factor for hypertension, hypercholesterolemia, type 2 diabetes mellitus, myocardial infarction, certain cancers, and osteoarthritis.

3. The National Institutes of Health defines overweight as _____ and obesity as _____.

4. Methods of assessing the percentage of body fat such as _____ and _____ are considered more valid means of diagnosing and quantifying obesity than actuarial tables.

5. A high waist-to-hip ratio, indicating a relative excess of fat in the abdomen as contrasted with the hips and buttocks, betokens a more serious risk of _____ and _____.

6. _____ is sometimes preferred to simple weight as a means of computing the ideal dosages of certain drugs, as well as for determining fluid, electrolyte, and caloric needs of infants and small children.

7. Calculating the length of the extremities and other body segments in proportion to height can aid in the diagnosis of _____ and _____.

8. Increased chest circumference and decrease in the degree of expansion are indicative of _____ in adults.

9. _____ measures the extent to which an examiner can move a joint in various standard directions, the limit of motion being the point at which the examiner feels resistance to further movement.

10. _____ testing is an objective, standardized method of testing the strength of various muscles and muscle groups.

11. In _____ testing of muscle strength, the subject exerts full force against a resistance that does not move appreciably, and the force is converted by a strain gauge into a measurable electronic signal.

12. One of the most common complications of childbirth is difficult or protracted labor, or _____.

13. Any procedure for the determination of certain critical dimensions of the maternal pelvis in order to ensure an adequate passage for normal childbirth is known as _____.

14. In clinical pelvimetry, the standard technique for estimating the adequacy of the pelvic inlet is to determine the _____.

Exercises

Multiple Choice: Circle the letter of the best answer from the choices given.

1. Anthropometric measurements are important in medicine in all of the following ways except
   A. To assess growth and development of children.
   B. To assess nutritional status of persons of all ages.
   C. To help in identifying acquired or hereditary deformities.
   D. To help in developing insurance actuarial tables
   E. In coordinating physical capacities of workers with ergonomic measurements of job requirements

2. Determination of weight is an important part of routine well-baby care because of all of the following reasons except
   A. Low birth weight or failure to gain may indicate a significant, even life-threatening disorder.
   B. To assess the level and competence of parental care.
   C. For comparison with standards or norms for sex, age, and weight.
   D. Excessive birth weight and excessive weight gain may signify serious abnormalities.
   E. To calculate therapeutic levels of medicine while avoiding toxic levels.

3. Dividing the subject's weight by the median desirable weight for a person of the same height and medium frame is a way to calculate
   A. Body mass index.
   B. Body surface area.
   C. Ponderal weight.
   D. Relative weight.
   E. Obesity.

4. Dividing the weight in kilograms by the square of the height in meters (kg/m^2) is a way to calculate
   A. Body mass index.
   B. Body surface area.
   C. Ponderal weight.
   D. Relative weight.
   E. Obesity.

5. Dividing the weight in kilograms by the cube of the height in meters (kg/m^3) is a way to calculate
   A. Obesity
   B. Body surface area.
   C. Ponderal weight.
   D. Relative weight.
   E. Body mass index.

Exercises

6. The essence of obesity is
   A. Body weight that is 20% or more in excess of ideal weight-for-height.
   B. BMI of 30 kg/m^2 or more.
   C. BMI between 25 and 30 kg/m^2.
   D. An excess of subcutaneous fat in proportion to lean body mass.
   E. Weighing more than the norms on insurance actuarial tables.

7. According to the text, which of the following methods is a reliable means of measuring subcutaneous body fat?
   A. "The pinch test," measuring the space between thumb and forefinger after pinching the skin.
   B. Underwater weighing.
   C. Galvanic skin response.
   D. Bioelectrical impedance analysis.
   E. DEXA (dual energy x-ray absorptiometry)

8. Factors affecting range of motion testing include all of the following except
   A. Anatomic structure of the joint and the type of motion tested.
   B. Gender and age of the subject.
   C. Swelling, inflammation, scarring, calcification.
   D. Laxity or damage of ligaments and other supporting structures.
   E. Overweight or obesity.

9. The most reliable way to quantify muscle strength is
   A. Have the subject squeeze the examiner's hand.
   B. Have the subject resist force applied by the examiner.
   C. Isotonic muscle testing.
   D. Isometric muscle testing.
   E. Bioelectrical impedance analysis.

10. One cause for dystocia discussed in the text is
    A. Cephalopelvic disproportion.
    B. Footling breech presentation.
    C. Desultory labor.
    D. Placental abruptio.
    E. Holiday approaching.

11. The measurement used to determine adequacy of the pelvic outlet in clinical pelvimetry is the
    A. Bony pelvis.
    B. Diagonal conjugate.
    C. Interspinous diameter.
    D. Intertuberous diameter.
    E. Pelvic brim.

Exercises

Short Answers

1. Define or explain:

   a. anthropometry _____
   _____

   b. dystocia _____
   _____

   c. goniometry _____
   _____

   d. isometric testing _____
   _____

   e. passive range of motion_____
   _____

   f. skinfold caliper _____
   _____

   g. waist-to-hip ratio _____
   _____

2. Why does a pediatrician measure the circumference of the child's head during a well-baby examination?
   _____
   _____
   _____

3. Give three reasons for performing goniometry.

   a. _____
   b. _____
   c. _____

4. Give three reasons for determining body surface area.

   a. _____
   b. _____
   c. _____

Exercises

5. What is the weight in kilograms of a person who weighs 186 lb?

   _____

6. Is the person in question 5 obese? Explain your answer.

   _____

   _____

   _____

Activities for Application and Further Study

1. Using one or more of the methods discussed in the text (body mass index, waist-to-hip ratio, skin fold caliper [a compass could probably suffice held parallel to the body rather than using the points], determine whether you and members of your family are overweight. If a bioelectrical impedance scale is available, compare the results from all the methods used. Which seems most reliable or accurate? (Note: BMI & W/H ratio calculators can be found on-line as well as body fat charts for skin fold caliper interpretation.)

2. Using cardboard or semirigid plastic, design and create a simple goniometer (a protractor and/or compass might be helpful). Perform range of motion tests on your classmates or family members using the description of the test from the textbook.

3. Survey mothers in your class and social circle. Ask them if they had a cesarean section and, if so, what was the reason for it. Ask them if they had a pelvimetry prior to the C-section and whether it was clinical, x-ray, or ultrasound. Summarize your findings (no names, please!) and discuss them in class.

Measurement of Vision and Hearing **3**

LEARNING OBJECTIVES

Upon completion of this chapter, the student should be able to

- Understand basic procedures for measuring visual acuity and visual fields;

- Discuss audiometry and its interpretation;

- Describe the balance system and explain how it is tested.

Ophthalmologic Measurements

Testing of visual acuity and visual fields, unlike most of the other measurements discussed in this section, demands the full cooperation of the patient and yields entirely subjective results, in that findings cannot be independently checked.

Vision testing is usually performed with standard charts containing letters or words of various sizes. The eyes are tested both separately and together. For children and illiterates, charts with pictures or symbols are used.

For the assessment of distant vision, the subject is placed 20 feet from the familiar Snellen chart and visual acuity is recorded as the smallest line of type in which the subject can read more than half the letters correctly. Each line is designated by the distance at which a person with normal vision can read it. Thus, 20/20 vision is normal, while 20/80 vision means that the subject must be as close as 20 feet to read a type size that a person with normal distant vision can read at 80 feet.

For near vision testing, lines or paragraphs are printed in various sizes of type (Jaeger test types) on a card that can be held in the hand. Testing may involve finding the smallest print that the subject can read at a standard distance, or finding the range of distances through which the subject can read a particular size of type.

Refraction is the use of an instrument containing lenses of various powers to measure deficiencies of near and distant vision more precisely than is possible with vision charts alone. This procedure enables the examiner to determine the strength of the corrective lens that must be prescribed to correct nearsightedness (myopia) or farsightedness (hypermetropia). By testing cylindrical lenses of various strengths at various angles, the examiner can also measure astigmatism (distortion of images by warping of the cornea out of the normal spherical shape) and prescribe appropriate correction.

The power of a refractive lens is measured in diopters. One diopter is the reciprocal of the focal length of the lens in meters. The stronger the lens, the shorter its radius of curvature and its focal length. Hence a higher diopter indicates a stronger lens.

$$\text{Focal length of 1 m:} \quad \frac{1}{1 \text{ m}} = 1 \text{ diopter}$$

$$\text{Focal length of 0.25 m:} \quad \frac{1}{0.25 \text{ m}} = 4 \text{ diopters}$$

Visual field testing is used to map areas of impaired or absent vision due to retinal disease or other ocular or neurologic abnormality. An Amsler grid consists of a network of lines, usually white on black, around a central point at which the subject is instructed to gaze while the examiner moves a small object through various parts of the visual field to detect defects. **Perimetry** is an assessment of peripheral vision, performed by testing the subject's ability to discern moving objects or flashing lights at the extreme periphery of the visual fields. **Tests for color-blindness** employ printed figures made up of variously sized dots in various colors and shades. Persons with normal color vision perceive numbers against a background of differently colored dots, but color-blind persons see only a random scattering of dots.

Otologic Measurements

Measurements of hearing, like those of vision, demand an alert and cooperative patient and yield results that, by and large, cannot be independently confirmed. Audiometry is the precise determination of hearing threshold—the faintest level of loudness that the subject can hear at any given pitch. In practice the subject's threshold of hearing is compared with an ideal threshold, and the difference expressed in decibels (*see box*).

What Is a Decibel?

The **decibel** (dB) is a dimensionless unit, a logarithmic expression of the ratio between two levels of intensity. It is one-tenth of a bel (B) and represents approximately the smallest difference in intensity between two sounds that can be appreciated by the human ear. The **bel** is named for Alexander Graham Bell (1847-1922), who was a teacher of the deaf and a professor of vocal physiology at Boston University before inventing the telephone in 1875.

Audiometry is performed to detect or measure hearing loss in persons complaining of deafness or other ear symptoms such as earache or tinnitus (ringing or other abnormal noise in one or both ears). Regular audiometric testing is required by federal law for workers exposed occupationally to high noise levels.

The basic instrument of audiometry is a finely calibrated tone generator capable of delivering pure tones of the required frequencies at a variety of intensity levels. The tones are presented to the examinee through earphones so that the ears can be tested separately and to minimize variations not related to the individual's hearing. Testing is carried out in an isolation chamber designed to exclude extraneous noise and vibration.

In conventional audiometry, each ear is tested at each of several standard pitches (usually 250, 500, 1000, 2000, 3000, 4000, 6000, and 8000 Hz). Testing can be performed manually by a technician or by automated machinery activated by the subject.

In the manual technique, the examinee gives the technician a visible signal when the tone is heard. The technician selects the frequencies and intensities of the tones presented. This method is more time-consuming and less precise than automatic audiometry, and requires a skilled technician. It may, however, be preferable with an examinee whose intelligence or ability to concentrate is limited, or who is unable to use the automatic equipment. Manual testing may also be of use to check questionable results of automatic testing and to detect malingerers.

An automatic audiometer presents the examinee with a programmed series of pure tones at various pitches. The intensity of each tone is gradually increased until the examinee signifies perception of it by pressing a button. This action causes the intensity of the tone to diminish, and the examinee releases the button again when the tone is no longer audible. Ordinarily the tones are pulsed (beeping), but a continuous tone may also be used.

The automatic audiometer produces a written result of test results. This record may be either a graph or a digital printout. The graphic record requires slightly more skill to interpret but is more precise and conveys more information. Digital records are highly reproducible and can be evaluated and compared by nonprofessional persons, but they round off decibel readings to the nearest multiple of 5, and give no information about the configuration of the response curves. They record no threshold when responses at any pitch are erratic.

Loss of hearing can be unilateral or bilateral, acute or chronic, fixed or progressive. It can occur at a single pitch level, at several adjacent pitches, or throughout the testing range. Hearing loss is divided clinically into two large classes, conduction and sensorineural. This classification depends on the anatomic site of the abnormality. Although audiometry alone cannot identify the anatomic origin of hearing loss, patterns of loss as shown by the audiometric record can provide important information to supplement data from history and physical examination.

Conductive hearing loss results from injury or disease of the conduction system, comprising the external ear (pinna and external auditory canal) and the middle ear (tympanic membrane and ossicles). Conductive hearing loss is frequently unilateral, and frequently reversible either spontaneously or with medical or surgical treatment. It tends to affect all pitch ranges to an equal degree.

Sensorineural hearing loss results from a lesion or malfunction of inner ear structures (cochlea, auditory nerve). Sensorineural loss includes presbycusis (hearing loss due to aging) and chronic acoustic trauma ("boilermaker's disease"). It is typically bilateral, and shows greater hearing loss at higher pitch levels. It is usually irreversible.

Significant hearing loss in the 500-2000 Hz range impairs the hearing of normal conversation. Hearing loss in the 3000-6000 Hz range impairs the hearing of music, telephone bells, and the voices of children and some women. A threshold shift of 50 dB or more in both ears throughout the lower range (250-2000 Hz) is usually perceived as severe deafness. With normal hearing in this range, a threshold shift of 50 dB or more at higher pitches may be only mildly disabling, or may even go unnoticed.

The eighth cranial (vestibulocochlear) nerve serves not only hearing but balance. Positional signals detected by structures in the vestibular division of the inner ear are carried by fibers of the eighth cranial nerve to the central nervous system. Disorders of the inner ear, the nerve, or the balance center can result in dysequilibrium (difficulty in maintaining balance), vertigo (a

sense of spinning), nystagmus (involuntary cyclical back-and-forth movement of the eyes), and nausea.

A standard technique to assess the integrity of the balance system involves stimulating the vestibules with warm or cool water instilled into the ear canals. For this procedure the patient reclines with the head at an angle of 30° so as to place the lateral semicircular canals in a vertical plane. The ears are irrigated, one at a time, first with warm water and then with cool water. During the irrigations the patient is instructed to engage in a mental task to provide distraction. Testing sessions are separated by rest periods.

The normal response to unilateral caloric stimulation of the vestibule is a transitory nystagmus (involuntary back-and-forth movements of the eyes). Nystagmus consists of alternating quick lateral movements in one direction (fast component or phase) followed by slower return movements (slow phase) in the opposite direction. A nystagmus is said to beat in the direction of the fast component. Nystagmus induced by cool water beats in the direction opposite to the ear being stimulated, while nystagmus induced by warm water beats in the same direction as the ear being stimulated. (Mnemonic: COWS = Cool Opposite, Warm Same)

Sometimes only warm water is used. Equivocal results of a standard test may be checked with ice water (not merely cool water). The vestibular caloric test cannot be performed if the patient has a perforated tympanic membrane or severe external otitis.

Exercises

Fill in the Blanks

1. Vision testing is usually performed with standard charts containing letters or words of various sizes, such as the _____ chart.

2. Near vision is tested using lines or paragraphs printed in various sizes of type (_____ test types) on a card that can be held in the hand.

3. _____ is the use of an instrument containing lenses of various powers to measure deficiencies of near and distant vision more precisely than is possible with vision charts alone.

4. The medical name for nearsightedness is _____.

5. The medical name for farsightedness is _____.

6. Distortion of images by warping of the cornea out of the normal spherical shape is known as _____.

7. One _____, the power of a refractive lens, is the reciprocal of the focal length of the lens in meters.

8. A _____ diopter indicates a stronger lens.

9. _____, used to map areas of impaired or absent vision due to retinal disease or other ocular or neurologic abnormality, is performed using an _____.

10. _____ is an assessment of peripheral vision, performed by testing the subject's ability to discern moving objects or flashing lights at the extreme periphery of the visual fields.

11. Tests for _____ employ printed figures made up of variously sized dots in various colors and shades.

12. _____ is the precise determination of hearing threshold—the faintest level of loudness that the subject can hear at any given pitch.

13. _____ is ringing or other abnormal noise in one or both ears.

14. _____ is used to testing a person's hearing.

15. _____ is usually reversible while _____ is not.

16. A threshold shift of 50 dB or more in both ears throughout the _____ is usually perceived as severe deafness.

Exercises

17. With normal hearing in the 250 to 2000 Hz range, a threshold shift of 50 dB or more at _____ may be only mildly disabling, or may even go unnoticed.

18. The nerve important to both hearing and balance is the _____.

19. The medical term for difficulty in maintaining balance is _____, while a sense of spinning is known as _____.

20. Involuntary cyclical back-and-forth movement of the eyes is called _____.

Multiple Choice: Circle the letter of the best answer from the choices given.

1. Refraction is determined in the following manner:
    A. Testing the subject's ability to discern moving objects or flashing lights at the extreme periphery of the visual fields.
    B. Instructing the subject to gaze at a central point in a network of lines, usually white on black, while the examiner moves a small object through various parts of the visual field.
    C. Having the patient identify letters or words of various sizes on a Snellen chart.
    D. Using an instrument containing lenses of various powers to measure deficiencies of near and distant vision more precisely than is possible with vision charts alone.
    E. Having patients read lines or paragraphs printed in various sizes of type printed on a Jaeger card.

2. Peripheral vision is tested by
    A. Testing the subject's ability to discern moving objects or flashing lights at the extreme limits of the visual fields.
    B. Instructing the subject to gaze at a central point in a network of lines, usually white on black, while the examiner moves a small object through various parts of the visual field.
    C. Having the patient identify letters or words of various sizes on a Snellen chart.
    D. Using an instrument containing lenses of various powers to measure deficiencies of near and distant vision more precisely than is possible with vision charts alone.
    E. Having patients read lines or paragraphs printed in various sizes of type printed on a Jaeger card.

3. Vision testing is usually performed by
    A. Testing the subject's ability to discern moving objects or flashing lights at the extreme limits of the visual fields.
    B. Instructing the subject to gaze at a central point in a network of lines, usually white on black, while the examiner moves a small object through various parts of the visual field.
    C. Having the patient identify letters or words of various sizes on a Snellen chart.
    D. Using an instrument containing lenses of various powers to measure deficiencies of near and distant vision more precisely than is possible with vision charts alone.
    E. Having patients read lines or paragraphs printed in various sizes of type printed on a Jaeger card.

Exercises

4. Myopia is also known as
   A. Color-blindness.
   B. Farsightedness.
   C. Astigmatism.
   D. Hypermetropia.
   E. Nearsightedness.

5. Hypermetropia is also known as
   A. Color-blindness.
   B. Farsightedness.
   C. Astigmatism.
   D. Myopia.
   E. Nearsightedness.

6. Astigmatism is best defined as
   A. The inability to distinguish colors.
   B. Blurring of images due to distortion of the cornea.
   C. The inability to see nearby objects clearly.
   D. The inability to see far objects clearly.
   E. The inability to see objects in the periphery of the vision.

7. The smallest difference in intensity between two sounds that can be appreciated by the human ear is the
   A. Diopter.
   B. Decibel.
   C. Perimetry.
   D. Bel.
   E. Audiometry.

8. All of the following apply to conductive hearing loss except
   A. It results from a lesion or malfunction of inner ear structures.
   B. It can result from disease or injury of the middle ear structures.
   C. It is frequently unilateral, and frequently reversible either spontaneously or with medical or surgical treatment.
   D. It tends to affect all pitch ranges to an equal degree.
   E. It can result from disease or injury of the external ear structures.

9. All of the following apply to sensorineural hearing loss except
   A. It results from a lesion or malfunction of inner ear structures.
   B. It includes hearing loss due to aging and chronic acoustic trauma.
   C. It is typically bilateral, and shows greater hearing loss at higher pitch levels.
   D. It is usually irreversible.
   E. It can result from disease or injury of the external ear structures.

Exercises

10. According to the text, in addition to deafness, disorders of the inner ear, the vestibulocochlear nerve, or the balance center can result in all of the following except
    A. Nystagmus.
    B. Vertigo.
    C. Nausea.
    D. Dysequilibrium.
    E. Astigmatism.

Short Answers

1. Define or explain:
   a. decibel _____
   _____

   b. diopter _____
   _____

   c. myopia _____
   _____

   d. nystagmus _____
   _____

   e. refraction_____
   _____

   f. COWS _____
   _____

2. How is it possible to test the vision of a person who cannot read?
   _____
   _____
   _____

3. List two tests mentioned in this chapter that are often used to screen persons without symptoms of abnormality or disease.
   a. _____
   b. _____

Exercises

4. What test described in this chapter does not depend on the patient's report of what is perceived or experienced?

   _____

5. What two functions are served by the eighth cranial nerve?

   a. _____

   b. _____

6. Discuss the advantages and disadvantages of automated audiometry as compared to that performed by a technician. Discuss the patient's performance, interpretation, and the limitations of each system.

   _____
   _____
   _____
   _____
   _____
   _____
   _____
   _____
   _____
   _____
   _____
   _____
   _____
   _____
   _____
   _____
   _____
   _____
   _____
   _____
   _____

Exercises

Activities for Application and Further Study

1. Find an Amsler grid on the Internet. Test your and your family's or classmates' visual fields using the instructions provided with the grid. (Realize that this is not a professional test, so any abnormalities should be verified by an optometrist or ophthalmologist.)

2. Testing of peripheral vision with visual field testing and perimetry is useful in assessing eye diseases or conditions. Describe the progressive effect of these conditions on a person's vision.

3. Hearing is important to medical transcriptionists. Find out if there is a university or clinic in your area that does audiometric testing and see if you can arrange a field trip for your class.

Measurement of Temperature, Rates, Pressures, and Volumes

4

Temperature

The phrase **vital signs** refers to four basic quantitative measurements that are part of every routine health assessment: temperature, pulse, respirations (respiratory rate), and blood pressure. In hospitalized patients these four measurements are performed and recorded at standard intervals.

Body heat is a by-product of metabolic reactions in tissues and is regulated within narrow limits by autonomic processes such as dilatation or constriction of superficial blood vessels and sweating. Body **temperature** is subject to wide individual variations from the oft-quoted normal level of 98.6° F (37.0° C). In addition, temperature varies diurnally by about 1.0° C from a low around 4:00 a.m. to a high around 4:00 p.m. In women of childbearing age, the average temperature is about 1.0° lower during the first two weeks of the menstrual cycle (before ovulation) than it is during the second two weeks.

A variety of devices are available for measuring body temperature in the clinical setting. These include the traditional mercury thermometer, disposable plastic strips that indicate temperature by color change, and electronic devices (thermistors) that provide digital readouts. The most accurate readings of the "core" or "true" temperature are obtained by using a rectal thermometer or placing a thermistor in a body cavity or in one of the great vessels. For practical purposes, however, temperatures are taken orally except in infants and small children. Electronic ear thermometers for use in children provide reliable readings.

Elevation of body temperature (fever, pyrexia), most often due to acute viral respiratory infection, is a universal human experience. The study of fevers, their causes, course, and treatment, made up a major part of ancient and medieval medicine. With the development of the thermometer around 1700, more precise observation of variations in body temperature became feasible (*see box*).

Inventors of Thermometers and Scales

The first thermometers were based on the principle that a fluid expands as its temperature rises and contracts as its temperature falls. Galileo Galilei (1564-1642) is credited with inventing an alcohol thermometer as early as 1595. Around 1710, Gabriel Fahrenheit (1686-1736) developed a mercury thermometer and devised the temperature scale that bears his name. On the Fahrenheit scale water freezes at 32° and boils at 212°.

Anders Celsius (1701-1744) created a revised temperature scale around 1743, based on 0° as the freezing point of water and 100° as its boiling point. Because each Celsius degree is 1/100 of the interval between freezing and boiling points, the Celsius scale is also called the centigrade scale. In 1848 William Thomson, Lord Kelvin (1824-1907) based a third scale on absolute zero, the temperature at which theoretically all molecular motion ceases. Degrees on the Kelvin scale are the same size as on the Celsius scale, but zero on this scale occurs at -273.15° C (-460° F).

Both Fahrenheit and Celsius scales are used in clinical medicine in the United States.

98.6° F = 37.0° C

To convert from Fahrenheit to Celsius, (1) subtract 32 and (2) multiply by 5/9 [0.555].

To convert from Celsius to Fahrenheit, (1) multiply by 9/5 [1.8] and (2) add 32.

Among the many causes of fever, the most common are infection, inflammation, toxemia, and malignant disease. Elevation of body temperature can also be due to derangement of heat regulating mechanisms, as in heat-stroke. Abnormally low body temperature can occur in hypothyroidism, hemorrhage, and terminal illness, and after prolonged exposure or severe trauma.

Certain illnesses, notably malaria, cause bouts of fever that recur at regular intervals as new generations of parasites are released into the circulation. A tertian fever recurs at intervals of 48 hours, a quartan fever at intervals of 72 hours. Fever that resolves suddenly is said to fall by crisis, while fever that gradually disappears over a period of two or three days is said to fall by lysis.

Fever of unknown origin (FUO) is a diagnostic category, sometimes defined as a documented fever (temperature of 101° F [38.3°C] or higher) lasting more than three weeks and not explainable by history or findings on physical examination and laboratory studies, including cultures. The most common causes eventually found for fever of unknown origin are infection (especially occult abscess, tuberculosis, cytomegalovirus or HIV infection, and endocarditis with negative cultures because of inappropriate antibiotic treatment), chronic inflammatory diseases (sarcoidosis, polymyositis, temporal arteritis, and inflammatory bowel disease), neoplasms (Hodgkin disease, other lymphomas, multiple myeloma, renal cell carcinoma), and drug reactions.

Ocular Tonometry

Routine measurement of the pressure within the eye is performed to detect glaucoma, a group of disorders characterized by increased intraocular pressure and risk of damage to the optic nerve, with resulting loss of vision. The normal intraocular pressure is less than 21 mmHg. Intraocular pressure can be measured by various non-invasive methods, all of which assess the resistance of the cornea to deformation by an externally applied force.

Indentation tonometry is performed with a simple hand-held device, the Schiøtz tonometer, which measures the depth to which a weighted plunger indents the cornea. The examiner then converts that figure to intraocular pressure in millimeters of mercury (mmHg) by consulting a table. Direct-reading electronic versions of this instrument are available. Applanation tonometry measures the amount of force necessary to flatten a fixed area of the cornea. This measurement requires instillation of fluorescein dye into the eye and observation of corneal flattening by the examiner with a slit lamp (discussed in Chapter 7). Pneumotonometry uses a puff of air to flatten the cornea.

Manometry of the Gastrointestinal Tract

The walls of the entire digestive tube from mouth to anus contain longitudinal and circular muscle fibers. Peristalsis is the coordinated action of these muscles, consisting of waves of alternating contraction and relaxation, by which the contents of the digestive tract are moved forward. In addition, the muscular action of some parts of the gastrointestinal tract aids digestion by promoting a mixing of foods with digestive juices.

A sphincter is a ring of muscle surrounding a normal bodily opening or passage and serving as a valve to control the release of material. While the anal sphincter is a true anatomic sphincter, most of the other so-called sphincters (for example, the lower esophageal sphincter between the esophagus and the stomach) are merely "physiologic," consisting of ill-defined or incomplete rings of muscle and providing only partial valve action.

Disturbances in peristalsis and in the function of gastrointestinal sphincters are features of many digestive tract disorders, both functional and organic, and are common causes of heartburn, colic (crampy abdominal pain), bloating, constipation, and diarrhea. The measurement of pressure within certain parts of the digestive tract, and particularly at anatomic and physiologic sphincters, provides information about the resting tone, contractile strength, and coordination of muscular activity at these levels. Gastrointestinal manometry may be based on direct measurement of pressure by a pressure transducer, on measurement of the resistance to flow from an opening in a water-perfused catheter, or on assessment of electrical impedance.

For esophageal studies a manometric catheter is passed through the nose or mouth, after application of topical anesthetic, and measurements are taken at rest and while the patient swallows. The pattern of peristalsis is followed with the catheter tip at various levels, and the tone and function of the lower esophageal sphincter are studied. For patients with symptoms of gastroesophageal reflux, continuous recording of luminal and sphincter pressure may be performed during several hours or overnight. Esophageal pH, a measure of acidity, can also be continuously monitored by a swallowed electrode.

The sphincter of Oddi controls the flow of bile and pancreatic juice into the duodenum. Disorders of this sphincter can be assessed with a manometer placed in the sphincter by means of a gastroduodenoscope (discussed in Chapter 8).

Anorectal manometry has been used to study patients with constipation and fecal incontinence. Its principal value is in the diagnosis of Hirschsprung disease (congenital megacolon), in which a deficiency in the innervation of the colon leads to chronic constipation and dilatation of the colon in children. The colon and rectum are emptied of stool by enemas before placement of the manometer.

Cardiovascular Measurements

The heart is a muscular pump—actually two pumps working side by side (see Fig.4.1). The right atrium receives venous blood from the systemic circulation and directs it into the right ventricle, which pumps it into the lungs for gas exchange. The left atrium receives freshly oxygenated blood from the lungs and directs it into the left ventricle, which pumps it through the aorta into the arteries of the systemic circulation. Systole is the contraction of a heart chamber

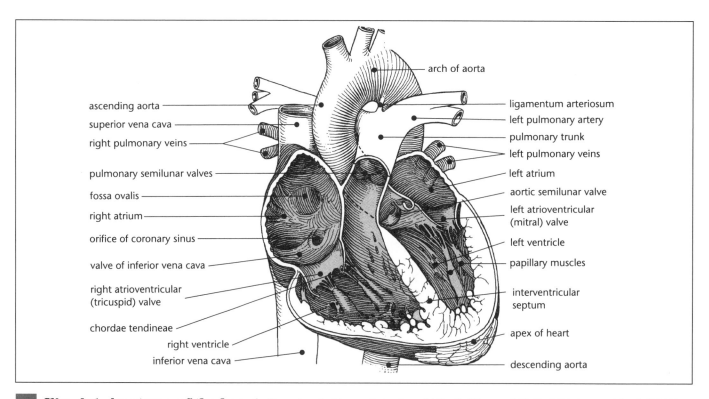

ascending aorta
superior vena cava
right pulmonary veins
pulmonary semilunar valves
fossa ovalis
right atrium
orifice of coronary sinus
valve of inferior vena cava
right atrioventricular (tricuspid) valve
chordae tendineae
right ventricle
inferior vena cava

arch of aorta
ligamentum arteriosum
left pulmonary artery
pulmonary trunk
left pulmonary veins
left atrium
aortic semilunar valve
left atrioventricular (mitral) valve
left ventricle
papillary muscles
interventricular septum
apex of heart
descending aorta

Fig. 4.1. Anatomy of the heart. Reproduced with permission from *Melloni's Illustrated Medical Dictionary*, 4th ed. (2002).

(atrium or ventricle) and diastole is the period of relaxation and refilling between systoles. The heart consists almost entirely of muscle tissue, which receives its blood supply from the coronary arteries, the first branches of the aorta.

Noninvasive Cardiac Measurements

The pulse is the regular thrusting sensation, synchronous with the heartbeat, that can be felt on palpation of any superficial artery. Feeling the pulse is one of the most ancient of all diagnostic procedures, antedating the earliest medical writings (*see box*).

Pulse

Palpation of the pulse is the single most important diagnostic technique in traditional Chinese medicine. Practitioners of this discipline use palpation to differentiate 31 pulse patterns at 18 positions on the right and left wrists, each with its diagnostic or prognostic significance. The widespread familiarity with the pulse at the wrist is attested by the words for 'wrist' in various languages (Italian *polso*, Portuguese *pulso*, Dutch *pols*). The Spanish for 'bracelet, cuff' is *pulsera*, and the corresponding German word is *Pulswärmer*. The anatomic term *temple* probably refers to the practice of measuring brief intervals of time (Latin *tempus*) by counting pulsations of the temporal artery in front of the ear.

The pulse rate can be measured by palpation of any superficial artery, and can also be detected by a cardiac monitor or pulse oximeter (described in Chapter 6) or determined from an electrocardiogram. In clinical practice it is usually taken on the volar surface of the wrist, where the radial artery can be compressed by the examining finger against the distal radius. The pulse is ordinarily taken with the examiner's index finger, never with the examiner's thumb, which has a prominent pulse of its own that may confound the reading. A standard technique is to count the pulse during a period of 15 or 30 seconds, as measured by the second hand of a watch, and to multiply the result by the appropriate factor to obtain the rate per minute.

The radial pulse rate is normally identical to the heart rate. In certain arrhythmias, however, some beats of the heart may not be sufficiently forceful to generate an impulse that can be felt in a peripheral artery. In such circumstances a more accurate estimate of the actual heart rate can be gained by auscultation over the cardiac apex with a stethoscope. Any difference between this **apical pulse** and the pulse taken at the wrist is called the **pulse deficit**.

The pulse rate varies widely from person to person, and is sometimes normal even when outside the usually quoted normal range of 60-100/min. The pulse is increased by exercise, emotional excitement, fever or high environmental temperature, many medicines and substances of abuse including alcohol and nicotine, and many circulatory or generalized disorders, such as shock, congestive heart failure, and myocardial infarction. The resting pulse may be less than 60/min in athletes as well as in persons with hypothermia or in the final stage of circulatory collapse, or as an effect of certain drugs (beta-blockers and others).

Apparent irregularity of the pulse, as determined at the wrist, can be due to extra beats (ventricular premature contractions), dropped beats, sinus arrhythmia (normal cyclical variations in heart rate with respirations), or any of a number of abnormal disturbances of rhythm.

In standard clinical parlance the term **pulse** is synonymous with **pulse rate** or **heart rate**. But arterial pulsations have features in addition to their simple frequency. Careful attention to the feeling imparted to the finger on palpation of a peripheral artery shows that the pulsations felt are not mere taps but rather waves, each rising rapidly to a peak of intensity and then falling away again. Nowadays the temporal configuration of the pulse can be detected by a pressure transducer, converted to an electrical signal, and displayed on a cathode ray tube. Before the modern era of sophisticated testing instruments, physicians learned to distinguish, by feel alone, waveforms of the pulse that were characteristic of various cardiac and systemic disorders.

A bounding pulse with a rapid rise and fall occurs in fever, a thready pulse in shock. Pulsus alternans, consisting of alternating strong and weak beats, usually indicates serious left ventricular dysfunction. In pulsus paradoxus, the amplitude of pulsations in peripheral arteries decreases with inspiration and increases with expiration— just the opposite of the expected response. This phenomenon is noted in disorders that reduce venous return to the heart during inspiration instead of increasing it, such as constrictive pericarditis and pericardial tamponade (blood or fluid under pressure within the pericardial sac preventing normal filling of the heart chambers).

Pulsations are not normally palpable in peripheral veins. They may be visible, however, in the jugular veins at the sides of the neck, and **jugular venous pulsations** can be detected by a pressure transducer and displayed on a cathode ray tube or a moving paper strip or tape. The normal jugular venous pulsation is a complex waveform consisting of three components, each coordinated with an event in the cardiac cycle.

Each component is a positive (upward) deflection, reflecting an increase of pressure in the vein. The a wave occurs with right atrial systole, the c wave with closure of the tricuspid valve, and the v wave with buildup of pressure in the right atrium at the end of atrial diastole. Abnormalities of the jugular venous waveform can result from valvular disease, arrhythmias, and other disorders affecting the function of the right side of the heart.

The pressure of the blood within the systemic arterial circulation has a major impact on health and well-being. When blood pressure is too low to maintain adequate perfusion of vital tissues such as the brain, the heart, and the kidneys, the condition is called **shock**. Whether due to acute blood loss, dehydration, severe burns, or toxic products of infection, shock is a life-threatening condition. Abnormal elevation of blood pressure (hypertension) by itself seldom creates an emergency, but when untreated for long periods it can overwork the heart and damage arteries, leading to heart failure, heart attack, stroke, and other severe consequences. It is estimated that one-fourth of the U.S. population, and one-half of those over age 60, have hypertension.

The measurement of **blood pressure** is one of the most frequently performed diagnostic procedures in medicine. The earliest research in this field involved connecting a manometer directly to the circulation (*see box*). Although such direct measurements are still performed during cardiac catheterization, a standardized indirect method is routinely used in clinical practice.

Blood Pressure

The first known experiments on direct measurement of blood pressure were made in the 18th century by Stephen Hales (1677-1761). An English clergyman with a scientific turn of mind, Hales studied gases, plant physiology, and the circulation of animals. To measure the blood pressure of a horse, he inserted a glass tube into its femoral artery and found that a column of blood rose in the tube to a height of about 11 feet.

Arterial blood pressure fluctuates substantially with each beat of the heart. Each contraction (systole) of the left ventricle sends a rush of blood into the aorta and its branches, causing a sharp rise in pressure. When the ventricle relaxes so as to refill for its next contraction, the blood pressure drops by 25-50% or more. If the arteries were rigid like metal pipes, the pressure would rise higher with systole and drop lower between beats of the heart. But because the arteries are elastic, they distend during systole and contract during diastole, thus moderating the changes in pressure due to alternating systole and diastole and tending to maintain a more even forward flow of blood.

The indirect method of determining blood pressure involves the use of a sphygmomanometer and a stethoscope. The sphygmomanometer is a gauge (either an aneroid manometer or a column of mercury in a glass tube) that measures the pressure of the air within an inflatable cuff that is placed around the subject's arm. The examiner inflates the cuff until pulsations of the heart can no longer be detected in the brachial artery below the cuff. This indicates that the pressure of air in the cuff exceeds the pressure of the blood.

While listening with the stethoscope over the brachial artery distal to the cuff, the examiner slowly deflates the cuff, noting the pressure, in millimeters of mercury (mmHg or torr), at which pulsations begin to be heard. This is the systolic pressure—the pressure at which jets of blood are able to overcome the pressure of the cuff during left ventricular systole. As air continues to escape from the cuff, pulsations become fainter and finally cease. The pressure within the cuff at the moment when pulsations are no longer audible is called the diastolic pressure, the lowest level to which the pressure drops between beats of the heart. By convention, these figures are reported as a fraction, with the higher number on top; e.g., 120/80, pronounced "one twenty over eighty." For a subject with very large arms, a larger cuff must be used to obtain an accurate reading. In certain circumstances blood pressure may be taken with the cuff applied to the thigh.

The difference between systolic and diastolic blood pressures is called the pulse pressure. If the blood pressure is 147/88, the pulse pressure is 59. The pulse pressure is increased in fever, thyrotoxicosis, arteriovenous fistula, and in persons with isolated systolic blood pressure. In the latter condition, an elevated pulse pressure may be more ominous than combined elevation of systolic and diastolic readings.

Automatic or electronic blood pressure devices of various kinds are available. Some of these are designed for self-testing by the patient. Some detect pulsations electronically and thus obviate the need for auscultation, which may not be feasible at an accident scene or in an ambulance or rescue helicopter.

Ideally the blood pressure is obtained with the subject comfortably seated, after a brief period of rest. Comparison of blood pressure readings in the two arms may indicate coarctation of the aorta (narrowing of the aorta between the origins of arteries to the right and left arms), and comparison of pressure determined in the lower extremities with pressure determined in the arms may indicate narrowing of the abdominal aorta or of one of its branches.

Hypertension is arbitrarily defined as a systolic blood pressure over 140, a diastolic blood pressure over 90, or both. In persons subject to the so-called white coat syndrome, the mere fact of having the blood pressure taken (or the mere presence of a physician or other health care provider) can cause transitory elevation of blood pressure above this level.

For such persons, **ambulatory blood pressure monitoring** may provide a more valid assessment of blood pressure. An ambulatory monitor consists of a blood pressure cuff that is worn continuously for 24-48 hours and a programmed recording unit that inflates the cuff and takes a reading every 15 minutes during the day and every 30 minutes during the night. After the testing period the data are downloaded from the electronic memory of the device for interpretation.

A **tilt table test** may be performed to assess the effect of assuming the erect posture on pulse and blood pressure. Although nonspecific, this test is simple and noninvasive, and is sometimes valuable in indicating incipient shock due to blood loss. It can also help to identify persons subject to orthostatic hypotension (significant drop in systemic blood pressure on assumption of the erect posture) due to certain drugs or inappropriate cardiovascular reflexes.

The patient lies horizontal on a motorized tilting table while baseline readings of pulse and blood pressure are obtained. Continuous electrocardiographic monitoring may also be performed. The table is then gradually tilted to a nearly vertical position, with the patient supported by a strap and a foot rest. Changes in cardiovascular measurements are noted and recorded.

Invasive Cardiovascular Procedures

In medicine, the term **invasive** refers to a diagnostic or therapeutic procedure that involves the insertion of instruments or appliances through a puncture or incision in the skin, most often into arteries or veins. Although all invasive cardiovascular procedures carry some risk of adverse consequences such as bleeding, clotting, severe injury to blood vessels or heart valves, and death, certain ones are used routinely because the precise information made available by them outweighs the risks.

Cardiac catheterization refers to any procedure in which a catheter (a small-caliber flexible tube) is inserted through a peripheral blood vessel and threaded into the heart (*see box*). Cardiac catheterization may be performed for purely diagnostic purposes, but nowadays it is often the first step in interventional procedures such as balloon angioplasty (stretching or breaking up atherosclerotic plaques in coronary arteries), placement of stents to maintain patency of coronary arteries, and radioablation of abnormal foci of electrical activity in the cardiac conduction system.

Cardiac Catheterization

Werner Forssmann (1904-1979) performed the first cardiac catheterization in 1929 in Eberswalde, Germany, using himself as the subject. He passed a catheter through his left antecubital vein and into his right atrium, observing the advance of the catheter on a fluoroscope screen by means of a mirror held by an assistant. Forssmann was so severely criticized by medical authorities for his rashness that he abandoned his study of cardiac physiology and specialized in urologic surgery. In subsequent decades, the technique of cardiac catheterization was developed and refined by André Cournand and D.W. Richards, with whom Forssmann shared the Nobel Prize in Medicine in 1956.

Diagnostic procedures that can be performed by means of a catheter in the heart include the measurement of pressures in the cardiac chambers, assessment of valve function, detection of septal defects and abnormal shunts, and sampling of blood for determination of oxygen concentration. Radiographic studies of cardiac chambers or coronary arteries require placement of a catheter for injection of contrast medium (discussed in Chapter 11).

Access to both right and left sides of the heart cannot be gained with a single catheter placed in a peripheral blood vessel, unless the patient has an abnormal communication between the two sides (septal defect) or the examiner creates such a communication by piercing the interventricular septum (not a standard procedure). The left ventricle is reached by a catheter inserted in a peripheral artery (usually either the brachial artery at the bend of the elbow or the femoral artery in the groin) and threaded through the aorta against the direction of blood flow. Access to the right atrium and right ventricle are gained from a peripheral vein (brachial or femoral). For both types of procedure, advancement of the catheter is monitored fluoroscopically (by continuous observation of x-ray images displayed on a television screen).

Placement of the catheter in a peripheral blood vessel can be performed through a small skin incision with direct visualization of the vessel, or by skin puncture. In either case the site is scrubbed with surgical disinfectant and a local anesthetic is injected. For catheterization of both the right and left sides of the heart, an adjacent artery and vein are entered through a single skin incision. The catheter may be passed into the vessel alone or it may be threaded through an outer sheath, which remains in place in the vessel wall and prevents friction at the puncture site during insertion and withdrawal of the catheter.

Catheters are made of various synthetic materials such as nylon, polyethylene, and Teflon, and manufactured in a wide variety of shapes and sizes. Some are straight while others have terminal curves (cobra, sidewinder, and headhunter catheters) or coils (pigtail catheter). The outer diameter of a catheter is measured in French (F) units; 1 F is 0.33 mm.

To improve rigidity and facilitate manipulation, a guidewire is placed inside the catheter. Guidewires are made to various designs depending on the applications for which they are intended. A standard guidewire consists of a single strand of stainless steel wire inside a tightly wound sheath, also of stainless steel. The core wire may be designed to move freely within the sheath, or may be fixed to the sheath near the distal end. A fixed guidewire may be used to direct the placement of the catheter tip within a narrow or tortuous vessel, to straighten out curves or coils in a catheter, or simply to assist in the initial insertion of a catheter. When it is necessary to change from one catheter to another during the course of a procedure such as coronary arteriography, a guidewire remains in place in the vessel while the first catheter is withdrawn and the second is threaded on it.

Cardiac catheterization is performed to identify and localize coronary artery disease and assess its severity, to measure left ventricular dysfunction (congestive heart failure, myocarditis), and to diagnose or assess congenital or acquired abnormalities of cardiac anatomy (septal defects, valvular stenosis or regurgitation). It is an important adjunct to other diagnostic techniques in the evaluation of patients with unexplained chest pain or other symptoms suggesting cardiac disease and in planning surgery to correct disease of coronary arteries or valves.

The measurement of the pressure within the vessel or cardiac chamber in which the tip of the catheter is placed is a principal function of cardiac catheterization. To measure pressure, the catheter is prefilled with saline solution mixed with heparin (an anticoagulant) to prevent clotting. The catheter is then attached to a transducer, a device that converts the pressure detected to an electrical signal that can be displayed on a cathode ray tube, as a digital readout, or as a continuous tracing on a strip of paper or tape. Two channels are provided for simultaneous measurement of pressure in two sites, as in measuring the pressure gradient and flow across a cardiac valve.

A multipurpose catheter may have five or more channels or lumens, each with its own function. These may include, besides pressure-measuring lines, a catheter to take blood specimens from various sites for gas analysis; electrode leads to permit performance of electrocardiography of cardiac chambers; a thermistor to monitor temperature after injection of chilled saline as a means of calculating cardiac output by the thermodilution technique; fiberoptic bundles to measure oxygen saturation; and a channel for injection of radiographic contrast medium.

For mechanical reasons it is seldom feasible to pass an arterial catheter through the aorta and left ventricle into the left atrium. A close estimate of left atrial pressure can, however, be obtained by measuring **pulmonary wedge pressure** (Ppw), also called pulmonary capillary wedge pressure (PCWP), with a Swan-Ganz catheter inserted through a peripheral vein. This type of catheter has a balloon near its tip, which can be inflated by injection of 1-2 mL of air through one of its lumens. The catheter is advanced through the right atrium and right ventricle into the pulmonary artery. Once the balloon is inflated, the forward flow of blood causes the catheter to become wedged in one of the smaller branches of the pulmonary artery.

The pressure reading taken from the port distal to the balloon is then essentially identical to the left atrial pressure and the left ventricular end-diastolic pressure (normally 8-10 mmHg). Elevation of this pressure above 15 mmHg suggests disease of the mitral or aortic valve or ventricular failure. Because placement of a flow-directed Swan-Ganz catheter is often feasible without fluoroscopic monitoring, this procedure can be performed at the bedside or in an emergency department rather than in a cardiac catheterization suite.

Another vascular catheterization procedure that is usually performed without fluoroscopic guidance is the placement of a central venous pressure line, often with access through an internal jugular or subclavian vein. **Central venous pressure** (CVP), that is, the pressure in the superior or inferior vena cava, closely reflects the volume of circulating blood and is therefore a useful index of the degree of shock and the response to its treatment. In an emergency setting the placement of a large-bore central venous catheter is often also useful for administering drugs or fluids.

Respiratory Measurements

The **respiratory rate** is one of the vital signs that are routinely determined during a physical examination and monitored in hospitalized patients and those receiving urgent care.

Breathing is an automatic function whose rate is governed principally by the concentrations of oxygen and carbon dioxide in the blood. The normal resting rate in healthy adults is 12-16 respirations/minute.

More rapid breathing (tachypnea) occurs in circumstances that increase the need for oxygen, such as exercise, emotional excitement, elevation of body temperature, and it can also be caused by most abnormal conditions that impair the ability of the heart and lungs to exchange oxygen and carbon dioxide (pneumonia, shock, congestive heart failure) or by metabolic acidosis (as in the Kussmaul respirations, both rapid and deep, of diabetic coma). Abnormally slow breathing (bradypnea) can result from respiratory depression due to drugs, stroke, head injury, or the terminal stage of any severe systemic or metabolic disorder. Cheyne-Stokes respirations are cyclic alternations between periods of apnea (cessation of breathing) or hypopnea (very shallow breathing) and periods of tachypnea.

If instructed to "breathe naturally," the average person finds it impossible to do so. Measurement of respiratory rate in the conscious patient is therefore performed surreptitiously—for example, by an examiner pretending to count the pulse or listen to the heartbeat. Ideally the respirations are counted for a full minute. Respiratory rate can be recorded automatically by various devices, most of them detecting respiratory movements of the thorax.

Acute and chronic disorders of the respiratory tract can impair the flow of air into and out of the lungs, reduce the amount of lung tissue available for gas exchange, or both. **Spirometry** is the measurement of lung volumes and inspiratory and expiratory flow rates with a precisely calibrated instrument (spirometer) according to a standard testing protocol.

Spirometry is indicated in respiratory disorders causing dyspnea, wheezing, or cough when a quantitative assessment of lung volumes and flow rates is needed for diagnosis or for judging the severity of the condition or the response to treatment. Testing of respiratory volumes and flow rates is also valuable in screening smokers for early chronic obstructive pulmonary disease, in planning surgery involving removal of lung tissue, and in quantifying pulmonary disability.

The testing procedure requires the patient to breathe through a disposable mouthpiece attached by flexible tubing to the spirometer. A padded clamp occludes the nostrils to ensure that air flow occurs only through the mouth. After inhaling as deeply as possible, the patient exhales into the mouthpiece as rapidly and forcefully as possible. Several repetitions of the test may be required in order to achieve maximal measurements. Ordinarily the results of various efforts are not averaged, but the best scores are assumed to be the most accurate. The validity of test results depends on close adherence to standard testing protocol, accurate calibration of the instrument, and good cooperation by the subject. Often the coaching provided by the technician performing the test is crucial in obtaining a maximal inspiration and expiratory effort.

The following measurements are performed during standard spirometry:

Tv (Vt) (tidal volume): the volume of air inhaled and exhaled during normal breathing, measured in liters (L).

FVC (forced vital capacity): the maximum volume of air that can be forcefully exhaled after a maximal inspiration, in liters.

FEV_1 (forced expiratory volume in 1 second): the volume of air that is exhaled during the first second of forceful exhalation, in liters.

FEV_1/FVC: the ratio of FEV_1 to FVC, expressed as a percent.

FEF_{25-75} (forced expiratory flow 25%-75%): the average flow rate during the midportion of a forced expiration, measured in liters per second (L/sec).

PEF (peak expiratory flow): the highest flow rate attained during forced expiration, measured in liters per second.

For patients believed to have asthma, in which the bronchi are subject to intermittent constriction with resulting reduction of airflow, the testing procedure may be modified by administration of pharmaceutical agents. Inhalation of histamine or methacholine causes sharp reduction of flow rates due to bronchospasm in persons with hyperreactive airways. Inhalation of a bronchodilator quickly improves flow rates in a person with naturally occurring bronchospasm, or after challenge with histamine or methacholine.

The range of normal spirometry findings for a given subject depends on height, age, gender, and race. The results obtained by testing are therefore reported not only as absolute numbers but also as percents of the patient's predicted performance, based on these variables. In addition, the spirometer generates a graph plotting inspiratory and flow rates against volumes (flow-volume loop).

Abnormal spirometric findings are basically of two types. In obstructive lung disease, a reduction in flow rate (FEV_1) occurs without a proportionate reduction in lung volume (FVC). This pattern is seen in emphysema and chronic bronchitis, which together constitute chronic obstructive pulmonary disease (COPD), as well as in asthma and acute bronchitis. In restrictive lung disease, both volume and flow rate are reduced in proportion. This type of spirometric finding occurs in pulmonary diseases causing scarring of the lungs or filling of air spaces with fluid or exudate, and also in diseases of the chest wall (pleura, ribs) impairing respiratory effort.

A compact, handheld personal spirometer to determine FEV_1 may be helpful for persons with asthma to judge the severity of acute airway compromise and the need for, or effectiveness of, medicines. The term **incentive spirometry** is applied to breathing exercises prescribed to prevent atelectasis and pneumonia due to inadequate lung expansion in postoperative patients, those with chest injuries, and others confined to bed. Exercises consist of periods of deep breathing at regular intervals throughout the day. Use of a personal spirometer enables the patient to measure pulmonary flow so as to meet goals established on the basis of age, gender, and height.

The following respiratory volumes cannot be measured by spirometry. They can, however, be determined indirectly by plethysmography (in which the subject sits in a sealed chamber while pressure and volume changes are noted during normal breathing, maximal inspiration and expiration, and panting respirations) or determination of total lung capacity by tracer gas studies (in which a known concentration of nonabsorbable gas is breathed for a period of time and its concentration in expired air is then determined).

TLC (total lung capacity): the volume of air in the lungs after maximal inspiration.

FRC (functional residual capacity): the volume of air remaining in the lungs after normal expiration.

RV (residual volume): the volume of air remaining in the lungs after maximal expiration.

The widely used expression **pulmonary function tests** (PFTs) does not apply, strictly speaking, to spirometry, since measurements of lung volumes and flow rates do not assess the function of the lungs, which is to exchange oxygen and carbon dioxide between the atmosphere and the blood. Some tests that may be performed in conjunction with spirometry do, however, measure gas exchange. The alveolar-capillary membrane, consisting of the walls of the pulmonary capillaries as they lie in apposition to the smallest pulmonary air sacs (the alveoli), is the anatomic site of gas exchange. Gas diffusion tests measure the passage of gases across this membrane.

In the carbon monoxide diffusion capacity ($D_L CO$) test, the patient takes a maximum inhalation of a mixture of air, helium, and carbon monoxide and holds it for ten seconds. The exhaled breath is then analyzed, and from the concentrations of gases present the diffusing capacity is calculated as the volume of gas transferred per minute per millimeter of mercury of difference between the gas pressure of alveolar air and capillary blood. Normally this value is at least 25mL/minute/mmHg.

Another way of assessing pulmonary gas diffusion is the nitrogen washout test. The air we breathe is approximately 80% nitrogen and 20% oxygen. Breathing 100% oxygen for a period of several minutes normally results in a gradual washing out of nitrogen from the lungs. For the nitrogen washout test, the subject breathes 100% oxygen and the nitrogen composition of exhaled air is determined serially. The finding of a nitrogen concentration greater than 2.5% after 7 minutes indicates erratic pulmonary gas diffusion. A variation of this test can be performed by graphing the nitrogen concentration of a single exhalation after maximal inhalation of 100% oxygen.

Pulmonary gas diffusing capacity may be significantly reduced in both restrictive and obstructive lung disease and in pulmonary embolism, and test results may also be abnormal in cardiac disease, anemia, and other conditions affecting respiratory physiology.

Exercises

Fill in the Blanks

1. The phrase _____ refers to temperature, pulse, respirations (respiratory rate), and blood pressure, four basic quantitative measurements that are part of every routine health assessment.

2. _____ is another word for fever.

3. A _____ fever recurs at intervals of 48 hours, a _____ fever at intervals of 72 hours.

4. Fever that resolves suddenly is said to fall by _____, while fever that gradually disappears over a period of two or three days is said to fall by _____.

5. Routine measurement of the _____ is performed to detect glaucoma.

6. Indentation tonometry is performed with a simple handheld device, the _____.

7. _____ measures the amount of force necessary to flatten a fixed area of the cornea.

8. _____ uses a puff of air to flatten the cornea.

9. _____ is the coordinated action of longitudinal and circular muscles, consisting of waves of alternating contraction and relaxation, by which the contents of the digestive tract are moved forward.

10. A _____ is a ring of muscle surrounding a normal bodily opening or passage and serving as a valve to control the release of material.

11. _____ provides information about the resting tone, contractile strength, and coordination of muscular activity at certain parts of the digestive tract, and particularly at anatomic and physiologic sphincters.

12. _____ is the contraction of a heart chamber, and _____ is the period of relaxation and refilling that follows.

13. A _____ is any difference between the pulse taken at the wrist and actual heart rate.

14. A _____ pulse with a rapid rise and fall occurs in fever, a _____ pulse in shock.

15. _____, consisting of alternating strong and weak beats, usually indicates serious left ventricular dysfunction.

Exercises

16. In _____, the amplitude of pulsations in peripheral arteries decreases with inspiration and increases with expiration—just the opposite of the expected response—noted in disorders such as _____ and _____.

17. When blood pressure is too low to maintain adequate perfusion of vital tissues such as the brain, the heart, and the kidneys, the condition is called _____.

18. When patients exhibit "white coat syndrome," alternative blood pressures readings may be obtained using _____ monitoring.

19. The term _____ refers to a diagnostic or therapeutic procedure that involves the insertion of instruments or appliances through a puncture or incision in the skin, most often into arteries or veins.

20. Any procedure in which a catheter is inserted through a peripheral blood vessel and threaded into the heart is called _____.

21. _____ is the measurement of lung volumes and inspiratory and expiratory flow rates with a precisely calibrated instrument according to a standard testing protocol.

22. Breathing exercises, consisting of periods of deep breathing at regular intervals throughout the day, prescribed to prevent atelectasis and pneumonia, are known as _____.

23. An indirect method of determining respiratory volumes is _____, in which the subject sits in a sealed chamber while pressure and volume changes are noted during normal breathing, maximal inspiration and expiration, and panting respirations.

24. Another indirect method of determining respiratory volumes is _____, in which a known concentration of nonabsorbable gas is breathed for a period of time and its concentration in expired air is then determined.

Multiple Choice: Circle the letter of the best answer from the choices given.

1. The most accurate readings of the "core" or "true" temperature are obtained
   A. With an oral mercury thermometer.
   B. With an electronic ear thermometer.
   C. With disposable plastic strips that indicate temperature by color change.
   D. Using a rectal thermometer or placing a thermistor in a body cavity or in one of the great vessels.
   E. Using a basal body temperature.

Exercises

2. A documented fever (temperature of 101° F [38.3°C] or higher) lasting more than three weeks and not explainable by history or findings on physical examination and laboratory studies is known as
    A. A tertian fever
    B. A quartan fever
    C. Pyrexia
    D. Malaria
    E. A fever of undetermined origin

3. Indentation tonometry, which measures the depth to which a weighted plunger indents the cornea, is used to measure
    A. Fever.
    B. Intraocular pressure.
    C. Blood pressure.
    D. Apical pulse.
    E. Peristalsis.

4. Gastrointestinal manometry may be based on all of the following except
    A. Applanation tonometry.
    B. Direct measurement of pressure by a pressure transducer.
    C. Measurement of the resistance to flow from an opening in a water-perfused catheter.
    D. Assessment of electrical impedance.

5. Gastrointestinal manometry may be used to evaluate all of the following conditions except
    A. Swallowing problems.
    B. Gastroesophageal reflux.
    C. Stomach emptying
    D. Sphincter of Oddi dysfunction.
    E. Constipation and fecal incontinence.

6. Important characteristics of pulses other than just simple frequency include all the following except
    A. Bounding pulse.
    B. Pulsus alternans.
    C. Peristaltic waveforms.
    D. Pulsus paradoxus.
    E. Thready pulse.

7. Characteristics of the jugular venous pulse include all the following except
    A. The a wave occurs with right atrial systole.
    B. The c wave with closure of the tricuspid valve.
    C. The v wave with buildup of pressure in the right atrium at the end of atrial diastole.
    D. Bounding pulse.
    E. It may be visible on the side of the neck.

Exercises

8. The pressure within the cuff at the moment when pulsations are no longer audible is called the
   A. Diastolic pressure.
   B. Systolic pressure.
   C. Jugular venous pressure.
   D. Pulse pressure.
   E. Interventricular pressure.

9. The pressure at which jets of blood are able to overcome the pressure of the cuff during left ventricular systole.
   A. Diastolic pressure.
   B. Systolic pressure.
   C. Jugular venous pressure.
   D. Pulse pressure.
   E. Interventricular pressure.

10. The difference between systolic and diastolic blood pressures is called
    A. Diastolic pressure.
    B. Systolic pressure.
    C. Jugular venous pressure.
    D. Pulse pressure.
    E. Interventricular pressure.

11. A simple, noninvasive test valuable in evaluating incipient shock or orthostatic hypotension is the
    A. Cardiac catheterization.
    B. Ambulatory blood pressure study.
    C. Tilt table test.
    D. Jugular venous pulse recording.
    E. Holter monitor study.

12. Diagnostic procedures that can be performed by means of a catheter in the heart include all of the following except
    A. The measurement of pressures in the cardiac chambers.
    B. Balloon angioplasty.
    C. Detection of septal defects and abnormal shunts.
    D. Sampling of blood for determination of oxygen concentration.
    E. Assessment of valve function.

Exercises

13. Rapid breathing, such as occurs in circumstances that increase the need for oxygen, such as exercise, emotional excitement, elevation of body temperature, is also known as
    A. Bradypnea.
    B. Cheyne-Stokes respirations.
    C. Kussmaul respirations.
    D. Hypopnea.
    E. Tachypnea.

14. Abnormally slow breathing is also called
    A. Bradypnea.
    B. Cheyne-Stokes respirations.
    C. Kussmaul respirations.
    D. Hypopnea.
    E. Tachypnea.

15. Rapid and deep respirations, such as occur in diabetic coma are
    A. Bradypnea.
    B. Cheyne-Stokes respirations.
    C. Hypopnea.
    D. Tachypnea.
    E. Kussmaul respirations.

16. Cyclic alternations between periods of apnea (cessation of breathing) or hypopnea (very shallow breathing) and periods of tachypnea are
    A. Bradypnea.
    B. Cheyne-Stokes respirations.
    C. Hypopnea.
    D. Tachypnea.
    E. Kussmaul respirations.

17. The volume of air inhaled and exhaled during normal breathing, measured in liters (L) is
    A. FVC (forced vital capacity).
    B. PEF (peak expiratory flow).
    C. Tv (Vt) (tidal volume).
    D. FEV_1 (forced expiratory volume in 1 second).
    E. FEF_{25-75} (forced expiratory flow 25%-75%).

Exercises

18. The maximum volume of air that can be forcefully exhaled after a maximal inspiration, in liters is
    A. FVC (forced vital capacity).
    B. PEF (peak expiratory flow).
    C. Tv (Vt) (tidal volume).
    D. FEV_1 (forced expiratory volume in 1 second).
    E. FEF_{25-75} (forced expiratory flow 25%-75%).

19. The volume of air that is exhaled during the first second of forceful exhalation, in liters is
    A. FVC (forced vital capacity).
    B. PEF (peak expiratory flow).
    C. Tv (Vt) (tidal volume).
    D. FEV_1 (forced expiratory volume in 1 second).
    E. FEF_{25-75} (forced expiratory flow 25%-75%).

20. The highest flow rate attained during forced expiration, measured in liters per second is
    A. FVC (forced vital capacity).
    B. PEF (peak expiratory flow).
    C. Tv (Vt) (tidal volume).
    D. FEV_1 (forced expiratory volume in 1 second).
    E. FEF_{25-75} (forced expiratory flow 25%-75%).

21. Respiratory volumes that cannot be measured by spirometry include all the following except
    A. RV (residual volume).
    B. FVC (forced vital capacity).
    C. FRC (functional residual capacity).
    D. TLC (total lung capacity).

22. The volume of air in the lungs after maximal inspiration is
    A. RV (residual volume).
    B. FVC (forced vital capacity).
    C. FRC (functional residual capacity).
    D. PEF (peak expiratory flow).
    E. TLC (total lung capacity).

23. The volume of air remaining in the lungs after normal expiration is
    A. RV (residual volume).
    B. FVC (forced vital capacity).
    C. FRC (functional residual capacity).
    D. PEF (peak expiratory flow).
    E. TLC (total lung capacity).

Exercises

24. The volume of air remaining in the lungs after maximal expiration.
    A. RV (residual volume).
    B. FVC (forced vital capacity).
    C. FRC (functional residual capacity).
    D. PEF (peak expiratory flow).
    E. TLC (total lung capacity).

Short Answers

1. Define or explain:

    a. apical pulse _____
        _____

    b. central venous pressure _____
        _____

    c. fever of unknown origin _____
        _____

    d. forced vital capacity _____
        _____

    e. peristalsis_____
        _____

    f. sphincter _____
        _____

    g. tilt table test _____
        _____

    h. Swan-Ganz catheter_____
        _____

    i. carbon monoxide diffusion capacity (D_LCO) test _____
        _____

    j. nitrogen washout test _____
        _____

Exercises

2. List and describe three methods for measuring intraocular pressure.

   a. _____

   b. _____

   c. _____

3. Which heart chamber is not readily accessible by cardiac catheterization? How are pressure readings for that chamber determined indirectly?

   _____

   _____

   _____

   _____

4. List five types of observation besides pressure recordings that may be performed during cardiac catheterization.

   a. _____

   b. _____

   c. _____

   d. _____

   e. _____

5. Give two examples of vascular catheterization procedures that may be performed without fluoroscopic guidance.

   a. _____

   _____

   b. _____

   _____

6. Give two examples of restrictive lung disease.

   a. _____

   _____

   b. _____

   _____

Exercises

7. Give two examples of obstructive lung disease.

    a. _____

    _____

    b. _____

    _____

8. Why does the term *pulmonary function tests* not apply to spirometry?

    _____

    _____

    _____

    _____

    _____

9. What tests are appropriately called pulmonary function tests?

    _____

    _____

    _____

    _____

    _____

Activities for Application and Further Study

1. With a basal body temperature thermometer, take your temperature just before arising using as little motion as possible and again at 4 p.m. for about a week. Graph the variations. What do you think is the cause for these variations? What is the significance of these variations for women of childbearing age?

2. Convert the so-called normal body temperature of 98.6°F to Celsius. Convert 17 Celsius to Fahrenheit. What is the current temperature in your area in both Celsius and Fahrenheit?

3. Using the blood pressure machine at your pharmacy or grocery, take your blood pressure on several occasions, such as (1) when you are rested and calm, (2) when you have just eaten a hearty meal, (3) after walking at a brisk pace for a few minutes, (4) while holding your breath. Graph the variations in blood pressure and discuss the cause and effect of changes you observe.

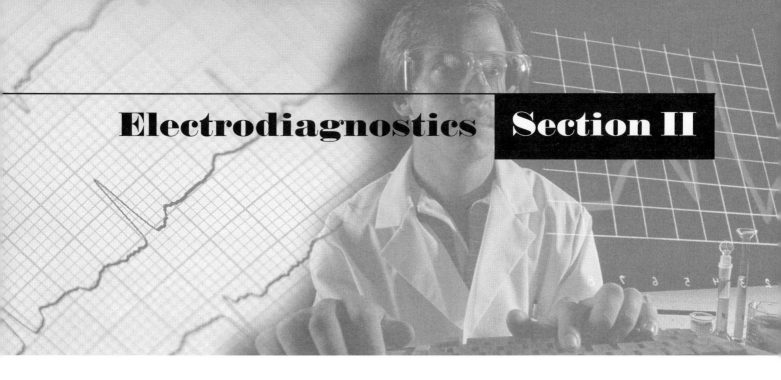

Electrodiagnostics

The normal activity of nerve and muscle tissue involves the generation and transmission of small currents of electricity (*see box on p. 62*). Many disorders that affect nerves and muscles change or impair the electrical activity of those tissues in predictable ways. That fact forms the basis of various standard diagnostic procedures used in modern medicine.

Although the propagation of a wave of electricity along a nerve or muscle fiber is a much more complex process than the flow of current through a metal wire (*see box*), it can be detected, measured, and recorded by suitably designed and calibrated instruments.

In virtually all electrodiagnostic techniques, the basic phenomenon studied is a difference in potential (voltage) between two points. This difference in potential is detected and measured by some form of galvanometer, which receives input from two electrodes placed at strategic points on or in the body. The difference in potential resulting from nerve or muscle activity is not static, like that between the two contacts of a battery, but constantly fluctuating. An electrodiagnostic technique must record these fluctuations in temporal sequence, either as a waveform displayed on a cathode ray tube or as a linear tracing on a strip of paper. Other forms of display, such as audible clicks in electromyography, may also be used. Data from electrodiagnostic procedures can be stored and transmitted digitally.

Current vs. Wave of Depolarization

Nerve and muscle tissue, including heart muscle and the highly specialized conducting system of the heart, consists of bundles or sheets of microscopic fibers, each of which is a living cell. A constant chemical pumping action performed by the cell membrane keeps it polarized—that is, the outside of the cell is electrically positive with respect to the inside.

The passage of an impulse along the course of a nerve or muscle fiber is a wave of depolarization, followed a fraction of a second later by a return to normal polarity (repolarization). This differs substantially from the longitudinal "flow" of electrons through an electric wire, and yet the effect is very similar: a physical, chemical, or electrical stimulus at one end of a nerve or muscle fiber is propagated or transmitted to the other end in a fraction of a second, where it elicits a response.

Frog Legs and Batteries

The Italian physician Luigi Galvani (1737-1798) is recognized as the father of electrophysiology. A lecturer in anatomy at the University of Bologna, Galvani did important research on bones and the kidney and in comparative anatomy. But he is chiefly remembered for his observations on the effects of the newly discovered electricity on living tissue.

There were no generators or batteries when he began his experiments, only devices for making static electricity by friction and crude capacitors (Leyden jars) for storing it. Galvani found that the leg muscles of a frog would twitch in response to electrical stimulation of the frog's spinal cord and also in response to direct stimulation even when severed from the frog's body. He obtained these results not only with static electricity but also by applying the natural electrical force of lightning and by creating small electrical currents with instruments made of different metals (copper and steel).

Galvani's pioneering work led to a gradually broadening understanding of the bioelectric function of nerve and muscle tissue, and hence indirectly to electrodiagnostic techniques such as electroencephalography and electrocardiography. Some of his observations also led to the development, by his colleague and rival, Alessandro Volta (1745-1827), professor of physics at the University of Pavia, of the voltaic pile, a primitive battery and the first artificial source of a continuous electrical current.

Galvani's name is preserved in the terms *galvanic* and *galvanometer*, Volta's in the *volt*, the metric and SI unit of electrical potential.

Electroencephalography, Electromyography, and Related Studies

5

Electroencephalography

Electroencephalography (EEG) is the recording of the electrical activity of the brain. First developed during the 1920s, this diagnostic technique gained acceptance slowly because of the difficulty of coordinating findings with symptoms and neurologic abnormalities. During the middle years of the 20th century, electroencephalography assumed increasing importance in the diagnosis of seizure disorders and in the identification and localization of intracranial neoplasms and vascular lesions.

In the past 20 years, sophisticated imaging techniques such as cerebral angiography, computed tomography (CT), magnetic resonance imaging (MRI), and positron emission tomography (PET) have proved to be more useful than EEG in the study of tumors and other local lesions. Electroencephalography remains the single most valuable diagnostic tool in identifying and classifying seizure disorders and certain dementias, sleep disorders, and toxic encephalopathies. Few EEG patterns are clearly diagnostic. Accurate interpretation of an EEG tracing demands intensive training and experience. In addition, the technician who performs the testing must adhere closely to established protocols in order to produce a diagnostically valid tracing.

The EEG is performed by attaching a number of electrodes (usually 8 or 16) to the scalp at standardized sites identified by bony landmarks (*see box*). Most of the electrodes are applied in pairs at corresponding sites on either side of the midline. Recordings are not taken from each electrode individually, but rather from certain standard combinations or arrays. These may be monopolar (comparing the activity detected by one or more electrodes with an indifferent electrode placed in the midline or on one ear) or bipolar (comparing the input from one electrode or group of electrodes with another electrode or group—for example, left frontal vs. left temporal electrodes, or left frontal vs. right frontal electrodes).

EEG Electrode Positions

Standard locations for the placement of EEG electrodes are designated by abbreviations according to the following scheme:

A – earlobe	N – nasion
C – central	(root of nose)
F – frontal	O – occipital
I – inion (external	P – parietal
occipital	T – temporal
protuberance)	

Locations are further specified by numerals. An odd number refers to the left side, an even number to the right side. The letter z (for *zero*) denotes the midline. Thus, P3 = left parietal electrode; Fz = midline frontal electrode. More complex designations may be used for special electrode positions.

The electrical activity detected in the underlying cerebral cortex by each selected combination of electrodes is amplified and displayed as up-and-down deflections in a continuous line on a monitor screen and recorded on a moving strip of paper. The standard 16-channel EEG produces tracings from 16 different arrays simultaneously. An EEG tracing records electrical activity in real time—that is, each electrical event is documented at the very instant it occurs, and the duration of the event can be determined by reference to the time scale of the record strip.

A standard EEG is recorded for at least 20-30 minutes while the subject rests quietly in the recumbent position, with eyes closed to reduce visual input. (In a sleep laboratory, an EEG may be recorded continuously for several hours.) In an ideal EEG session, the subject falls asleep during the recording. In order to increase the likelihood that this will occur, the subject may be deprived of sleep before the EEG is recorded, or a short-acting barbiturate or other hypnotic may be administered before the beginning of the session.

Various measures may be used to elicit significant responses in the tracing. Standard provocative measures are hyperventilation (deep and rapid breathing, which lowers the subject's plasma carbon dioxide concentration) and photic stimulation by exposure to a rapidly flashing light. Besides entering the exact nature and time of such maneuvers on the tracing, the technician supervising the recording of an EEG notes any other factors or events that can affect the tracing, such as movement of the subject (even eye opening) and sudden loud noises or other distractions.

Interpretation of the EEG is based on a consideration of the amplitude, frequency, and configuration of waves, the observation of differences from one part of the cerebral cortex to another (focal changes), the occurrence of specific wave forms (spikes, spindles), and responses to provocative maneuvers.

The amplitude (height or depth) of each wave or spike in the tracing reflects the voltage of electrical activity detected by the electrode or electrodes in question. This voltage is the sum of the action potentials of millions of cortical neurons. (Electrical activity of brain centers below the level of the cerebral cortex is not reflected in the EEG.) The normal voltage range in the waking adult is 25-75 mcV (microvolts, i.e., millionths of a volt). Higher voltages (above 75 mcV) are normal in children and in sleeping adults.

Waves or up-and-down deflections from the baseline in an EEG tracing do not occur with perfect regularity, but rather at a rate that varies slightly within certain limits. Four such ranges or rhythms of EEG wave frequency are distinguished by Greek letters. (Note that in EEG nomenclature the names of the letters are written out; thus, theta wave.)

Alpha waves, which are characteristic of the resting state in the normal waking adult, have a frequency of 8-13 Hz (hertz, or cycles per second). The faster **beta waves**, with a frequency between 13.5 and 35 Hz, are seen in a state of heightened alertness. The very slow **delta waves** (0.5-4.0 Hz) normally occur only in the deeper (third and fourth) stages of sleep, but may also be seen in certain metabolic, circulatory, or neoplastic disorders of the central nervous system and in dementia. **Theta waves** (4.5-7.5 Hz) are seen in normal children and adolescents, but in adults they occur only during sleep or near-sleep.

Focal variations in the amplitude or frequency of wave patterns, or asymmetry between right and left cortical areas, may indicate local lesions (tumors, injury, sites of origin of partial seizures). Paroxysmal bursts of abnormal rhythm may coincide with seizure activity but can also occur in metabolic and space-occupying lesions of the brain. Certain configurations or wave patterns of the EEG tracing have been found to correspond to specific types of electrical activity. **Sleep spindles** are brief spindle-shaped bursts of low-voltage activity, with a frequency of 12-14 Hz, which occur in light (stage 2) sleep. Also characteristic of stage 2 sleep is the **K-complex**, a negative (downward) spike followed by a high-voltage slow (delta) wave.

A spike in an EEG tracing is an extremely narrow wave, that is, one consisting of a brief deflection and a rapid return to the baseline—by convention, one lasting less than 80 msec (milliseconds). Series of spike-and-wave (spike-and-dome) complexes occurring at a rate of 3/second are highly characteristic of petit mal epilepsy but are noted only during seizure activity. Spike-and-wave complexes with a frequency of 10/second are seen during a grand mal seizure. Between seizures, the EEG of a person with grand mal epilepsy may show widespread paroxysmal bursts of irregular spikes and spike-wave complexes.

Besides assisting in the diagnosis of epilepsy, the EEG is an important resource for monitoring the course of the disease. Periodic EEG tracings can assist in judging the efficacy of therapy and in deciding whether to discontinue treatment after a long period of freedom from seizures. In secondary epilepsy due to a space-occupying lesion, serial EEGs can sometimes show whether the lesion is remaining stable or expanding.

Sleep Studies (Polysomnography)

A sleep laboratory is a facility in which persons with sleep disorders undergo diagnostic evaluation while sleeping or trying to sleep. The patient rests in bed in a dark, quiet environment while electroencephalographic tracings and other diagnostic studies are performed. Polysomnography is the simultaneous performance of several monitoring activities during sleep. In addition to electroencephalography, these studies may include electrocardiography; electronic recording of eye, chin, and limb movements; monitoring of nasal and oral air flow, the rate and depth of respirations, and arterial oxygen saturation; and videorecording of body position and movement. Indications for sleep studies are chronic insomnia, obstructive sleep apnea, narcolepsy, sleep pattern disorders, and parasomnias such as sleepwalking.

Four stages or levels of normal sleep have been identified on the basis of EEG changes. In the waking state, the EEG typically shows low-voltage waves of moderate frequency (alpha waves) or high frequency (beta waves). In contrast, the EEG during most of the time spent in sleep is characterized by slower waves of higher voltage. After falling asleep, one passes gradually from stage 1 to stage 4 over a period of about 45 minutes, each stage being characterized by waves of lower frequency and higher voltage than the preceding one. After about 30 minutes in stage 4, the sleeper gradually passes back through stage 3 to stage 2. A full night's sleep typically includes five to seven such cycles, but only the first one or two of these may reach stage 4.

During stage 1 sleep, the EEG shows theta waves, which have a frequency of 4-7 Hz. In stage 2, so-called **sleep spindles** occur—brief intermittent bursts of faster (12-14 Hz) activity. Very slow (1-2 Hz) high-voltage delta waves occur during stages 3 and 4. The deeper the stage of sleep, the more difficult it is for the sleeper to be aroused by external stimuli. About 50% of normal sleep is spent in stage 2.

During the four stages of sleep thus far described, the parasympathetic division of the autonomic nervous system is dominant. Pulse, blood pressure, and respiratory rates gradually decline, and gastrointestinal motility is increased. Voluntary muscles are relaxed but not inhibited; a normal sleeper changes position every 5-20 minutes.

Upon the return to stage 2 after an interval at deeper stages, a series of striking alterations occur. The sleeper passes into an entirely different state, in which many of the features characterizing stages 1-4 are sharply reversed. The EEG now shows low-voltage, high-frequency activity, as in the waking state. Cerebral blood flow and oxygen consumption are increased, and the sympathetic division of the autonomic nervous system becomes activated, with increases in pulse, blood pressure, and respiratory rate, and inhibition of gastrointestinal motility.

A profound loss of tone, amounting almost to paralysis, affects all the voluntary muscles except those controlling eye movements. While the rest of the sleeper's body lies immobile and inert, the eyes undergo spells of rapid, irregular movement. Hence this phase of sleep is called **rapid-eye-movement (REM) sleep**. In contrast, the four stages previously described are said to pertain to non-REM or NREM sleep.

Periods of REM sleep typically occur with each return to stage 2—hence five to seven times during a full night's sleep—and they make up about 25% of the total period of sleep. The longer one sleeps, the more frequently periods of REM sleep occur, and the longer they last.

During REM sleep, the subject is even less susceptible to arousal by external stimuli than in stage 4 sleep, but is more likely to awaken spontaneously.

Alcohol and barbiturates suppress REM sleep, while reserpine and lysergic acid diethylamide (LSD) increase it. After selective deprivation of REM sleep, experimental subjects experience a rebound period of increased REM sleep, which may persist for more than one night. REM sleep cycles also increase in frequency and duration during withdrawal from barbiturates, amphetamines, and narcotics.

Electroretinography, Electrooculography

Electrodiagnostic studies of the eye, first performed experimentally in the late nineteenth century, led to the development of two techniques currently used to evaluate the response of the eye to light.

Electroretinography (ERG) records electrical activity in the retina after photic stimulation. A detecting electrode is placed in contact with the topically anesthetized cornea, and one or more neutral electrodes are placed on the skin around the eye. Flashes of light, of standardized color, intensity, and frequency, are then presented to the eye, and the amplitude and shape of the evoked electrical response in the retina are recorded. Instead of light flashes, the stimulus may consist of an alternating checkerboard pattern.

Ordinarily stimuli are presented throughout the entire visual field; this is called *ganzfeld* (German, 'whole field') stimulation. A focal stimulus can be applied to evaluate a limited area of the retina (e.g., the macula, the highly sensitive zone corresponding to the center of the visual field). Manipulating background luminosity and altering the color of the light and the rate of flicker makes it possible to narrow the response to a particular type of retinal cell (i.e., rods vs. cones). Electroretinography is useful in the diagnosis of retinitis pigmentosa, cone dystrophy, diabetic retinopathy, and central retinal vein occlusion.

Electrooculography (EOG), often performed in conjunction with electroretinography, evaluates the ability of the retinal pigment layer to adapt to changes in light intensity. (Somewhat confusingly, the term *electrooculography* is also applied to a diagnostic study of eye movements, performed with electrical recording equipment while the subject reads and watches a swinging pendulum.)

Electromyography and Nerve Conduction Velocity (NCV) Studies

Detection and measurement of electrical impulses associated with the action of voluntary (skeletal) muscles by **electromyography** (EMG) provides diagnostic information in various disorders affecting the muscles themselves (muscular dystrophy, myositis, myasthenia gravis) or the central or peripheral nervous system (amyotrophic lateral sclerosis, Guillain-Barré syndrome, spinal stenosis, nerve entrapment). The usual indication for the procedure is unexplained local or general muscle weakness.

The device used to perform electromyography consists of various types of recording electrodes, an amplifier that magnifies the very small electrical signals generated by neuromuscular activity and detected by these electrodes, a cathode ray oscilloscope that provides a visual display of electrical activity, and a speaker that converts that activity into an audible signal. Findings can be printed on a moving strip or stored digitally.

The electrodes used to detect nerve and muscle activity are of several types. Fine needle electrodes are inserted through the skin and into skeletal muscle to detect muscle action potentials. A monopolar needle electrode is insulated except at its tip. One or more indifferent electrodes must be used in conjunction with it. A coaxial needle electrode also has an insulated tip but uses the barrel through which it passes as the indifferent electrode. Surface electrodes, which do not penetrate the skin, are used as reference or ground electrodes in electromyography, and in studies of nerve conduction velocity, discussed below. Electrode paste is applied to the skin before application to a surface electrode to ensure good electrical contact.

The EMG procedure consists in inserting one or several needle electrodes into voluntary muscles in the area under study. Because this is painful, the subject may be premedicated with a sedative or even a narcotic analgesic. Any spontaneous electrical activity of resting muscle is first noted. Spontaneous activity is abnormal and usually indicates a disease affecting muscle tissue (as opposed to its nerve supply), such as muscular dystrophy.

A recording is then made of action potentials generated as the subject contracts the muscle at various levels of force from minimal to maximal. The intensity, duration, and frequency of the wave forms generated by voluntary muscle contraction supply information as to the presence, type, and severity of neuromuscular disease. The quality of the audible signal (clicks, regular or irregular bursts of noise) may also provide valuable diagnostic clues.

Nerve conduction velocity (NCV) studies are often performed in conjunction with electromyography. A small electrical stimulus is delivered by a surface electrode placed over a nerve trunk in an extremity, and the rate and amplitude of transmission of the electrical impulse through the nerve are detected by other surface electrodes placed along the course of the nerve. Needle electrodes may be used for these studies also, but they are inserted into muscles, not nerves. The results of several tests are averaged. Nerve conduction velocity is not affected by intrinsic muscular disease but may be altered by conditions affecting nerve tissue (Guillain-Barré syndrome, nerve entrapment syndromes).

Exercises

Fill in the Blanks

1. _____ is the recording of the electrical activity of the brain, important in the diagnosis of seizure disorders.

2. A _____ array of electrodes in an EEG is one that compares the activity detected by one or more electrodes with an indifferent electrode placed in the midline or on one ear.

3. A _____ array of electrodes in an EEG is one that compares the input from one electrode or group of electrodes with another electrode or group—for example, left frontal vs. left temporal electrodes, or left frontal vs. right frontal electrodes.

4. Provocative measures of _____ and _____ may be used to elicit significant responses in the tracing.

5. _____ are brief spindle-shaped bursts of low-voltage activity, with a frequency of 12-14 Hz, which occur in light (stage 2) sleep.

6. A negative (downward) spike followed by a high-voltage slow (delta) wave, characteristic of stage 2 sleep, is the _____.

7. A _____ in an EEG tracing is an extremely narrow wave, that is, one consisting of a brief deflection and a rapid return to the baseline—by convention, one lasting less than 80 msec (milliseconds).

8. _____ is the simultaneous performance of several monitoring activities during sleep.

9. In electroretinogram, stimuli presented throughout the entire visual field are called _____ (German, 'whole field') stimulation.

10. Detection and measurement of electrical impulses associated with the action of voluntary muscles by _____ provides diagnostic information in various disorders affecting the muscles themselves or the central or peripheral nervous system.

Multiple Choice: Circle the letter of the best answer from the choices given.

1. Electroencephalography remains the single most valuable diagnostic tool in identifying and classifying all of the following except
   A. Seizure disorders.
   B. Sleep disorders.
   C. Toxic encephalopathies.
   D. Intracranial neoplasms and vascular lesions.
   E. Certain dementias.

Exercises

2. Waves of 4.5-7.5 Hz are seen in normal children and adolescents, but in adults they occur only during sleep or near-sleep and are called
   A. Alpha waves.
   B. Spike waves.
   C. Beta waves.
   D. Delta waves.
   E. Theta waves.

3. On an EEG, waves characteristic of the resting state in the normal waking adult that have a frequency of 8-13 Hz are called
   A. Alpha waves.
   B. Spike waves.
   C. Beta waves.
   D. Spindle waves.
   E. Theta waves.

4. Very slow waves of 0.5-4.0 Hz that normally occur only in the deeper (third and fourth) stages of sleep, but may also be seen in certain metabolic, circulatory, or neoplastic disorders of the central nervous system and in dementia are
   A. Alpha waves.
   B. Spike waves.
   C. Beta waves.
   D. Delta waves.
   E. Theta waves.

5. On an EEG, faster waves, with a frequency between 13.5 and 35 Hz, seen in a state of heightened alertness, are
   A. Alpha waves.
   B. Spike waves.
   C. Beta waves.
   D. Spindle waves.
   E. Theta waves.

6. Polysomnography consists of all the following studies except
   A. Electrocardiography.
   B. Electromyography.
   C. Electronic recording of eye, chin, and limb movements, videorecording of body position and movement.
   D. Monitoring of nasal and oral air flow, rate and depth of respirations, and arterial oxygen saturation.
   E. Electroencephalography.

Exercises

7. Electroretinography is useful in the diagnosis of all of the following except
    A. Corneal dystrophy.
    B. Cone dystrophy.
    C. Diabetic retinopathy
    D. Central retinal vein occlusion.
    E. Retinitis pigmentosa.

Short Answers

1. Define or explain:

    a. alpha rhythm_____

    _____

    b. coaxial needle electrode _____

    _____

    c. photic stimulation_____

    _____

    d. polysomnography _____

    _____

    e. REM sleep _____

    _____

    f. electromyogram _____

    _____

    g. nerve conduction study _____

    _____

2. What are some reasons for performing an electroencephalogram?

    a. _____

    b. _____

    c. _____

    d. _____

Exercises

3. What measures may be used to evoke particular responses during the performance of an electroencephalogram?

_____

_____

_____

_____

_____

_____

4. Describe the findings of an EEG positive for petit male and grand mal seizures.

_____

_____

_____

_____

5. List five indications for a polysomnogram.

a. _____

b. _____

c. _____

d. _____

e. _____

6. Distinguish between an electrooculogram and an electroretinogram.

a. electrooculogram _____

_____

b. electroretinogram _____

_____

7. Distinguish between the two meanings of electrooculography.

_____

_____

_____

_____

Exercises

8. List five disorders in which an electromyogram might yield abnormal results.

   a. _____

   b. _____

   c. _____

   d. _____

   e. _____

Activities for Application and Further Study

1. Find a polysomnogram report on the Internet. Summarize the different sections and relate them to the discussion in the text. Do the different parts of the report correlate to the different studies listed in the text?

2. Carpal tunnel syndrome, which may be diagnosed with an electromyogram, is a common job-related condition among medical transcriptionists. Survey people you know who have or had this condition to find out if they had an EMG. Ask them to describe the procedure and whether it was painful. Summarize your findings in a short report.

Electrocardiography 6

Upon completion of this chapter, the student should be able to

- Describe the conduction system of the heart;

- Explain how electrocardiography is performed and what diagnostic information it provides;

- Discuss ambulatory electrocardiography, stress testing, and pulse oximetry.

Electrocardiography

Electrocardiography (ECG, EKG) is the measurement and recording of the electrical activity of the heart (*see box*). Electrodes placed at standard sites on the chest and extremities detect voltage differences that are shown as waves or deflections from a baseline in a cathode-ray tube display or in a linear tracing on a strip of paper. Data can also be stored digitally and analyzed by a computer. The electrocardiogram permits precise determination of heart rate and rhythm and can detect abnormalities of cardiac size, shape, conduction, and function as well as ischemia (diminished blood supply) or infarction (tissue death due to diminished blood supply).

Electrocardiography

Electrocardiography was developed by the Dutch physician and physiologist Willem Einthoven (1860-1927) around 1900. Einthoven devised a highly responsive voltage detector called a string galvanometer to measure the electrical activity of the heart. In order to make a permanent record of the rapidly shifting electrical potentials, he arranged for the movements of the galvanometer needle to deflect a beam of light as it fell on a moving strip of photographic film. When the film was developed it showed a linear tracing whose up-and-down deviations corresponded to electrical events in the cardiac cycle. Because the tracings had to be developed in a darkroom, electrocardiography developed in close association with another fledgling diagnostic specialty, radiology. In fact, many of the first ECG experts were radiologists.

The principal uses of electrocardiography are in identifying and analyzing abnormalities in heart rate and rhythm, abnormalities in the size

or shape of the heart or one or more of its chambers, and transitory or permanent effects of impairment of the coronary circulation. In addition, electrocardiography is of value in the diagnosis of pericarditis, in verifying the function of an artificial pacemaker, and in assessing various systemic and metabolic disorders that affect heart function.

Before proceeding further in this chapter, you may wish to review the anatomy of the heart as depicted and briefly described in Chapter 4.

The conducting system of the heart (*see Fig.6.1*) consists of highly specialized tissue capable of initiating and transmitting the electrical impulses that cause the heart to beat. The pacemaker of the heart is the sinoatrial (SA) node, a small nubbin of tissue in the upper part of the right atrium. Although nerves of the autonomic nervous system and circulating substances such as epinephrine and certain drugs can affect the rate and rhythm of the heart, the SA node continues to function as a pacemaker, stimulating regular cardiac contractions, even if all nerves to the heart are severed. In medical jargon, the SA node is almost universally called simply the sinus.

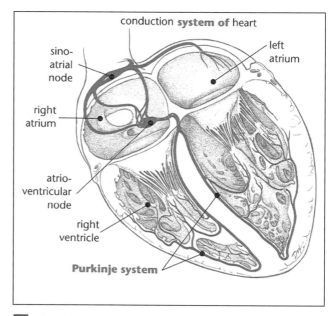

Fig. 6.1. Conducting system of the heart
Reproduced with permission from *Melloni's Illustrated Medical Dictionary*, 4th ed. (2002).

Each electrical impulse generated by the SA node triggers a wave of depolarization that spreads over both atria, causing them to contract. Located low in the right atrium is another mass of specialized tissue, the atrioventricular (AV) node (usually called simply the node). When the wave of depolarization set off by the SA node reaches the AV node, it is picked up and transmitted down the bundle of His to the septum between the two ventricles. In the septum the bundle of His divides into right and left bundle branches, of which the left further divides into anterior and posterior fascicles. All of these tracts of conducting tissue eventually break up into a network of Purkinje fibers, which penetrate the walls of the ventricles. The outward passage of the wave of depolarization through the muscular ventricular walls causes them to contract.

A pair of electrodes placed at any two points on the body surface and connected to a sufficiently sensitive galvanometer will detect some of the electrical activity of the heart, as damped and diffused by the body tissues intervening between the heart and the electrodes. One of Einthoven's most important contributions was his development of standard locations for electrode placement (*see box*). These standard locations provide precise information not only about heart rate and rhythm but also about the shape and size of the heart chambers and the state of health of the heart muscle.

Ordinarily an ECG is performed with the subject lying supine in bed or on an examining table. The technician attaches an electrode to each forearm just above the wrist and to each leg just above the ankle, and connects each electrode to a correspondingly marked wire leading into the machine. Electrodes are small disks or cups of highly conductive, corrosion-resistant metal and are held in place with elastic bands or spring clips or by suction.

To ensure good electrical contact, a film of gel or paste containing common salt or another suitable electrolyte is spread between each elec-

Electrode Placement

Willem Einthoven's original equipment was primitive and cumbersome by comparison with what is available today, and his methods were correspondingly crude. The subject sat with both arms and the left leg immersed in large jars of saline solution, which served as detecting electrodes. By setting his machine to record potential differences between each pair of electrodes in turn, Einthoven produced three bipolar tracings, each "looking at" the heart from a different angle.

Although the jars of saline were long ago replaced by metal electrodes applied to the skin of the arms and the left leg, the standard limb electrodes (or "leads"—the term refers to the wires connecting the electrodes to the machine) still retain the designations Einthoven gave them:

Lead I: Right Arm, Left Arm
Lead II: Right Arm, Left Leg
Lead III: Left Arm, Left Leg

(Mnemonic: The Roman numeral gives the number of *L*s.)

Following Dutch and German practice, Einthoven spelled the name of his invention "Elektrokardiogramm." That is the source of the K in EKG, still widely used today as an alternative to ECG. For his pioneering work in electrocardiography he received the Nobel Prize for Medicine or Physiology in 1924.

trode and the skin. Alternatively a thin strip of fabric impregnated with electrolyte may be used. A single suction-type electrode, having its own lead wire, is used to record chest leads, and is moved from one position to the next between tracings. For some applications (stress testing, monitoring during resuscitation or in an acute-care setting) disposable electrodes with adhesive backing may be used.

As waves of depolarization and repolarization move through the heart, they cause fluctuations in the potential or voltage that can be detected by the electrodes. Various combinations of electrodes sample the electrical activity in a regular sequence so as to build up a three-dimensional "picture" of cardiac activity.

Recordings taken from leads I, II, and III are **bipolar**. That is, for each of these leads the instrument measures the difference of potential between two electrodes. By convention, one of these is called the recording electrode. When a wave of depolarization or repolarization passing through the heart moves toward the recording electrode and away from the other electrode, the tracing shows an upward deflection from the baseline. When a wave of depolarization or repolarization moves away from the recording electrode and toward the other electrode, the tracing shows a downward deflection from the baseline. If a wave of electrical activity moves transversely, keeping the same distance from both electrodes, the tracing shows no deflection.

Any given recording electrode can supply information about the rate and rhythm of ventricular contractions, and may also show abnormalities of impulse formation or conduction or evidence of ischemia or infarction. But a single pair of leads can provide only limited data about the size, shape, and position of the heart, and may not show any sign of disease affecting parts of the heart other than those facing the recording electrode.

The three **unipolar** limb leads (aVR, aVL, and aVF) are obtained by simply changing the electrical connections between the electrodes and the galvanometer in the ECG machine. Instead of measuring the difference in potential between the recording electrode and one other

electrode (as is done for leads I, II, and III), the unipolar limb leads compare the potential of the recording electrode against that of all the other electrodes together. (This includes a fourth electrode on the right leg, which is never used as a recording electrode.)

Because the electrical sum of these three other electrodes is zero, the recording electrode picks up a smaller voltage than in the standard limb leads, and deflections in the tracing are therefore smaller. In order to make these deflections comparable in amplitude to those of the standard limb leads, the unipolar limb leads are "augmented" by the ECG machine. All this means is that the machine automatically increases the sensitivity of its galvanometer when these leads are being recorded.

Whereas the recording axis of each bipolar lead is fixed by the positions of the two electrodes, the recording electrode of a unipolar lead registers a true vector. (A vector is a quantity having both magnitude and direction.) In the following nomenclature, a stands for augmented and V for vector. The third letter in each abbreviation refers to the site of the recording electrode.

aVR: Right Arm
aVL: Left Arm
aVF: Left Leg (F for 'foot')

The **precordial** or chest leads are obtained by placing electrodes on the chest in front of the heart. The standard electrode positions for the six chest leads occur at approximately equal intervals around the anterior chest starting from the right sternal border and ending in the left midaxillary line. These too are vector leads, with the recording electrode balanced against all four of the limb electrodes together. They are numbered V_1 through V_6.

A standard 12-lead electrocardiogram consists of the standard limb leads, I, II, and III; the augmented (bipolar) limb leads, aVR, aVL, and aVF; and precordial leads V_1 through V_6, in that order. The bipolar and unipolar limb leads taken together give a composite view of the heart in the frontal plane, as it appears in a standard chest x-ray. The precordial leads yield a composite view of the heart in cross-section, as it is seen in a CT scan or MRI projection.

After attaching the electrodes, the technician makes a tracing by setting the recording paper in motion. Most electrocardiograph machines are programmed to record the first six leads (I, II, III, aVR, aVL, and aVF) automatically. Between recordings made from the chest lead, the paper drive is stopped to permit shifting of the electrode from one position to the next. The paper moves at a constant speed under a needle or stylus that inscribes a continuous line showing fluctuations in potential. For a standard tracing the paper moves at a rate of 25 mm/sec. The paper drive can also be set to run at 50 mm/sec. to expand the tracing and permit finer analysis of small deviations or to produce a more informative tracing when the heart rate is very rapid and complexes are close together.

To facilitate measurements of time and voltage, the paper has a grid imprinted on it. The larger squares of the grid are 1 cm on each side, and each of these squares is subdivided into 25 smaller squares 2 mm on a side. At a paper speed of 25 mm/sec., each larger square thus represents 0.2 sec., and each smaller square represents 0.04 sec. In a standard ECG tracing, an upward or downward deviation of 2 cm (2 large squares) corresponds to a difference in potential of 1 millivolt (mV). When voltages are very high, the machine can be set at half standard (1 cm = 1 mV).

Every tracing includes a record of the deviation from the baseline obtained by presenting a difference of potential of exactly 1 mV to the galvanometer while the paper is moving but the galvanometer is disconnected from the subject. This standardization wave, inserted by the technician at the touch of a button, verifies the sensitivity setting of the machine at the time the tracing was made. The machine also includes a device for identifying the lead that is being recorded by marking the edge of the moving paper with a code consisting of dots and dashes.

A complete tracing consists of samples of each of the twelve standard leads. Most of these are 10-12 cm in length, corresponding to a recording time of 2 sec, and typically including 2-3 cardiac cycles. The strip for lead II, however, is 30 cm in length, corresponding to a recording time of 6 sec. Because this is done to provide a broader overview of cardiac rhythm than is feasible with a 2-sec tracing, the longer lead II strip is called a **rhythm strip**.

The electrical events of the normal cardiac cycle cause a series of characteristic deflections, or waves, to appear in the ECG tracing (*see Fig. 6.2*). Note that the ECG detects electrical activity, not muscular contraction or movement as such. Figure 6.2 shows the waves of the normal ECG and indicates the cardiac event to which each corresponds.

P wave: atrial depolarization

Q wave: septal depolarization

R wave: ventricular depolarization moving toward recording electrode

S wave: ventricular depolarization moving away from recording electrode

T wave: ventricular repolarization

U wave: origin unknown

Atrial rate: The number of P waves/minute.

Ventricular rate: The number of R waves/minute.

(With normal cardiac function, atrial and ventricular rates are identical.)

PR interval: The time elapsed between the beginning of the P wave and the beginning of the R wave, representing the interval between the beginning of atrial depolarization and the beginning of ventricular depolarization.

QRS interval: The time duration of a typical QRS complex, which represents the whole process of ventricular depolarization.

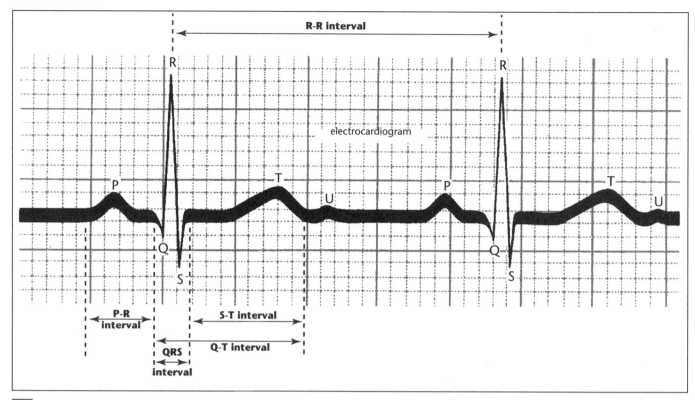

Fig. 6.2. Sample electrocardiogram with intervals.
Reproduced with permission from *Melloni's Illustrated Medical Dictionary*, 4th ed. (2002).

Not all of these waves necessarily appear in every lead. Moreover, some of them typically vary in amplitude (size) and polarity (above or below the baseline) from one lead to another. For example, the P wave is always upright in leads I, II, and aVF, as it appears in the figure. In lead aVR, however, it is always inverted (dips below the baseline). In V_1, the chest lead whose electrode faces the right side of the heart, the S wave is typically larger (goes further from the baseline) than the R wave. (This is designated an rS pattern.) As the chest leads progress around the heart to its left side, this relation gradually changes. In V_3 or V_4 the R and S waves will be found to be approximately equiphasic (that is, the R wave goes about as far above the baseline as the S wave goes below it—an RS pattern), while in V_6 the R wave predominates (Rs).

In addition, the waves of the ECG can vary in amplitude, polarity, and shape as a reflection of various cardiac abnormalities. For example, inverted T waves in lead I or lead II usually indicate myocardial ischemia (deficient blood supply to heart muscle). Deep, wide Q waves in any lead are generally evidence of myocardial infarction. The total absence of P waves from all leads indicates that the sinoatrial node is not functioning as a pacemaker.

The mean electrical axis of the heart in the frontal plane, usually called simply the electrical axis, or still more simply the axis, is an imaginary line representing the direction along which the mean or maximum electrical activity passes down through the heart during each cardiac cycle. The axis as projected in the frontal plane is determined by a comparison of the heights of the R waves in the first six leads of the ECG. Axis deviation to right or left can indicate asymmetric enlargement of a heart chamber, aberrant conduction of cardiac impulses, or other abnormality.

In modern practice, many modifications and variations of the standard ECG are used for specialized applications. An esophageal lead, using a swallowed electrode, can explore the posterior surface of the heart electrically; a cardiac catheter with an ECG electrode at its tip can make recordings from within cardiac chambers; during surgery, electrodes can be applied directly to the heart. Vectorcardiography is a specialized branch of electrocardiography based on analysis of vector "loops" as displayed on a cathode ray tube.

A continuous cathode ray tube display of lead II is used to monitor heart action in emergency departments and intensive care units. Cardiac monitors used in emergency departments, coronary care units, and operating rooms can be set to sound an alarm upon the occurrence of various electrocardiographically detectable abnormalities in rate, rhythm, conduction, or waveform.

Telemetry (radio transmission of an ECG signal from a monitor worn by the patient to a nearby receiving station) allows maximum mobility of patients in coronary care units. The ECG signal can be digitized and transmitted by radio waves or telephone wires for recording and interpretation at a site remote from the patient's location.

Ambulatory ECG Monitoring

A patient with intermittent symptoms such as cardiac palpitation or sudden loss of consciousness often has a normal ECG tracing between episodes. Ambulatory monitoring can help to record and diagnose unpredictable alterations in cardiac rate or rhythm and correlate ECG findings with events such as meals, effort, chest pain, and palpitation. A **Holter monitor** is a compact ECG machine worn by a patient for 24-48 hours to provide continuous recording of cardiac electrical activity. Stored on tape, the data are analyzed by a computer at the end of the testing period.

For a patient with symptoms occurring only at long intervals, an event monitor may be more appropriate. This type of instrument monitors the ECG constantly but stores data for only 1-2 minutes, except when the patient activates a memory function upon the occurrence of chest pain, palpitation, or near-syncope.

Stress Testing

Stress testing refers to any standardized diagnostic measure designed to assess the effects of stress on the function of the heart. Stress may be induced by physical exercise on a motorized treadmill or bicycle ergometer, or by injection of a drug. Although the principal diagnostic procedure used during stress testing is a continuous electrocardiogram, blood pressure and oxygen consumption are also routinely monitored. Studies such as echocardiography, nuclear imaging, and cardiac catheterization may also be carried out during the test period.

Stress testing is a standard method of identifying and grading coronary artery disease in patients with angina pectoris or a history of myocardial infarction. It is also widely used to predict future cardiac events, to monitor rehabilitation after myocardial infarction, and to judge the need for coronary artery bypass surgery or balloon angioplasty.

In standard exercise testing, the subject walks on an electrically driven treadmill whose speed and angle of inclination can be varied according to a standard protocol. The Bruce protocol begins with a treadmill speed of 1.7 mph and a grade of 10° and increases both speed and grade every 3 minutes. A test session usually lasts 6-10 minutes.

The unit of measure for an exercise workload is the metabolic equivalent (MET), defined as the amount of oxygen consumed at bedrest (3.5 mL/kg/min). In maximal or symptom-limited testing, the subject keeps on exercising with increasing workloads until the session must be stopped because of chest pain, physical exhaustion, or significant changes in blood pressure, heart rhythm, or ECG findings. In submaximal (pulse-limited) stress testing, exercise continues only until a target heart rate (based on the subject's age, health history, and physical condition) has been reached.

Electrocardiographic changes during exercise that suggest coronary artery disease include elevation or depression of ST segments by more than 1 mm, T-wave inversion, significant arrhythmias, a fall in systolic blood pressure, and a marked rise in diastolic blood pressure. Exercise stress testing is about 90% accurate in identifying persons without coronary artery disease. Exercise testing is contraindicated in severe obesity or late pregnancy and in the presence of acute myocardial infarction or other significant cardiac or systemic disease.

As an alternative to exercise, the effect of intravenous infusion of certain drugs may be observed. Dobutamine, an adrenergic agonist, increases heart rate and blood pressure in a fashion similar to physical exertion. Dipyridamole and adenosine dilate normal coronary arteries but do not increase blood flow through vessels narrowed by atherosclerosis.

Pulse Oximetry

This is a method of monitoring the oxygen saturation of circulating hemoglobin, as detected by a probe attached to the patient's finger or ear-lobe. The probe emits two beams of light at different wavelengths and records the differential absorption of these beams by hemoglobin in the capillary circulation. This provides an estimate of oxygen saturation. Data gathered by the probe are analyzed by a computer and displayed audibly and graphically. Each pulse beat is marked by a beep and the rate per minute is shown digitally. The oximeter is programmed to sound an alarm when pulse, blood flow, or oxygen saturation fall outside of established safe limits.

Normal oxygen saturation is 95-100%. Levels below 90% can indicate serious respiratory or circulatory deficiency, but may not be reflected by clinical signs such as dyspnea, tachypnea, or cyanosis (bluish color of lips and nailbeds). Pulse oximetry is widely used in acute care settings and in monitoring cardiopulmonary function in anesthetized and comatose patients and those with severe chronic respiratory disease requiring artificial or assisted ventilation or oxygen therapy. This technique depends on a normal flow of blood through the skin to which the probe is attached. It does not assess the carbon dioxide level of the blood.

Exercises

Fill in the Blanks

1. _____ is the measurement and recording of the electrical activity of the heart.

2. In electrocardiograms, _____ placed at standard sites on the chest and extremities detect voltage differences that are shown as _____ or _____ from a baseline in a cathode-ray tube display or in a linear tracing on a strip of paper.

3. The electrocardiogram permits precise determination of _____ and _____ and can detect abnormalities of cardiac size, shape, _____, and function as well as _____.

4. Infarction is _____ due to diminished blood supply, or _____.

5. The _____, a small nubbin of tissue in the upper part of the right atrium, is known as the pacemaker of the heart.

6. When the wave of depolarization set off by the SA node reaches the _____, a mass of specialized tissue located low in the right atrium, it is picked up and transmitted down the _____ to the septum between the two ventricles.

7. In the septum, the bundle of His divides into right and left bundle branches, of which the left further divides into anterior and posterior fascicles which eventually break up into a network of _____, which penetrate the walls of the ventricles.

8. The outward passage of the wave of depolarization (that began in the _____) through the muscular ventricular walls causes them to contract.

9. As waves of _____ and _____ move through the heart, they cause fluctuations in the potential or voltage that can be detected by ECG electrodes.

10. When the difference of potential between two limb lead electrodes (I, II, and III) is measured, these recordings are called _____.

11. The tracing shows an upward deflection from the baseline when a wave of depolarization or repolarization passing through the heart moves toward the _____ and away from the other electrode.

12. The tracing shows a downward deflection from the baseline when a wave of _____ or _____ moves away from the recording electrode and toward the other electrode.

13. If a wave of electrical activity moves transversely, keeping the same distance from both electrodes, the tracing shows no _____.

Exercises

14. The three _____ limb leads (aVR, aVL, and aVF) are obtained by simply changing the electrical connections between the electrodes and the galvanometer in the ECG machine.

15. Because the amplitude of the unipolar limb leads is less than that of the bipolar limb leads, the machine automatically increases the sensitivity of its galvanometer when these leads are being recorded; thus the unipolar leads are _____.

16. The _____ or chest leads are obtained by placing electrodes on the chest in front of the heart, numbered _____.

17. The bipolar and unipolar limb leads taken together give a composite view of the heart in _____, as it appears in a standard chest x-ray. The precordial leads yield a composite view of the heart in _____, as it is seen in a CT scan or MRI projection.

18. The strip for lead II, called a _____, is 30 cm in length, corresponding to a recording time of 6 seconds, and provides a broader overview of cardiac rhythm than is feasible with a 2-sec tracing.

19. With normal cardiac function, _____ and ventricular rates are identical.

20. On an ECG, _____ refers to the size of the waves and _____ to whether the wave extends above or below the baseline.

21. A treadmill exercise stress test may be performed using the _____ protocol.

22. The unit of measure for an exercise workload is the _____ defined as the amount of oxygen consumed at bedrest (3.5 mL/kg/min).

23. In patients unable to exercise, the drug _____ may be used to perform stress testing because it increases heart rate and blood pressure in a fashion similar to physical exertion.

Multiple Choice: Circle the letter of the best answer from the choices given.

1. The uses of electrocardiography include all of the following except
   A. Identifying and analyzing abnormalities in heart rate and rhythm or in the size or shape of the heart or one or more of its chambers.
   B. Assessing valve deformities or malfunction.
   C. Identifying transitory or permanent effects of impairment of the coronary circulation.
   D. Diagnosing pericarditis.
   E. Verifying the function of an artificial pacemaker.

Exercises

2. Even if all nerves to the heart are severed, this structure continues to function as a pacemaker, stimulating regular cardiac contractions.
   A. Bundle of His.
   B. Atrioventricular node.
   C. Sinoatrial node.
   D. Interventricular septum.
   E. Purkinje fibers.

3. By convention, in medical jargon, this structure is known simply as the "sinus."
   A. Purkinje fibers.
   B. Sinoatrial (SA) node.
   C. Interventricular septum.
   D. Atrioventricular (AV) node.
   E. Bundle of His.

4. By convention, in medical jargon, this structure is known simply as the "node."
   A. Purkinje fibers.
   B. Sinoatrial (SA) node.
   C. Interventricular septum.
   D. Atrioventricular (AV) node.
   E. Bundle of His.

5. Recordings measuring the difference of potential between two electrodes taken from leads I, II, and III are _____.
   A. Bipolar.
   B. Depolarization.
   C. Precordial.
   D. Unipolar.
   E. Sinus.

6. Instead of measuring the difference in potential between the recording electrode and one other electrode (as is done for leads I, II, and III), these leads compare the potential of the recording electrode against that of all the other electrodes together.
   A. Bipolar.
   B. Precordial.
   C. Depolarization.
   D. Sinus.
   E. Unipolar.

Exercises

7. On an ECG, atrial depolarization is represented by the
    A. P wave.
    B. Q wave.
    C. R wave.
    D. S wave.
    E. T wave.

8. On an ECG, ventricular depolarization moving away from the recording electrode is represented by the
    A. P wave.
    B. Q wave.
    C. R wave.
    D. S wave.
    E. T wave.

9. On an ECG, ventricular repolarization is represented by the
    A. P wave.
    B. Q wave.
    C. R wave.
    D. S wave.
    E. T wave.

10. On an ECG, ventricular depolarization moving toward the recording electrode is represented by the
    A. P wave.
    B. Q wave.
    C. R wave.
    D. S wave.
    E. T wave.

11. On an ECG, septal depolarization is represented by the
    A. P wave.
    B. Q wave.
    C. R wave.
    D. S wave.
    E. T wave.

12. A U wave on an ECG represents an event of
    A. Atrial depolarization.
    B. Septal depolarization.
    C. Unknown origin.
    D. Ventricular depolarization.
    E. Ventricular repolarization.

Exercises

13. On an ECG, the number of P waves/minute is the
    A. Atrial rate.
    B. Ventricular rate.
    C. PR interval.
    D. QRS interval.
    E. QRS complex.

14. On an ECG, the number of R waves/minute is the
    A. Atrial rate.
    B. QRS interval.
    C. QRS complex.
    D. Ventricular rate.
    E. PR interval.

15. In V_1, the chest lead whose electrode faces the right side of the heart, the S wave is typically larger (goes further from the baseline) than the R wave. This is designated as _____.
    A. A QRS interval.
    B. An rS pattern.
    C. A PR interval.
    D. An Rs pattern.
    E. An RS pattern.

16. On an ECG, when the R wave goes about as far above the baseline as the S wave goes below it, this is known as _____.
    A. A QRS interval.
    B. An rS pattern.
    C. A PR interval.
    D. An Rs pattern.
    E. An RS pattern.

17. On an ECG, in lead V_6, when the R wave pre-dominates over the S wave, this is known as _____.
    A. A QRS interval.
    B. An rS pattern.
    C. A PR interval.
    D. An Rs pattern.
    E. An RS pattern.

Exercises

18. On an ECG, inverted T waves in lead I or lead II usually indicate evidence of
    A. Myocardial ischemia.
    B. Atrial depolarization.
    C. Myocardial infarction.
    D. Ventricular depolarization.
    E. The sinoatrial node is not functioning as a pacemaker.

19. Deep, wide Q waves in any lead are generally evidence of
    A. Myocardial ischemia.
    B. Atrial depolarization.
    C. Myocardial infarction.
    D. Ventricular depolarization.
    E. The sinoatrial node is not functioning as a pacemaker.

20. The total absence of P waves from all leads indicates
    A. Myocardial ischemia.
    B. Atrial depolarization.
    C. Myocardial infarction.
    D. Ventricular depolarization.
    E. The sinoatrial node is not functioning as a pacemaker.

21. According to the text, electrocardiographic changes during exercise that suggest coronary artery disease include all of the following except
    A. Elevation or depression of ST segments by more than 1 mm.
    B. A prolonged PR interval.
    C. Significant arrhythmias.
    D. A fall in systolic blood pressure or a marked rise in diastolic blood pressure.
    E. T-wave inversion.

Exercises

Short Answers

1. Define or explain:

   a. Holter monitor _____

   _____

   b. PR interval _____

   _____

   c. precordial leads _____

   _____

   d. pulse oximeter _____

   _____

   e. SA node _____

   _____

   f. stress testing _____

   _____

   g. AV node _____

   _____

   h. bundle of His _____

   _____

   i. Purkinje fibers _____

   j. QRS interval _____

   _____

2. List three reasons for performing electrocardiography.

   a. _____

   b. _____

   c. _____

3. List three reasons for performing stress testing.

   a. _____

   b. _____

   c. _____

Exercises

4. What kind of information about heart function can be learned from any ECG lead?

_____

_____

_____

5. What kind of information may require examination or comparison of several leads?

_____

_____

_____

6. What is the significance of deep, wide Q waves in an ECG lead?

_____

_____

_____

7. Explain the mnemonic for remembering the limb leads, I, II, and III.

_____

_____

_____

8. In the leads denoted by the letters aVR, aVL, aVF, what do the letters "a" and "V" stand for? What does the third letter stand for?

_____

_____

_____

9. What is the axis of the heart? How is it determined on an ECG? What does deviation of the axis indicate?

_____

_____

_____

_____

_____

Exercises

Activities for Application and Further Study

1. What is the origin of the abbreviation *EKG* for electrocardiogram? Which abbreviation is preferred—EKG or ECG? Support your answers.

2. Find examples of the following types of EKGs on the Internet and bring to class for discussion. Use the advanced search features to specify pages that include images.
   a. ECG showing myocardial ischemia.
   b. ECG showing myocardial infarction.
   c. ECG showing arrhythmia.
   d. Holter monitor tracing report.
   e. Pulse oximetry tracing.
   f. Other abnormal ECG tracings.

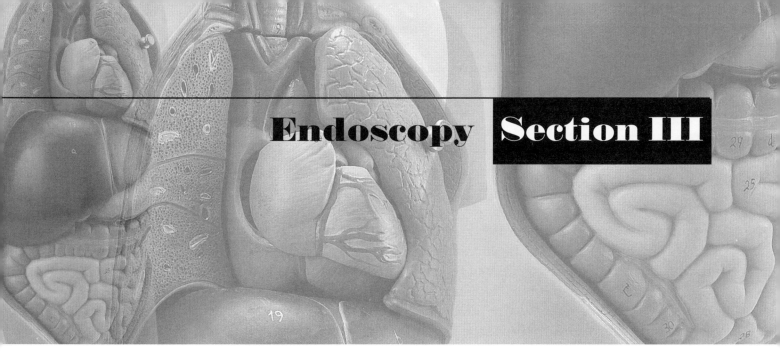

Endoscopy Section III

Endoscopy is the visual inspection of structures inside the body by means of an instrument (endoscope) inserted either through a natural orifice such as the mouth or the anus or through an incision made for the purpose. We know from archaeologic evidence and from surviving medical writings of ancient cultures that even in antiquity physicians examined body regions such as the rectum and the vagina with instruments called specula.

A speculum is a simple device that dilates the opening of a body passage or cavity and may also direct or reflect light into it. Specula in routine use in modern medicine include the nasal speculum, the otoscope, the vaginal speculum, and the anoscope. The slit-lamp and ophthalmoscope may also be included here although no part of them enters the patient's body. No sharp distinction can be made between endoscopy and speculum examinations. This section discusses routine examinations belonging to both categories.

The earliest practicable endoscopes were developed in the nineteenth century. By the middle of the twentieth century, endoscopic examinations of the esophagus and stomach, and rectum and sigmoid colon, and the urinary bladder were part of standard medical practice. Early endoscopes were straight metal tubes equipped with magnifying lenses and some kind of light

source. Some were adapted for special purposes, such as obtaining biopsies, performing minor surgery, or taking photographs. Because they were rigid, their usefulness was limited. For example, they could not be advanced more than 25-30 cm into the lower intestinal tract. In addition, many kinds of endoscopic examination (e.g., cystoscopy, examination of the inside of the urinary bladder) were so painful that general or spinal anesthesia was usually required.

With the development of fiberoptics, flexible endoscopes became possible. A fiberoptic endoscope (fiberscope) contains a compact bundle of 25-50,000 flexible rods of fibrous glass that direct a beam of light to the tip of the instrument and convey images back to the examiner. The thousands of individual images are reconstituted as a mosaic by a viewing lens, somewhat like the image on a television or computer screen. Even when the fibers are bent to a right angle, light rays and images pass through them as if they were traveling in a straight line.

The flexibility of fiberoptic instruments has greatly increased the range of endoscopy. The small intestine can now be examined with an instrument introduced through the nose, and the entire colon can be visualized with an instrument introduced through the anus. In addition, flexible endoscopes have reduced the discomfort and inconvenience of being examined. Cystoscopy is now practicable with only a topical anesthetic.

A further advantage of fiberoptics is that light can be directed through the instrument from a source outside the patient. Early instruments had light bulbs at their inner ends, which became hot within a short time and could injure tissues. If a bulb burned out, the endoscope had to be removed and then reinserted after the bulb had been replaced. Endoscopes with fiberoptic systems use halogen, xenon, or diode light sources located proximally (outside the patient), which provide intensely bright white light with a minimum of heat.

Not only are modern endoscopes flexible, but the development of miniaturized lens systems has permitted their caliber to be much reduced from what was necessary fifty years ago. Modern endoscopes are highly specialized to meet particular needs. Most of them are furnished with television cameras permitting video display (either panoramic or zoom) of the examination as it is performed and digital recording of images for future reference. The small caliber of an endoscope does not, however, permit binocular vision (simultaneous inspection of a structure or region with both eyes), and hence true depth perception is not possible.

Although flexible endoscopes are available for the examination of most bodily areas, rigid endoscopes are still widely used. A major consideration in the choice of instrument may be cost and availability. A flexible endoscope with its fiberoptic and special lighting systems costs more than ten times as much as the corresponding rigid instrument with conventional lenses and lighting.

An endoscopic procedure is performed when direct visual examination of an internal structure or region is expected to provide information useful in the evaluation of symptoms or in the elucidation of abnormal findings on physical examination or with laboratory or imaging studies. Some types of endoscopy (e.g., colonoscopy in persons at risk of colorectal cancer because of age or family history) are performed as screening procedures.

General anesthesia is required for some endoscopic procedures, such as mediastinoscopy. For others (e.g., esophagoscopy) local anesthesia may be routine, and for still others no anesthesia at all is required. The patient may receive a sedative before the procedure, or a drug may be administered to suppress excessive respiratory tract secretions or digestive tract movement. Endoscopy of the lower bowel requires preliminary emptying of the colon with laxatives or enemas. Most endoscopic procedures are quite safe, and adverse effects such as bleeding, infection, and perforation are uncommon.

Nowadays endoscopes such as the arthroscope and the laparoscope are routinely used not only for examination but also to perform surgery. These instruments are equipped with irrigation and suction apparatus to flush secretions, blood, and other materials away from the inspection or surgical site. A wide variety of ancillary devices, including biopsy brushes and forceps, laser cutting and cautery apparatus, snares to remove polyps, and cutting and suturing instruments, are available for the performance of endoscopic surgery.

Visual Examinations of the Eyes, Ears, Nose, and Respiratory Tract

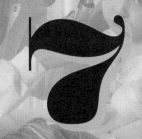

7

Examination of the Eye

Slit Lamp Examination

A slit lamp is a low-power binocular microscope mounted on a stand, with which an ophthalmologist examines the eyes of the seated subject. The instrument directs a beam of bright light through a narrow slit, giving the examiner a magnified cross-sectional image of structures in the anterior portion of the eye. Mydriatic drops are instilled before the examination to dilate the pupil so as to provide maximal visualization of structures behind the iris. For examination of the conjunctiva and anterior cornea, fluorescein dye may also be instilled.

Slit-lamp examination is part of a routine ophthalmologic evaluation and is also used to investigate disorders of the eyelids, conjunctiva, cornea, iris, and lens, including conjunctivitis, keratitis and corneal ulcers, ocular trauma, glaucoma, cataract, and iritis. A slit-lamp is used in fitting contact lenses. Many slit-lamps are equipped for the performance of applanation tonometry (described in Chapter 3) and for recording findings with a digital camera or videocamera.

Clouding of the aqueous humor due to the presence of inflammatory cells causes blurring and diffusion of the light as it passes through the anterior chamber, a phenomenon called "flare and cells." Keratic precipitates (KPs) are opaque deposits on the posterior surface of the cornea, also due to local inflammation.

Funduscopy

Funduscopy (not "fundoscopy") is examination of the ocular fundus, the curving inner surface of the posterior portion of the eyeball as visualized through the pupil with an instrument called an ophthalmoscope. The fundus includes the retina (the light-sensitive layer of specialized sensory cells on which the lens of the eye focuses its images), the optic disk (the bundle of nerve fibers carrying visual information from the retina to the brain), and the retinal arteries and veins.

The ophthalmoscope is a handheld instrument with a light source and a set of lenses mounted on a wheel-like diaphragm that permits rapid change of magnification. Since the examiner is looking at the retina through the patient's own ocular lens, any visual deficiency must be compensated with one of the lenses in the instrument. The strength of the lens in use, measured in diopters (see Chapter 3), appears in a window on the instrument and gives a rough measure of how far the patient's vision varies from normal.

The ophthalmoscope also includes red and green filters to emphasize certain features of the fundus, a grid for estimating distances, and a means of adjusting the intensity of the light and the size of the aperture through which it is projected into the eye. For a thorough ophthalmoscopic examination, the pupil is dilated with a topical mydriatic to give maximum exposure of the fundus and to minimize constriction of the pupil in response to the examining light. Funduscopy may not be practicable if the examiner's view is blocked by an opacified lens (cataract) or hemorrhage within the eye.

Funduscopy is performed as part of a routine adult physical examination because it provides a unique view of the retinal arterioles, whose condition is usually representative of arteries in the rest of the body. The effects of systemic diseases such as arteriosclerosis, hypertension, and diabetes mellitus may be reflected more clearly in the retina than elsewhere. Diabetic retinopathy and certain other disorders of the retina may cause neovascularization (abnormal growth of capillaries).

Ophthalmoscopic examination is also performed to evaluate eye pain, visual disorders, retinal disease (retinitis pigmentosa, macular degeneration), and ocular trauma. Swelling of the optic disk may be due to inflammation (papillitis) or to an increase of intracranial pressure ("choked disk"). It is sometimes measured by the difference between lens settings needed to focus on the disk and on the rest of the fundus ("2-diopter choke").

Funduscopically observed changes in the vessels in hypertension are graded according to the Keith-Wagener-Barker classification:

Grade I: Focal or diffuse narrowing of retinal arterioles, with reduction of the A-V (arteriole-venule) ratio. Narrowed arterioles may be described as having a copper-wire or silver-wire appearance.

Grade II: Further narrowing of arterioles. Crossing phenomena (apparent nicking or narrowing of a venule where an arteriole crosses it).

Grade III: All of the above and retinal flame (i.e., flame-shaped) hemorrhages and/or exudates (opaque zones of local infarction and degeneration).

Grade IV: All of the above and papilledema (swelling of the optic nerve).

Examination of the Nose

Nasal Speculum Examination

The anterior naris (nostril) can be examined with a Vienna speculum, a simple bivalve instrument without a light source. The examiner holds the instrument in the nondominant hand and introduces it into the naris with the blades closed. While gently spreading the blades of the instrument apart by squeezing the handles together, the examiner inspects the interior of the nose by means of a lamp held in the dominant hand or with a head-mounted lamp or reflector. Visibility is limited, but speculum examination often suffices for the evaluation of epistaxis (nosebleed), local inflammation, ulceration, polyps (lumpy swellings of mucous membrane, usually due to nasal allergy) or other tumors, foreign bodies, trauma, or septal deviation or perforation. Most nosebleeds result from erosion of small blood vessels in the K (for

Kiesselbach) area on the anterior septum (the dividing wall between the nostrils).

The naris may be sprayed with a vasoconstrictor to reduce swelling before the examination. Minor procedures such as extraction of a foreign body or cautery of a varicosity can be performed by means of the nasal speculum. Disposable specula of plastic or other synthetic materials are often used.

Anterior Rhinoscopy

A rhinoscope is a rigid or flexible endoscope inserted through a nostril and designed to enable the examiner to see both the anterior and the posterior naris. The term anterior rhinoscopy is used to distinguish this type of examination from inspection of the choanae with an angled mirror placed in the pharynx (see Posterior Rhinoscopy, below). A rhinoscope permits a more complete examination of the turbinates and septum than is possible with a speculum. In particular, the instrument gives access to the middle meatus, into which the frontal, maxillary, and anterior ethmoidal sinuses and the nasolacrimal duct all drain. Topical anesthetic and topical vasoconstrictor may be applied before the examination. Some instruments are equipped with digital or video cameras or both.

Posterior Rhinoscopy

When swelling within the nasal passages prevents satisfactory insertion of a rhinoscope, or when the site of clinical interest is one or both of the posterior nares, posterior rhinoscopy may be used. This is an indirect examination performed with an angled mirror so placed in the oropharynx that it reflects light upward into the nasopharynx and gives a view of the posterior nares, also called the choanae (singular, choana). (Avoid the common but redundant and incorrect phrase "posterior choanae.")

The light source is a head-mounted lamp or reflector worn by the examiner. The mirror is warmed so that moisture in the patient's breath will not fog it. Although the mirror does not ordinarily touch any part of the pharynx, patients often have difficulty holding still enough to prevent some contact, with resultant gagging. Hence a topical anesthetic may be sprayed into the throat before the examination.

The examination is undertaken to investigate nasal obstruction, bleeding sites, tumors, and foreign bodies.

Examination of the Ear

Otoscopic Examination

An otoscope is a handheld diagnostic instrument with a light source, a magnifying lens, and cone-shaped specula of various sizes, which are usually disposable.

Otoscopy gives a view of the external auditory meatus and the tympanic membrane. The examination is part of a general health assessment and is also undertaken to investigate earache, hearing loss, bleeding or discharge from the ear, foreign body, and otic trauma. In order to get an adequate view of the tympanic membrane, the examiner must straighten the ear canal by pulling the pinna (the shell-like, sound-collecting portion of the external ear) back and up with one hand while positioning the otoscope with the other. Cerumen (earwax), exudate, or swelling may prevent adequate visualization of ear structures. It may be necessary to remove cerumen with an instrument or by lavage (washing with warm water) before the examination can be performed.

The normal tympanic membrane is pearly gray and translucent, so that the malleus (hammer, one of the sound-transmitting bones of the middle ear) can just be seen behind it. The membrane is not perfectly flat, and its profile reflects the light of the otoscope in a typical triangular pattern ("light reflex"). Otoscopic examination may disclose bulging, retraction, perforation, or

scarring of the membrane or the presence of fluid (with or without bubbles of air or gas) or blood in the middle ear.

An otoscope may be equipped with a digital or video camera or both. Some otoscopes are so constructed that small instruments can be passed through them into the ear canal to remove cerumen or foreign bodies, perform myringotomy (incision of the tympanic membrane), or place a ventilation tube in the membrane. These instruments are often called operating otoscopes. They should not be confused with the operating microscope, a stationary and much more elaborate instrument with binocular magnification used to perform delicate operations such as tympanoplasty and stapedotomy on the middle ear.

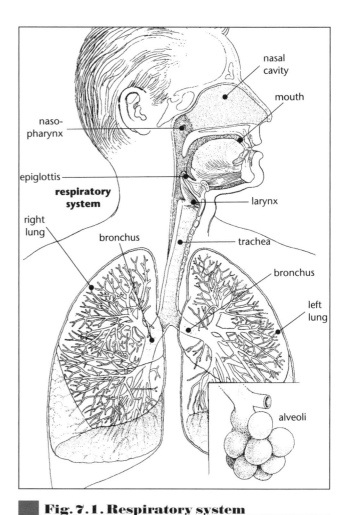

Fig. 7.1. Respiratory system

Reproduced with permission from *Melloni's Illustrated Medical Dictionary,* 4th ed. (2002).

Examination of the Larynx

Direct Laryngoscopy

Direct laryngoscopy refers to visual examination of the vocal cords and surrounding structures with an endoscope, in contrast to indirect laryngoscopy, which involves use of an angled mirror placed in the oropharynx (see below). Laryngoscopy is performed to evaluate acute respiratory obstruction, hoarseness, chronic cough, and trauma, benign or malignant tumors, or foreign bodies of the larynx. It is also necessary for intubation of the trachea with an oral endotracheal tube and, usually, for placement of a nasotracheal tube.

A rigid laryngoscope is a hand-held instrument with a self-contained light source and a long, slightly curved blade to retract the tongue. When the instrument is in use the blade makes a right angle with the handle, but for storage it folds down to lie parallel to the handle. For examination with this instrument the patient lies supine, with the head extended. The examiner stands or sits at the patient's head. With the handle of the instrument in the left (nondominant) hand, the examiner inserts the blade in the patient's mouth and lifts the tongue up and forward. As the blade advances, its tip raises the epiglottis (a fold behind the base of the tongue that forms a lid over the respiratory tract during swallowing), exposing the larynx. Instruments (suction apparatus, biopsy forceps, endotracheal tube) held in the examiner's dominant hand can be passed alongside the blade and into the larynx.

A flexible fiberoptic laryngoscope (nasolaryngoscope) is used for elective rather than emergency evaluation of the larynx. This instrument is passed through a nostril after application of anesthetic spray to the nostril and the pharynx. It provides visualization of the nasopharynx and proximal trachea (just distal to the vocal cords). Flexible laryngoscopes are equipped with video cameras to provide immediate display and digital storage of findings.

Indirect Laryngoscopy

This is a simple inspection of the vocal cords and surrounding structures with an angled mirror placed in the oropharynx. Topical anesthetic is applied to the pharynx in the form of spray or troches to prevent gagging. The instrument is warmed so that moisture from the patient's breath will not condense on the reflecting surface and fog the image. The seated patient extends the tongue and grasps it with a fold of gauze. The mirror is then placed in the oropharynx and the vocal cords visualized with light from a head-mounted lamp or mirror. The patient is asked to say, "Ee-ee-ee" in as high-pitched a voice as possible while the examiner observes the motion of the vocal cords.

Examination of the Lower Respiratory Tract

Rigid Bronchoscopy

Indications for bronchoscopy are acute or chronic inflammation, obstruction, hemorrhage, tumor, and foreign bodies of the lower respiratory tract. The first instruments used to visualize the trachea and bronchi were rigid tubes developed more than a century ago, primarily for use in removing foreign bodies. Although flexible bronchoscopes (bronchofiberscopes) are now in wide use, rigid bronchoscopy may still be preferred for some applications. Extension of the neck adequately for this procedure may not be possible in some patients.

The instrument is introduced through the mouth of the supine and anesthetized patient. Usually anesthesia is administered intravenously and oxygen is supplied by nasal cannula. In addition, topical anesthetic is applied to the pharynx and larynx to reduce gagging during the procedure. The instrument is advanced beyond the larynx and into the trachea, and manipulated into the main bronchi, one at a time.

Rigid bronchoscopes are available with viewing tips set at various angles, but the straight-viewing bronchoscope is most versatile. Available accessories include video imaging and storage, suction apparatus, equipment to perform cytologic washing or brushing, forceps for taking biopsies and removing foreign bodies, and laser and electrocautery devices.

Fiberoptic Bronchoscopy

The indications for this procedure are essentially the same as for rigid bronchoscopy. General anesthesia is usually not needed in adults, but sedation is administered and the airway is sprayed with topical anesthetic. The bronchofiberscope is introduced through a nostril (see Fig. 7.2). The instrument can be passed into individual segmental bronchi for visual inspection, bronchoalveolar lavage (BAL), or instillation of contrast medium for local bronchography.

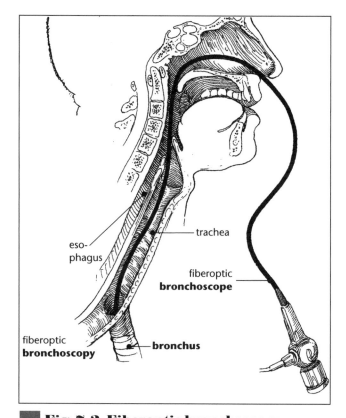

Fig. 7.2. Fiberoptic bronchoscopy
Reproduced with permission from *Melloni's Illustrated Medical Dictionary*, 4th ed. (2002).

Exercises

Fill in the Blanks

1. A _____ is a microscope which directs a beam of bright light through a narrow slit, giving the examiner a magnified cross-sectional image of structures in the anterior portion of the eye.

2. Clouding of the aqueous humor due to the presence of inflammatory cells causes blurring and diffusion of the light as it passes through the anterior chamber, a phenomenon called _____.

3. _____ are opaque deposits on the posterior surface of the cornea, also due to local inflammation.

4. _____ is examination of the ocular fundus, the curving inner surface of the posterior portion of the eyeball as visualized through the pupil with an instrument called an ophthalmoscope.

5. Another word for funduscopy is _____.

6. The light-sensitive layer of specialized sensory cells on which the lens of the eye focuses its images is known as the _____.

7. The bundle of nerve fibers carrying visual information from the retina is known as the _____.

8. _____ is a condition of abnormal growth of capillaries of the retina.

9. An increase of intracranial pressure may cause a type of swelling of the optic disk known as _____.

10. The medical word for nostril is _____; both nostrils are called the _____.

11. _____ is the medical word for nosebleed.

12. _____ allows examination of the middle meatus, into which the frontal, maxillary, and anterior ethmoidal sinuses and the nasolacrimal duct all drain.

13. Indirect examination of the posterior nares performed with an angled mirror so placed in the oropharynx that it reflects light upward into the nasopharynx is called _____.

14. _____ gives a view of the external auditory meatus and the tympanic membrane.

15. The medical term for the shell-like, sound-collecting portion of the external ear is _____.

16. The _____ refers to the typical triangular pattern of reflected light from the tympanic membrane on otoscopic examination.

Exercises

17. _____ may be so constructed that small instruments can be passed through them into the ear canal to remove cerumen or foreign bodies, perform myringotomy or place a ventilation tube in the membrane.

18. _____ refers to visual examination of the vocal cords and surrounding structures with an endoscope, in contrast to _____, which involves use of an angled mirror placed in the oropharynx.

19. The fold behind the base of the tongue that forms a lid over the respiratory tract during swallowing is the _____.

20. Inspection of the vocal cords and surrounding structures with an angled mirror placed in the oropharynx after topical anesthetic is applied to the pharynx is done using _____.

21. Examination of the lower respiratory tract for acute or chronic inflammation, obstruction, hemorrhage, tumor, and foreign bodies is performed by means of _____.

Multiple Choice: Circle the letter of the best answer from the choices given.

1. A slit lamp may be used to investigate all of the following except
   A. Conjunctivitis, keratitis, and corneal ulcers.
   B. Ocular trauma, glaucoma, cataract, and iritis.
   C. Fitting contact lenses.
   D. Glaucoma.
   E. Papilledema.

2. The funduscopic examination includes all of the following structures in the eye except
   A. The retina.
   B. The optic disk.
   C. The retinal arteries and veins.
   D. The cornea.
   E. The macula.

3. Ophthalmoscopic examination is performed for all of the following reasons except
   A. To evaluate the retinal arterioles whose condition usually reflects the rest of the arteries in the body.
   B. To evaluate cataracts.
   C. To evaluate eye pain and ocular trauma.
   D. To evaluate retinal disease (retinitis pigmentosa, macular degeneration).
   E. To evaluate swelling of the optic disk.

Exercises

4. Speculum examination of the nose can be used to evaluate all of the following except
    A. Tinnitus.
    B. Local inflammation or ulceration.
    C. Polyps (lumpy swellings of mucous membrane, usually due to nasal allergy) or other tumors.
    D. Foreign bodies, trauma, or septal deviation or perforation.
    E. Epistaxis (nosebleed).

5. An otoscopy examination is performed to evaluate all of the following except
    A. Earache.
    B. Hearing loss.
    C. Bleeding or discharge from the ear
    D. Foreign body or otic trauma.
    E. Sinusitis.

6. Examination of the eyes is performed with the
    A. Bronchoscope.
    B. Laryngoscope.
    C. Ophthalmoscope.
    D. Otoscope.
    E. Rhinoscope.

7. Examination of the ears is performed with the
    A. Bronchoscope.
    B. Laryngoscope.
    C. Ophthalmoscope.
    D. Otoscope.
    E. Rhinoscope.

8. Examination of the lower respiratory tract is performed with the
    A. Bronchoscope.
    B. Laryngoscope.
    C. Ophthalmoscope.
    D. Otoscope.
    E. Rhinoscope.

9. Examination of the nose is performed with the
    A. Bronchoscope.
    B. Laryngoscope.
    C. Ophthalmoscope.
    D. Otoscope.
    E. Rhinoscope.

Exercises

10. Examination of the upper respiratory tract is performed with the
    A. Bronchoscope.
    B. Laryngoscope.
    C. Ophthalmoscope.
    D. Otoscope.
    E. Rhinoscope.

Short Answers

1. Define or explain:

    a. cerumen _____

    _____

    b. choana _____

    _____

    c. fiberscope _____

    _____

    d. mydriatic _____

    _____

    e. ocular fundus _____

    _____

    f. speculum _____

    _____

2. Compare advantages and disadvantages of rigid and flexible laryngoscopy.

    _____

    _____

    _____

    _____

3. What kind of information about a patient's general health can be learned from funduscopy.

    _____

    _____

    _____

Exercises

4. What type of examination mentioned in this chapter requires the cooperation and participation of the patient?

    _____

    _____

    _____

    _____

5. Which examinations described in this chapter might be performed as emergency procedures?

    _____

    _____

    _____

    _____

6. Describe the features of the ophthalmoscope and the purpose of each.

    _____

    _____

    _____

    _____

7. What is meant by a "2-diopter choke"?

    _____

    _____

    _____

    _____

8. What are the limitations and advantages of nasal speculum examination, anterior rhinoscopy, and posterior rhinoscopy?

    _____

    _____

    _____

    _____

Exercises

9. Compare and contrast rigid and flexible bronchoscopy.

_____

_____

_____

Activities for Application and Further Study

1. On the Internet, find color images of diseased retinas (hypertensive retinopathy, diabetic retinopathy, optic disk in hypertension, and other terms used in your textbook). Go to the Web sites where these images appear and look for descriptions that fit the Keith-Wagener-Barker classifications. Print or download these to disk for later reference. Summarize your research in writing. (A Google image search is a good way to begin your research.)

2. On the Internet, find images of the various instruments discussed in this chapter. Save to disk or print for your notebook. Share your findings with the class.

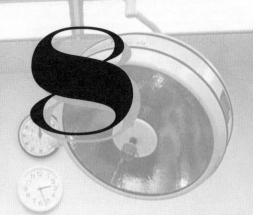

Endoscopy of the Digestive Tract and Genitourinary System

8

Endoscopy of the Upper Digestive Tract

Esophagoscopy

Indications for endoscopy of the esophagus include pain or difficulty in swallowing, hematemesis (vomiting of blood), chronic heartburn and other upper digestive complaints, and swallowed foreign body. The examination can be performed with either a rigid instrument passed through the mouth or a fiberoptic instrument passed through the nose. A flexible instrument is used when the

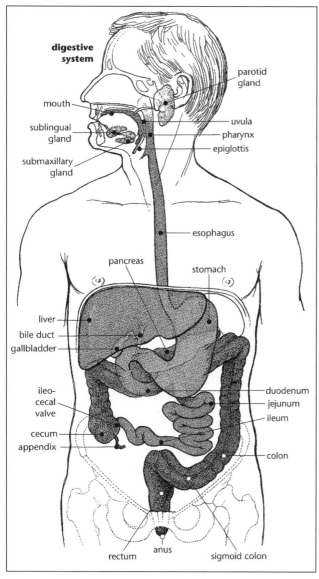

digestive system

parotid gland

mouth

sublingual gland

submaxillary gland

uvula
pharynx
epiglottis

esophagus

pancreas

stomach

liver
bile duct
gallbladder

ileocecal valve

cecum
appendix

duodenum
jejunum
ileum

colon

rectum   anus   sigmoid colon

Fig. 8.1. Digestive system
Reproduced with permission from *Melloni's Illustrated Medical Dictionary*, 4th ed. (2002).

examination includes the stomach and duodenum. The throat is anesthetized with topical spray and the patient lies on the right or left side. Findings are displayed on a television screen and can be digitally recorded. Instruments for taking biopsies, cauterizing bleeding lesions, or removing foreign bodies can be passed through the endoscope. Esophagoscopy can reveal ulceration, stricture, or Barrett metaplasia associated with gastroesophageal reflux, esophageal varices or diverticula, and benign or malignant tumors.

Esophagogastroscopy

Endoscopic examination of the stomach can be carried out with either a rigid or a flexible instrument, but the flexible gastroscope (*see Fig. 8.2*) yields superior visualization with less discomfort for the patient and less risk of perforation. Indications for this type of examination are similar to those for esophagoscopy but also include problems peculiar to the stomach, such as acute or chronic gastritis, ulceration, hiatal hernia, and benign or malignant tumors. The examiner may distend the stomach with air injected through the gastroscope to improve visualization if the gastric walls are folded.

Esophagogastroduodenoscopy (Gastroduodenoscopy)

An esophagogastroduodenoscope is a flexible instrument that is introduced through the nose and advanced through the pharynx, esophagus, and stomach into the duodenum, the first part of the small intestine. Indications for this examination are similar to those for esophagogastroscopy, but include disorders pertaining specifically to the duodenum such as peptic ulcer, stenosis due to scarring, diverticulum, or tumor. Placement of an endoscope in the duodenum is also necessary for endoscopic retrograde cholangiopancreatography (ERCP), a radiographic study of the biliary and pancreatic ducts after injection of contrast medium (described in Chapter 11).

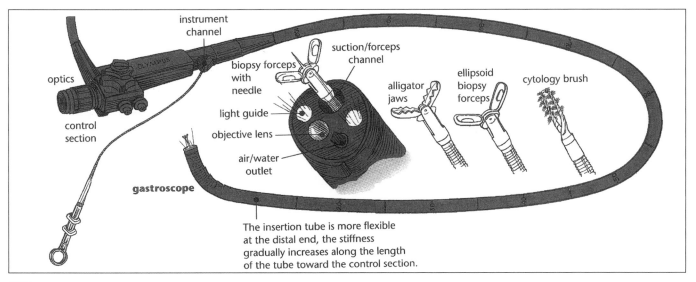

Fig. 8.2. Gastroscope. Reproduced with permission from *Melloni's Illustrated Medical Dictionary*, 4th ed. (2002).

Endoscopy of the Lower Digestive Tract

Examination of the interior of the rectum by means of a tube inserted through the anus is one of the oldest endoscopic procedures in medical history. Before the availability of flexible instruments, however, such examinations could seldom be carried out to a distance of more than 30 cm (12 in) above the anus because of the coiling, irregular course of the sigmoid colon. Nowadays the physician can select from a wide range of flexible instruments in various lengths, depending on the part of the lower digestive tract that is the site of clinical interest.

Anoscopy

An anoscope is essentially an anal speculum, a simple handheld tubular instrument designed to give visual access to the anal canal. Because an anoscope is a straight metal tube with an open end, an obturator (a metal plug with a rounded, cone-shaped tip) must be placed inside it for insertion. Some instruments have their own fiberoptic lighting systems, while others require an external light source. An operating anoscope has a cutaway portion to allow surgical procedures such as cautery to be performed while the instrument is in place. Disposable plastic anoscopes are available.

Anoscopy is performed to evaluate pain, bleeding, swelling, or other anal complaints. The patient lies on the left side with the hips and knees flexed, the right hip more than the left (Sims position). The instrument, warmed and lubricated with a water-soluble gel, is inserted with the obturator in place. The obturator is withdrawn and the examiner evaluates the anal canal and the distal rectum. Abnormal findings may include hemorrhoids (dilated anal veins), fissure (a linear tear in the mucous membrane of the anal canal), fistula in ano (an abnormal passage through tissues, ending in the anal canal), trauma, infection, inflammatory bowel disease (Crohn disease), and tumors.

Proctoscopy

With a slightly longer barrel than an anoscope, a proctoscope permits inspection of the interior of the rectum. The instrument may be a simple tube with an obturator, or it may be equipped with accessories for taking biopsies and performing minor surgical procedures. It may also have an insufflator, a device with which air is pumped into the rectum so as to distend it for full examination. Disposable plastic proctoscopes are available.

Indications for this examination are the same as for anoscopy, and also include masses or swellings felt on digital examination of the rectum and rectal foreign body.

The examination procedure is as for anoscopy, except that the genupectoral (knee-chest) position may be preferred because it allows gravity to expand and unfold the rectum. Under ideal conditions the rectum is emptied of stool before the examination by the use of laxatives, enemas, or both.

Sigmoidoscopy (Proctosigmoidoscopy)

As mentioned above, 30 cm from the anus is the approximate upper limit for examination with a rigid endoscope. With an instrument of that length, the examiner can reach the sigmoid colon, the zig-zag portion of the colon just above the rectum. Indications for sigmoidoscopy are rectal bleeding, change in bowel habits, tumor or other abnormality noted on abdominal palpation or imaging studies, and surveillance for colorectal cancer in persons at heightened risk because of age or personal or family history.

The examination can be performed in the left lateral position, but the knee-chest position allows better visualization. Preparation includes emptying of the colon with laxatives or enemas. Accessories that may be used with the sigmoidoscope include an insufflator, long-handled cotton swabs, saline irrigation, a suction device to remove secretions or saline, and biopsy forceps. Rigid sigmoidoscopy has largely been supplanted by colonoscopy with a flexible fiberoptic instrument, which not only permits better visualization of the sigmoid colon with less discomfort for the patient, but also can be used to evaluate the rest of the colon.

Colonoscopy

Indications for colonoscopy are essentially the same as for sigmoidoscopy. A fiberoptic colonoscope can be advanced all the way to the cecum, the most proximal part of the large intestine. The instrument is equipped with video display and with provision for performance of biopsy and minor surgery. The left lateral position is generally satisfactory. Sedation may be administered before the examination, which many patients find moderately painful. The procedure is contraindicated in late pregnancy.

Endoscopy of the Urinary Tract

Passage of a suitably designed endoscope through the urethra permits examination of virtually the entire urinary tract. Indications for endoscopy are hematuria (blood in the urine), chronic or recurrent urinary tract infection, urinary calculi, tumor, and other symptoms or disorders referable to the urinary tract.

Urethroscopy

A rigid urethroscope is a short tubular instrument designed to provide a view of the interior of the urethra. It is principally of use in examining the male urethra for prostatic enlargement or infection, urethral stricture (local narrowing due to scarring), varices, infectious lesions, and foreign bodies. Urethroscopy is routinely performed as well in the course of cystoscopy. Instruments of different lengths are available for the two sexes. The examination is performed with the male patient supine and the female patient in the lithotomy position—supine, with the hips flexed, the thighs abducted, and the feet supported in stirrups. Usually only topical anesthesia (applied as a gel) is required.

Cystoscopy

A cystoscope is a rigid or flexible instrument inserted into the bladder through the urethra. Fiberoptic instruments are more usual nowadays because they provide better visualization with

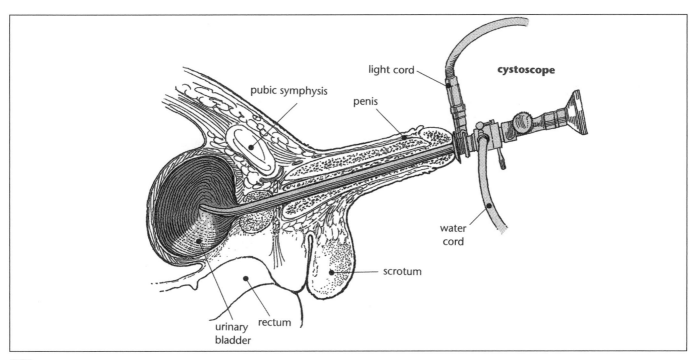

Fig. 8.3. Cystoscope. Reproduced with permission from *Melloni's Illustrated Medical Dictionary*, 4th ed. (2002).

less discomfort for the patient. Cystoscopy is used to evaluate hematuria, acute or chronic cystitis, vesical calculi, and ulcerative lesions or tumors of the bladder. It is also used for placement of ureteral catheters in the investigation of ureteral obstruction and to instill contrast medium for retrograde pyelography.

The examination is performed with the patient in the lithotomy position. It may be necessary to dilate the urethra before inserting the instrument, or even to perform meatotomy (one or more slits to enlarge the external urethral meatus). Most cystoscopes are adaptable for the performance of surgical procedures (biopsy, cautery or removal of polyps) and are equipped for continuous irrigation of the bladder with physiologic saline solution. A resectoscope is a cystoscope equipped with a cutting device with which a urologist can excise strips of tissue from a hyperplastic prostate under direct vision.

Ureteroscopy

The interior of a ureter can be examined with a fine-caliber flexible endoscope introduced through a cystoscope and threaded into the ureter. A ureteroscope is used in the evaluation of ureteral obstruction or malfunction, to guide removal of ureteral calculi, and for the placement of a ureteral stent to correct stricture.

Nephroscopy

A ureteroscope that is of sufficient length and maneuverability to reach the renal pelvis is called a nephroscope. Direct examination of the renal pelvis can provide information about hematuria, calculous disease, tumors, and other disorders of the kidney.

Endoscopy of the Female Reproductive System

Vaginal Speculum Examination

Speculum examination of the vagina and cervix is part of the routine health evaluation of women, and is a necessary prelude to the performance of a Pap smear, colposcopy, or cervical biopsy. This procedure is indicated in the evaluation of abnormal vaginal bleeding, discharge, pain, masses, and other gynecologic disorders.

A vaginal speculum is a simple bivalve instrument of metal or rigid plastic. Disposable vaginal specula are in wide use. The examination is performed with the patient in the lithotomy position. The speculum, warmed and lubricated with water-soluble gel, is inserted into the vagina with the blades together. Spreading and locking the blades gives the examiner a view of the vaginal walls and the uterine cervix.

Colposcopy

The colposcope is a stationary low-power (2X to 20X) binocular microscope with self-contained lighting, which is used in conjunction with a vaginal speculum to provide a magnified view of the cervix and the vaginal mucosa. The instrument is equipped with a green filter to enhance visibility of blood vessels and abnormal vascular patterns.

Colposcopy is indicated for evaluation of lesions or abnormal zones of the cervix, in identifying areas of cervical dysplasia in a patient with an abnormal Pap smear, and as an aid in biopsy or minor surgical procedures. Acetic acid solution or Lugol solution may be applied to the cervix before examination to accentuate zones of squamous cell change and indicate likely areas for biopsy.

Hysteroscopy

This is visual inspection of the interior of the uterus with an endoscope inserted through the cervix. Hysteroscopy is indicated in the study of abnormal uterine bleeding, uterine masses (fibroids, polyps), infertility, habitual abortion (repeated miscarriage), and congenital malformations of the reproductive system. It can also be used to direct chorionic villus biopsy. Hysteroscopy has largely replaced D&C (dilatation of the cervix and curettage of the endometrium) for many diagnostic applications.

A hysteroscope consists of an outer sheath or sleeve that fits within the cervix and an inner barrel. In a nulliparous subject (one who has never given birth) the cervix may have to be dilated as a preliminary to insertion of the sheath. During the examination the uterine cavity is distended with physiologic saline solution, carbon dioxide gas, or some other medium. A continuous flow of saline flushes away blood and tissue debris for better visibility. Both rigid and flexible hysteroscopes are used, and with either type provision is usually made for the performance of biopsy and other surgical procedures.

The patient is examined in the lithotomy position under either general or local (paracervical block) anesthesia. The procedure is performed shortly after the end of a menstrual period, when endometrial proliferation is minimal. A preliminary pregnancy test must be negative, except when the procedure is performed for chorionic villus sampling.

Exercises

Fill in the Blanks

1. The flexible gastroscope is preferable to the rigid because it provides superior _____ with less _____ for the patient and less risk of _____.

2. An _____ is a flexible instrument that is introduced through the nose and advanced through the pharynx, esophagus, and stomach into the duodenum.

3. Use of a rigid scope for examination of the lower GI tract is limited to no more than 30 cm (12 in) above the anus because _____.

4. A _____ is a dilated anal vein.

5. A _____ is a linear tear in the mucous membrane of the anal canal.

6. A _____ is an abnormal passage through tissues, ending in the anal canal.

7. For proctoscopy, the genupectoral (knee-chest) position may be preferred over the Sims position used for anoscopy because _____.

8. Rigid sigmoidoscopy has largely been supplanted by _____ with a flexible fiberoptic instrument.

9. The most proximal part of the large intestine is the _____.

10. A _____ is a cystoscope equipped with a cutting device with which a urologist can excise strips of tissue from a hyperplastic prostate under direct vision.

11. A _____ is indicated in the evaluation of abnormal vaginal bleeding, discharge, pain, masses, and other gynecologic disorders.

12. During colposcopy, _____ solution or _____ solution may be applied to the cervix before examination to accentuate zones of squamous cell change and indicate likely areas for biopsy.

Exercises

Multiple Choice: Circle the letter of the best answer from the choices given.

1. Indications for endoscopy of the esophagus include all of the following except
   A. Peptic ulcer.
   B. Hematemesis.
   C. Chronic heartburn and other upper digestive complaints.
   D. Swallowed foreign body.
   E. Pain or difficulty in swallowing.

2. Findings on esophagoscopy may include all of the following except
   A. Ulceration, stricture, or Barrett metaplasia associated with gastroesophageal reflux.
   B. Esophageal varices.
   C. Diverticula of the esophagus.
   D. Benign or malignant tumors.
   E. Duodenal stenosis.

3. Indications for esophagogastroscopy include all of the following except
   A. Acute or chronic gastritis.
   B. Gastric ulceration.
   C. Hematuria.
   D. Hiatal hernia.
   E. Benign or malignant tumors.

4. A finding that may appear on esophagogastroduodenoscopy that would not be apparent on simple esophagoscopy or esophagogastroscopy would be which of the following?
   A. Acute or chronic gastritis.
   B. Gastric ulceration.
   C. Duodenal diverticulum.
   D. Hiatal hernia.
   E. Peptic ulcer.

5. Anoscopy is performed to evaluate all of the following except
   A. Pain.
   B. Bleeding.
   C. Fissures.
   D. Diverticula.
   E. Internal hemorrhoids.

Exercises

6. The position in which the patient lies on the left side with the hips and knees flexed, the right hip more than the left is the
   A. Lithotomy position.
   B. Sims position.
   C. Left lateral position.
   D. Genupectoral.
   E. Supine position.

7. According to the text, findings on anoscopy could include all of the following except
   A. Fistula in ano.
   B. Fissures.
   C. Crohn's disease.
   D. Diverticula.
   E. Hemorrhoids.

8. Indications for sigmoidoscopy or proctosigmoidoscopy include all the following except
   A. Rectal bleeding.
   B. Change in bowel habits.
   C. Tumor or other abnormality noted on abdominal palpation or imaging studies.
   D. Surveillance for colorectal cancer.
   E. Gastric ulceration.

9. Which of the following endoscopic procedures would be used to examine the cecum?
   A. Anoscopy.
   B. Colonoscopy.
   C. Colposcopy.
   D. Proctoscopy.
   E. Proctosigmoidoscopy.

10. Endoscopy of the urinary may be done for all of the following reasons except
    A. Hernia.
    B. Hematuria.
    C. Chronic or recurrent infection.
    D. Calculi.
    E. Tumor.

Exercises

11. The position in which the patient lies supine, with the hips flexed, the thighs abducted, and the feet supported in stirrups is the
    A. Genupectoral.
    B. Left lateral position.
    C. Lithotomy position.
    D. Sims position.
    E. Supine position.

12. Excision of strips of tissue from a hyperplastic prostate under direct vision can be performed during which of the following endoscopic examinations?
    A. Esophagogastroduodenoscopy.
    B. Colposcopy.
    C. Colonoscopy.
    D. Cystoscopy.
    E. Hysteroscopy.

13. A ureteroscopy is an examination performed on the
    A. Upper gastrointestinal system.
    B. Lower gastrointestinal system.
    C. Female reproductive tract.
    D. Lower genitourinary system.
    E. Upper genitourinary system.

14. Which of the following procedures is indicated for evaluation of lesions or abnormal zones of the cervix and in identifying areas of cervical dysplasia in a patient with an abnormal Pap smear?
    A. Speculum exam of vagina and cervix.
    B. Colposcopy.
    C. Colonoscopy.
    D. Cystoscopy.
    E. Nephroscopy.

15. Fibroids are likely to be discovered during which of the following endoscopic procedures?
    A. Colposcopy.
    B. Colonoscopy.
    C. Cystoscopy.
    D. Hysteroscopy.
    E. Speculum exam.

Exercises

Short Answers

1. Define or explain:

    a. colposcopy _____

    _____

    b. hematemesis _____

    _____

    c. lithotomy position _____

    _____

    d. meatotomy _____

    _____

    e. obturator _____

    _____

    f. sigmoid colon _____

    _____

2. List three indications for each of the following procedures:

    a. cystoscopy _____

    _____

    _____

    b. gastroduodenoscopy _____

    _____

    _____

    c. hysteroscopy _____

    _____

    _____

    d. proctoscopy _____

    _____

    _____

Exercises

3. List four examination positions mentioned in this chapter and indicate some types of examination for which each is appropriate.

    a. _____

    b. _____

    c. _____

    d. _____

4. Which examinations discussed in this chapter might be done to discover a source of bleeding?

    _____

    _____

    _____

    _____

5. Which examinations discussed in this chapter might be part of a routine health examination for certain patients?

    _____

    _____

    _____

    _____

Activities for Application and Further Study

1. Find pictures in a medical dictionary or on the Internet of the examination positions mentioned in this chapter. Explain how the different positions might facilitate the examinations for which they are used.

2. Would the procedures described in this chapter be considered invasive (look up the definition or find it explained in another chapter)? Why or why not?

3. Find on the Internet a sample report of an esophagogastroduodenoscopy, colonoscopy, cystoscopy, or hysteroscopy. What were the indications for the procedure (preoperative diagnosis); what were the findings (postoperative diagnosis, findings paragraph)?

Endoscopic Examinations Requiring Incisions

9

Incisional Endoscopy

The availability of small-caliber flexible endoscopes has been a major factor in the development of minimal-access surgery, also called keyhole, buttonhole, or Band-Aid surgery. These terms refer to surgical procedures that are carried out through incisions so small that they do not require suturing. Many types of surgery on the abdominal and pelvic organs that were formerly performed through large incisions are now done with a laparoscope. Similarly, operations on joints, particularly the knee, that formerly required an open procedure are now often done arthroscopically.

Although these and other types of endoscope are widely used nowadays to facilitate surgical procedures, they are all basically diagnostic instruments. For an endoscopic examination performed through an incision in skin or mucous membrane, disinfection of the skin as for surgery, and local or general anesthesia, are necessary. The aperture may be created by cutting with a surgical knife (scalpel) or by puncturing the surface with a trocar and cannula. A cannula is a hollow metal tube of small caliber, used for various diagnostic and therapeutic purposes. A trocar is a sharp-pointed obturator that fits inside the cannula and is used to pierce the skin and introduce the cannula into the resulting opening, after which the trocar is removed.

Thoracoscopy

Diagnostic evaluation of the outer (pleural) surface of the lung and the pleural cavity surrounding it formerly required an open surgical procedure. Nowadays endoscopy is often used for direct investigation of these structures. Thoracoscopy can provide valuable diagnostic or staging information in cancer of the lung and is also indicated in disorders of the pleura such as pleural effusion (presence of fluid in the pleural cavity), empyema (pus in the pleural cavity), and pleural thickening or calcification seen on chest x-ray. Lung and pleural biopsies can be taken during the procedure.

A thoracoscope is a small-caliber endoscope that is inserted through a skin incision between two ribs to provide a view of the interior of the pleural cavity. For an extensive examination, the instrument may be introduced at several points, each requiring a separate incision. The procedure is performed under general anesthesia. In addition, endotracheal intubation and ventilatory support are necessary because during the examination the lung on the side under examination is partially collapsed. At the end of the procedure, a drain is placed in one of the incisions to permit evacuation of air and fluid from the pleural space.

Mediastinoscopy

The mediastinum is the middle portion of the chest cavity, the anatomic region between the lungs that contains the heart and great vessels, the trachea, and the esophagus. Lymph nodes and the thymus gland also occupy this region. Mediastinoscopy is direct visual examination of these structures with an endoscope inserted through an incision in the midline just above the sternum (breastbone). For this procedure, as for thoracoscopy, the patient is given a general anesthetic and is intubated for ventilatory support.

Because the mediastinal lymph nodes receive drainage from the lungs, examination and biopsy of these structures is important in the diagnosis and staging of lung cancer. These nodes are also often involved in other disorders, such as Hodgkin disease and sarcoidosis. Mediastinoscopy may also be indicated for the investigation of disorders of the trachea, esophagus, and pericardium.

Laparoscopy

Examination of structures in the abdomen by means of an endoscope inserted through a small incision in the abdominal wall has virtually replaced open procedures (exploratory laparotomy) undertaken for purely diagnostic reasons. In addition, many surgical procedures formerly requiring laparotomy, such as appendectomy, cholecystectomy, inguinal herniorrhaphy, and oophorectomy, are now routinely performed laparoscopically.

The patient undergoing laparoscopy is first given a general anesthetic. A Veress needle is then inserted through a skin puncture, usually just below the umbilicus, and carbon dioxide gas is introduced into the peritoneal cavity under pressure. This process is called **insufflation**, and the condition it creates—the presence of air or gas in the peritoneal cavity—is called **pneumoperitoneum**. The purpose of creating a pneumoperitoneum is to distend the abdominal cavity so as to permit manipulation of the laparoscope and visualization of abdominal and pelvic structures. An incision or port is then made through the abdominal wall at a location most suitable for the intended investigation, and the laparoscope is introduced. Further incisions may be made as needed. For surgical procedures, other instruments may be inserted through these incisions. Carbon dioxide gas is released from the abdomen at the end of the procedure.

Culdoscopy

The rectouterine pouch of Douglas, also called the cul-de-sac, is a pocket of peritoneum lying between the rectum and the uterus. Because it is the lowest point in the female pelvic cavity, pus from pelvic infections tends to gravitate to this point, where it can be drained through an incision in the posterior fornix of the vagina by a procedure called culdocentesis.

One of the earliest endoscopic procedures to be performed through an incision was culdoscopy. Originally this examination involved insertion of a rigid endoscope through an incision in the posterior fornix with the patient, under general anesthesia, in the knee-chest position. This position was required to permit the pelvic organs to drop forward by gravity. Nowadays the procedure can be performed in the lithotomy position with carbon dioxide gas insufflation. Both rigid and flexible instruments are available. Sometimes only local anesthesia is needed.

Although culdoscopy provides less visualization of the pelvic organs than pelvic laparoscopy, some minor surgical procedures and biopsy are feasible by this technique. Culdoscopy finds its widest application in the evaluation of ovarian masses, endometriosis and other sources of chronic pelvic pain, and infertility.

Arthroscopy

Radiographic studies of joints, even after the injection of a contrast medium (arthrography), provide only limited information about disorders of cartilage and ligaments. Arthroscopy (*see Fig. 9.1*), the direct inspection of the interior of a joint with an endoscope introduced through a skin puncture, has become a routine procedure for the evaluation of acute and chronic joint problems (pain, swelling, instability, locking), particularly in the knee. In addition, arthroscopic (not "orthoscopic") surgery has largely replaced open procedures for the repair of ligament and cartilage injuries in the knee and other joints.

Arthroscopy is usually performed under local anesthesia. The rigid fiberoptic instrument is inserted through a small skin puncture and the joint is distended with saline solution for the examination. A flow of saline carries blood and, for surgical procedures, fragments of soft tissue and cartilage away from the site.

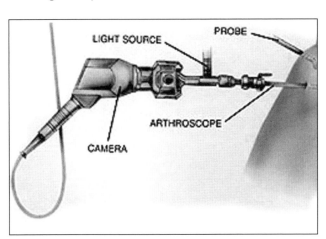

Fig. 9.1. Arthroscope
Reproduced with permission from Mitek and Stryker. .

Exercises

Fill in the Blanks

1. Surgical procedures that are carried out through incisions so small that they do not require suturing are called by a variety of names including _____, _____, _____, or _____.

2. A _____ is a hollow metal tube of small caliber, used for various diagnostic and therapeutic purposes.

3. A _____ is a sharp-pointed obturator that fits inside the cannula and is used to pierce the skin and introduce the cannula into the resulting opening, after which the trocar is removed.

4. _____ is the presence of fluid in the pleural cavity.

5. The medical term for pus in the pleural cavity is _____.

6. A _____ is a small-caliber endoscope that is inserted through a skin incision between two ribs to provide a view of the interior of the pleural cavity.

7. The _____ is the anatomic region between the lungs that contains the heart and great vessels, the trachea, and the esophagus.

8. The outer surface of the lung is the _____.

9. _____ is direct visual examination of the structures of the middle portion of the chest cavity with an endoscope inserted through an incision in the midline just above the sternum.

10. A _____ is a small-caliber endoscope that is inserted through a skin incision between two ribs to provide a view of the interior of the pleural cavity.

11. _____ is examination of structures in the abdomen by means of an endoscope inserted through a small incision in the abdominal wall.

12. The presence of air or gas in the peritoneal cavity achieved by insufflation is called _____.

13. An incision in the posterior fornix of the vagina is called _____.

14. The direct inspection of the interior of a joint with an endoscope introduced through a skin puncture is _____.

Exercises

Multiple Choice: Circle the letter of the best answer from the choices given.

1. The indications for thoracoscopy include all of the following except
   A. Diagnostic or staging information in cancer of the lung, including lung and pleural biopsies.
   B. Biopsies of mediastinal lymph nodes.
   C. Pleural effusion.
   D. Empyema.
   E. Pleural thickening or calcification seen on chest x-ray.

2. Pneumoperitoneum is
   A. Pleural thickening or calcification seen on chest x-ray.
   B. The presence of fluid in the chest cavity.
   C. The presence of pus in the chest cavity.
   D. The insufflation of carbon dioxide gas to distend the abdomen.
   E. The presence of air in the chest cavity.

3. According to the text, indications for culdoscopy include all of the following except
   A. Drainage of pus from the cul-de-sac.
   B. Evaluation of ovarian masses.
   C. Evaluation of endometriosis and other sources of chronic pelvic pain.
   D. Evaluation of infertility.
   E. Investigation of uterine fibroids.

4. Endoscopic inspection of the interior of joints is
   A. Arthroscopy.
   B. Culdoscopy.
   C. Orthoscopy.
   D. Mediastinoscopy.
   E. Arthrography.

5. Endoscopic inspection of the surface of the lung and the area surrounding the lungs is
   A. Arthroscopy.
   B. Culdoscopy.
   C. Laparoscopy.
   D. Mediastinoscopy.
   E. Thoracoscopy.

Exercises

6. Endoscopic inspection of the rectouterine pouch of Douglas, the area between the uterus and the rectum is
   A. Arthroscopy.
   B. Culdoscopy.
   C. Laparoscopy.
   D. Mediastinoscopy.
   E. Thoracoscopy.

7. Endoscopic inspection of the area between the lungs including the heart and great vessels, the trachea, thymus, lymph nodes, and the esophagus is
   A. Arthroscopy.
   B. Culdoscopy.
   C. Mediastinoscopy.
   D. Thoracoscopy.
   E. Peritoneoscopy.

8. Endoscopic examination of the abdomen using insufflation of carbon dioxide to create a pneumoperitoneum is
   A. Arthroscopy.
   B. Culdoscopy.
   C. Laparoscopy.
   D. Mediastinoscopy.
   E. Peritoneoscopy.

Short Answers

1. Define or explain:
   a. cul-de-sac _____

   _____

   b. empyema _____

   _____

   c. insufflation_____

   _____

   d. mediastinum _____

   _____

   e. trocar _____

   _____

   f. Veress needle _____

   _____

Exercises

2. List five reasons for performing mediastinoscopy.

   a. _____

   b. _____

   c. _____

   d. _____

   e. _____

3. What procedures discussed in this chapter might be performed in emergency situations?

   _____

   _____

   _____

   _____

   _____

4. What two procedures discussed in this chapter provide access to the same bodily region by different anatomic approaches?

   _____

   _____

   _____

   _____

Activities for Application and Further Study

1. List some circumstances in which an open surgical procedure might be preferred to endoscopic surgery.

2. Research and list as many procedures as you can find that are done by laparoscopic technique (beyond those listed in the text). Which are diagnostic? Which are therapeutic?

3. Find at least one case study or sample report for each of the procedures discussed in this chapter. What were the indications for the procedure? What were the findings?

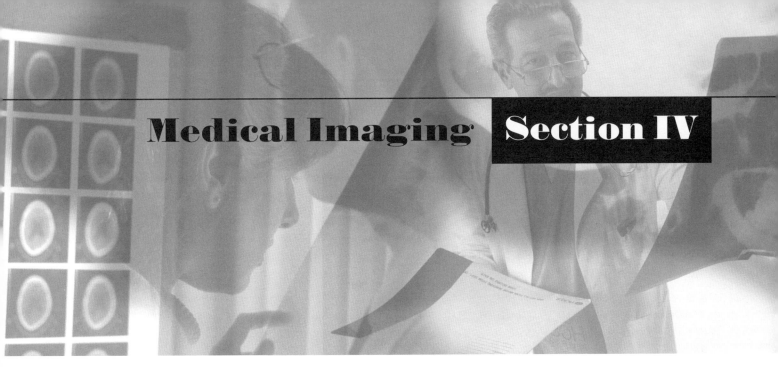

Medical Imaging   Section IV

Diagnostic imaging is the production of a likeness or graphic representation of some part of the human body (occasionally, the whole body) for the purpose of identifying, locating, characterizing, measuring, or otherwise assessing abnormalities of structure or function due to developmental disorders, injury, disease, or other causes. Usually the image produced is preserved for storage and future reference in some durable form—on paper or photographic film, or in digital form on tape, CD, or another medium. Medical imaging is a highly complex and diversified field, making use of a broad range of sophisticated technology and constantly developing new methods and applications.

The most elementary medical image is a drawing prepared by an artist. From remote antiquity, drawings and three-dimensional models of parts of the normal body in stone, plaster, wax, or other media have been used to teach anatomy. Medical illustration is an extension of this activity to abnormal structures. Paintings and sculptures by some of the world's greatest artists include images of deformity and disease.

Before the development of color photography, a careful drawing was the most accurate way to preserve the visual appearance of abnormal changes or findings due to maldevelopment,

disease, or injury, both for future reference by the treating physician and for purposes of medical education. Most of the illustrations in 19th- and early 20th-century medical textbooks were pen-and-ink drawings, lithographs, or engravings prepared by skilled artists. As with depictions of normal anatomy, a major advantage of medical illustration is that the artist can create a cutaway, schematic, or idealized view that emphasizes elements worthy of special attention while suppressing irrelevant details. Nowadays medical illustration is used primarily in health care education.

Medical photography has taken over many of the functions once performed by medical illustration. Given adequate lighting and a cooperative patient, any intelligent adult can produce a photograph of acceptable quality for medical purposes quickly and without elaborate equipment. Medical photography is particularly valuable in preserving evidence of injury in forensic medicine (automobile accidents, child abuse, criminal assault), in recording before-and-after views in plastic and reconstructive surgery, and in objectively documenting the effects of treatment in clinical trials. Images recorded by a digital camera can be stored, retrieved, edited, and transmitted electronically by means of equipment and methodologies that are readily available to all. For special photographic techniques or applications, such as stereoscopic views of the retina, more sophisticated equipment and special skills are required.

Videography (recording motion pictures on television tape) also plays an important role in medicine. It is especially useful in following the steps of a complex surgical procedure that only one or two persons at the operating table can observe at first hand. A skillful videographer can often make a record that shows structures and surgical techniques in close-up with greater clarity and fidelity than any human observer could match. Videographic recording is widely used in conjunction with other imaging techniques, such as fluoroscopy and angiography, to be discussed below.

Medical illustration and medical photography are not limited to recording the surface features of the living patient. Images of specimens removed during surgery or at autopsy can also be recorded, and photomicrographs of slides and smears prepared for microscopic examination can also be preserved with appropriate equipment. But all of these methods depend ultimately on the ability of the human eye to observe light rays.

In 1895, the German physicist Wilhelm Conrad Röntgen discovered and reported a previously unknown form of radiation. While working in his laboratory at the University of Würzburg, he noted that a Hittorf-Crookes tube, recognized as a source of cathode rays, was emitting other rays as well, which could penetrate solid objects of wood or metal and induce phosphorescence in crystals at a distance. By a series of well-conceived experiments, he quickly determined the basic properties of these rays, which (using the mathematician's traditional symbol for something unknown) he called x-rays.

He found that the internal structure of objects that are opaque to light rays, including the human body, could be projected on a screen coated with phosphorescent crystals when the object of study was placed between the x-ray source and the screen. Of even greater importance, such images could also be preserved permanently by being recorded on the same light-sensitive glass plates that were used in those days instead of film to make photographic negatives.

The discovery of x-rays completely revolutionized many aspects of medicine during the first half of the 20th century. It now became possible to see with the eye many structural features and abnormalities that had formerly defied visual observation. Broken bones, foreign bodies such as bullets, and infectious and neoplastic processes in the lungs could be clearly seen and sharply localized in a manner that would have been dismissed as magic or science fiction a few years earlier.

But it soon became evident that x-rays are capable of inducing harmful changes in tissues after intense or prolonged exposure—nonhealing inflammatory conditions of the skin, malignant tumors, injury to germ cells that can affect offspring, and fetal damage. In this respect, as well as in their ability to penetrate objects that are opaque to light, x-rays closely resemble the gamma rays produced by radioactive substances. (The first radioactive element, radium, was discovered and studied by Marie and Pierre Curie in France less than a decade after the discovery of x-rays.) The application of safety precautions in the use of diagnostic radiation became a major concern (see box). Meanwhile, the discovery of the toxic effects of x-rays on certain types of tissue, particularly cancers, led to their use in radiotherapy.

Until the 1960s, developments in radiology (sometimes called röntgenology or roentgenology) dominated the field of medical imaging. Steady improvements in techniques and materials led to the production of sharper images and a broad range of specialized examinations while reducing the amount of radiation exposure. Contrast media (liquids that block x-rays and

Radiographic Safety

Elaborate regulations for the protection of both patients and workers have been enacted at both state and federal levels. Work areas with radiation hazards must be posted and access to them must be restricted to authorized personnel. X-ray machines must be recalibrated regularly and their shielding checked to make sure that it provides proper protection to both medical personnel and patients.

Radiographic technicians are trained to use the minimum machine settings (voltage and exposure time) for the examination needed, to restrict the radiation beam to the area of clinical interest, and to check settings carefully so as to avoid the need for repeat exposures. Women who are or may be pregnant do not undergo any x-ray examination unless it has been determined that the expected benefit of the examination outweighs the risk of fetal harm. For certain types of examination, gonadal shielding (protection of testes or ovaries with lead-impregnated rubber sheeting) may be used.

Radiologists and radiographic technicians use protective equipment (lead aprons, lead gloves, stationary or movable shields) to avoid excessive exposure to radiation. Anyone who is exposed occupationally to x-ray and other forms of ionizing radiation is required to wear a radiation dosimeter, colloquially called a film badge. This is a small receptacle, worn attached to the clothing, that contains a strip of photographic film protected by various materials (plastic, aluminum, cadmium) or by different thicknesses of material. The cumulative x-ray exposure of the wearer is indicated by the degree to which the film has been affected by radiation. The film in the badge is developed and "read" once a month and replaced with fresh film. Each person's exposure records are preserved permanently in a national registry.

therefore create an image in an x-ray picture) were used to outline structures such as parts of the digestive tract and the circulatory system. Motion picture photography made it possible to record the flow of swallowed contrast medium through the esophagus, stomach, and intestine and of injected medium in the arteries and veins.

During the second half of the 20th century, the field of medical imaging experienced an explosion of new developments. The usefulness of x-ray studies was enormously enhanced by computed (axial) tomography (CT or CAT scanning), in which a group of x-ray images are combined and analyzed by a computer so as to produce a series of cuts or sectional views.

In addition, entirely new physical principles were discovered and adapted for purposes of diagnostic imaging. Ultrasonic waves (high-frequency sound waves, far above the pitch audible to the human ear) were found able to penetrate tissues and generate echoes that could be captured by suitable equipment and converted into visual images. Magnetic resonance imaging (MRI) is based on the behavior of protons (hydrogen atoms) in a strong magnetic field. Nuclear imaging, the use of radioactive isotopes to create visual images of certain changes in living tissues, provides yet another type of diagnostic information. Ultrasound has the advantage that it does not expose the subject to x-rays or, so far as is known, to any other potentially harmful form of energy. Hence it can be used with safety during pregnancy, and examinations can be repeated as often as necessary without the risk of cumulative harm from radiation.

Much of the basic work in radiology is performed by radiographic technicians who have been trained and certified in radiographic technique, the maintenance and use of diagnostic equipment, film processing, patient care, and radiologic safety precautions. Most imaging studies are performed according to established routines that specify patient preparation, patient positioning and placement of film, selection of equipment (film type and size, grids, filters) and equipment settings (voltage, exposure time, distance from x-ray source to patient).

An imaging study, or group of studies, is ordinarily ordered by a physician to aid in the diagnostic evaluation of symptoms or abnormal findings. Before ordering an examination the physician may consult with a radiologist to determine the most appropriate studies for the intended purpose. In some settings (for routine health evaluations, before certain types of surgery, or in workers exposed to certain hazardous airborne substances), a chest x-ray or other radiologic study may be performed as a screening procedure in a person without symptoms or suspected abnormalities.

Orders for imaging studies are transmitted in writing to the radiologic department or laboratory. Ordinarily an imaging requisition contains information for the radiographic technician and radiologist about significant medical history and physical findings. Any history of allergy, particularly to radiographic contrast media, is noted. When previous imaging studies have been performed, they are made available to the radiologist for comparison with current studies and perhaps to guide the choice of further examinations.

Some types of diagnostic procedure (chest x-ray, IVP, obstetrical ultrasound examination) are performed by a radiographic technician working independently of a radiologist. Others (fluoroscopy, angiography) are conducted largely by the radiologist. Many examinations require special preparation of the patient, such as fasting, laxatives, enemas, withholding of regular medicines, administration of premedication, local or general anesthesia, and placement of endoscopes or catheters.

A radiologist dictates a report of findings observed during an examination and after review of films, with conclusions or radio-

graphic diagnoses as appropriate, and the report is then sent to the ordering physician. (For mammography, federal law requires that a report in nontechnical language also be transmitted to the patient.)

Radiologic diagnoses may be quite specific ("Left pneumothorax with 30% collapse of the lung and no mediastinal shift," "Solitary Lincoln cent in the ascending colon with no evidence of bowel obstruction"). Often, however, only very general observations or conclusions can be recorded, with a note recommending clinical correlation (that is, interpretation of radiographic findings, or the lack thereof, in the light of the patient's history and findings on physical examination and other diagnostic testing).

The radiologist's report may include comments about the quality of images obtained by a technician (improper patient positioning, faulty developing technique), patient preparation (necklace left in place for chest x-ray, stool in the colon during barium enema examination), or other factors that may adversely affect the diagnostic accuracy of the study (poor patient cooperation or movement during exposure of films).

The modern imaging laboratory, whether a free-standing operation or a department in a hospital, may employ dozens of radiologists and technicians, perform thousands of procedures each month, and have a capital investment of many millions of dollars in equipment. Besides devices used to perform imaging studies, the furnishings of an x-ray department include apparatus for the administration of contrast agents, supplies for the medical support of patients including emergency resuscitation equipment, and specialized examining tables capable of being adjusted to any desired position and equipped with necessary supports, restraints, and padding. A diagnostic suite and its equipment may be adaptable for a broad variety of examinations, or may be "dedicated"—that is, designed specifically, or used exclusively, for a single type of procedure such as mammography or cerebral angiography.

A radiologist often specializes in one type of procedure or in the examination of one bodily region or system. The radiologist may work closely with an interventional cardiologist, a neurosurgeon, or a vascular surgeon, and may even perform interventional procedures. Technicians, too, are often specialists in one type of procedure.

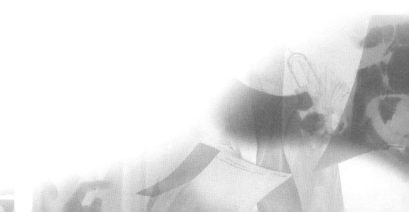

Plain Radiography

10

LEARNING OBJECTIVES

Upon completion of this chapter, the student should be able to

- Discuss the basic principles of diagnostic radiography;

- Discuss the diagnostic value of the standard PA chest x-ray;

- Describe the values and limitations of plain radiographic studies of the abdomen and extremities;

- Explain the importance of mammography and bone densitometry as screening procedures for healthy women.

Plain Radiography

Although ultrasound and MRI have replaced conventional x-ray examinations for many applications, radiology is still the mainstay of diagnostic imaging. This chapter discusses standard x-ray procedures performed without contrast media, including fluoroscopy, mammography, and bone densitometry.

X-rays are a form of electromagnetic radiation having a wavelength between that of gamma rays and that of ultraviolet rays. The importance of x-rays in medicine arises from their ability to penetrate most of the tissues of the human body and to expose photographic film in a manner similar to light.

In modern diagnostic radiology, x-rays are produced in a high-voltage electron tube (Coolidge tube) with equipment that controls the intensity of the beam, its direction and shape, and the duration of emission. X-rays pass through the part of the body under study and create an image on a sheet of film that is protected from light in a film holder or cassette. Since no lenses are used to focus x-rays, the image is about the same size as the subject, and correspondingly large sheets of film must be used. The standard film size for chest x-rays is 14 x 17 inches (35.5 x 43 cm).

Most x-ray equipment is permanently installed in a properly equipped and shielded radiographic suite. Portable x-ray machines are available to perform certain types of examination in an emergency department, at the bedside, in the patient's home, intraoperatively (during the course of a surgical procedure), or for mass screening in a nursing home, factory, or correctional facility.

Units of Measurement Used in Radiography

Since the early days of diagnostic radiology, efforts have been made to measure the amount of radiation transferred to the subject during an examination. Such measurement was considered important as a means of monitoring the effects of radiation on living tissue. The first unit established, the *roentgen*, was based on the electrical effects of radiation. One roentgen is defined as the amount of x-ray or gamma radiation that produces 0.333×10^{-9} coulomb of electrical charge in 1.0 cc of dry air at standard conditions of temperature and pressure.

In order to adapt this purely physical measurement to human biology, the rem (an acronym for *roentgen equivalent in man*) was developed. The rem introduced the concept of relative biological effectiveness and established coefficients for various types of radiation (alpha, beta, gamma, x-ray) and for different tissues (skin, bone marrow, gonads).

Later the roentgen was replaced by the *rad* (an acronym for *radiation absorbed dose*), which was defined as an amount of radiation equivalent to 0.01 J (joule) per kg of irradiated material. The joule, named for James Joule (1818-1889), the British physicist who discovered the first law of thermodynamics, is the SI unit of electrical, mechanical, and thermal energy.

Nowadays roentgens, rems, and rads have been replaced by the gray and the sievert, chiefly because the earlier units weren't congruent with units in the International System of Units. One gray (Gy) corresponds to an absorbed dose of 1 joule per kilogram. Obviously, then, 1 Gy equals 100 rads. The gray is named for the pioneering British radiobiologist Louis H. Gray (1905-1965), who defined the rad in 1940.

The new, SI-compatible unit corresponding to the rem is the sievert (Sv), named for the Swedish medical physicist Rolf M. Sievert (1896-1966). Since the sievert is an absorbed dose of 1 joule per kilogram as modified by the same biological coefficients as in the calculation of the rem, 1 Sv equals 100 rems.

Radiographic equipment includes a provision for incorporating the patient's name, identifying numbers, and the date of the examination into the image on the film. Usually the institution or laboratory performing the study is also identified. Radiopaque markers may be placed on the film to distinguish right from left, to indicate that the study was performed before or after a certain procedure (e.g., reduction of a dislocation), with or without weights or stress applied to an extremity, and so forth. Markers may also be placed on the subject, for example to show the exact site of a skin wound in a search for an imbedded foreign body.

X-ray film is developed in an automatic processing machine similar to those used in conventional photography. A developing solution reacts chemically with the silver-containing emulsion on the film in proportion to the amount of radiation that has reached each area of the film. An area that has received a large amount of radiation turns deep gray or black, while an area that has been protected from radiation by an opaque object, such as bone or a ring worn on a finger, does not darken but remains transparent or translucent. After a timed exposure to the developer, the film passes through a fixative or "hypo" bath that arrests all further chemical reaction. Finally the film is rinsed with water and dried by a current of warm air. A film processor yields a dry, finished film ready for viewing less than five minutes after the exposure was made.

Videographic (TV) equipment is used to record moving pictures of internal organs such as the heart and to trace the flow of contrast medium through blood vessels (angiography) and the digestive system.

In fluoroscopy, a continuous stream of x-rays passing through a part of the body is made to create an image on a sensitive screen. Fluoroscopy was widely used during the first half of the 20th century to examine the heart and lungs, to monitor the reduction of fractures, and for other applications. Older fluoroscopic equipment exposed both physician and patient to a dangerous amount of radiation. Modern equipment electronically enhances the radiographic image and projects it on a television screen so that the dose of radiation can be kept to a minimum (*see box on p. 129*). Nowadays fluoroscopic monitoring is used extensively in studies with contrast media (gastrointestinal series, angiography) and in invasive and interventional cardiology to track the position of catheters, stents, and other devices.

Although modern picture archiving and communicating systems make it possible to store and retrieve x-ray images digitally and to transmit them instantly anywhere in the world, much of the day-by-day diagnostic work in radiology (chest x-rays, examinations of injured extremities) involves the production of one or more negative images on sheets of film. By long-established convention, these negatives are not printed on paper, as is done in conventional photography. Instead, the negative itself serves as the picture. For examination or "reading," the film is placed on a backlighted view box that provides bright, even illumination.

For most x-ray examinations the patient is asked to remove clothing, jewelry, and other personal articles that could cause confusion or lead to a misdiagnosis by introducing extraneous features into the image. Nearly all garments have zippers, buttons, buckles, grommets, or other fasteners or decorations that will appear in an x-ray image. Such clothing must be exchanged for a plain cloth gown or sheet. For an individual x-ray picture (as opposed to fluoroscopy or videoradiography) the patient must remain motionless for the brief duration of the exposure. For studies of the upper trunk, breath-holding is required.

The fact that x-ray images are made by rays that have passed through the subject accounts for several important differences between x-ray and conventional photography. Different tissues offer different amounts of resistance to the passage of x-rays and, as already mentioned, produce correspondingly lighter or darker images on film. A structure or body area that allows x-rays to pass freely, resulting in a darker or black area on the film, is said to be *radiolucent* (by analogy with *translucent*). A structure or object that blocks x-rays, resulting in less exposure of the film and a lighter or white area, is said to be *radiopaque*.

The radiologist can distinguish only four degrees of density in tissue: metal density (bone, gallstones, urinary calculi, metallic foreign bodies including orthopedic hardware); water density (body fluids and most soft tissues other than fat); fat density; and air or gas density (air in respiratory passages, gas in digestive passages, or either of these in inappropriate places). Shapes or outlines appear in an x-ray image only where two zones of contrasting density touch or overlap.

The radiologist can see the outline of a bone (which is of metal density) because it is silhouetted against surrounding soft tissues of water density. A bubble of air in the stomach is visible because it, too, is surrounded by, and contrasts with, water-density tissue. But where two structures of like density (e.g., two muscles, or the spleen and the pancreas) are contiguous, no silhouette is produced, and the border or interface between them is not represented in the image.

This limitation of radiography has been overcome to some extent by the use of contrast media (singular, *medium*)—solutions of metallic salts or iodides that are radiopaque. Introduced into the body, these can outline a hollow structure such as the stomach or the colon, or a tubular system such as the circulation, the bile ducts, or the urinary tract. Contrast media can be swallowed, injected, or introduced through a tube, catheter, or enema apparatus. Air or gas can be introduced into a hollow structure to serve as a negative contrast medium. Contrast radiography is discussed in the next chapter.

Unlike a photograph, an x-ray picture gives no information about the depth or contours of the subject. An x-ray picture is literally just a shadow or group of shadows. Everything is represented in an absolutely flat, two-dimensional image. An

x-ray film of a right hand, when turned over, cannot be distinguished from an x-ray of a left hand. For that reason, an x-ray picture of any part of an extremity is normally labeled R or L at the time of exposure. A metal letter clipped to the corner of the filmholder becomes a part of the image.

When x-rays leave their source they tend to radiate in all directions. Their direction and lateral spread can be controlled with metal housings, deflectors, and cones, but any x-ray beam (like any beam of light), no manner how narrow, will tend to spread out the farther it gets from its source. This has an effect on the fidelity with which an x-ray picture reproduces the internal structures through which the rays have passed. The closer an object is to the source of x-rays (and the farther from the film), the larger and less distinct it will appear (*see box*). Hence for maximum clarity the zone of clinical interest is placed as close to the x-ray film as possible. A standard chest x-ray is taken with the front of the patient's chest against the film holder and the x-ray source behind the patient. (This is called a postero-anterior or PA view.) This technique gives maximum definition to the heart shadow while blurring and dulling the shadow of the spinal

Where's That Flashlight?

You can easily demonstrate, with a flashlight in a darkened room, the effect of distance from the radiation source on the size and clarity of an image. Shine the flashlight toward a blank wall from a distance of 2-3 feet. While holding the light source steady in one hand, move your other hand between it and the wall. As your hand approaches the light source, its image becomes large and fuzzy; as it approaches the wall, its image becomes smaller and sharper.

column. When the thoracic spine is the center of interest, the same part of the body is x-rayed with the patient's back nearest the film holder (anteroposterior or AP view).

As x-rays pass through tissue they tend to be deflected to some extent from their straight course, much as light waves are when passing through murky fluid. This phenomenon (soft-tissue scatter) causes some blurring of images, which may limit the value of a study performed on an obese subject or in certain body regions. In order to reduce soft-tissue scatter and the effects of lateral spreading (radiation), a Bucky grid may be placed between the subject and the film. This grid consists of dozens of very thin metal strips arranged in parallel with very narrow spaces between them. Rays that are still traveling comparatively straight after passing through the subject get through the grid and expose the film. Deflected rays, traveling at an oblique angle, cannot get through to add their blurring effect to the image. During the fraction of a second that the film is being exposed, the grid is set in motion by an automatic mechanism so that the grid itself will not appear in the image.

Tomography (also called laminography) is a technique for focusing on a particular site or level within the subject. The x-ray source and the filmholder, both mounted on a rigid frame that maintains an exact distance between them, rotate simultaneously in an arc, in opposite directions, with the subject between them. The point within the subject about which this rotation occurs will produce an image of maximum clarity on the film, while tissues closer to and farther away from that point will be blurred or invisible. In effect, a tomogram is an x-ray of a narrow slice of the subject. Typically a series of tomograms or "cuts" are made, each focused at a different plane. Tomography is used primarily in defining and localizing abnormal masses and foreign bodies. The term *tomography* can also refer to cut or slice type images produced by computer analysis and reconstruction of radiographic data in computed tomography (CT) (discussed in Chapter 12) and in other imaging methods.

In dual-energy imaging, two images of the same structure are recorded, one after the other, with different levels of x-ray energy. Because the second image is made only a fraction of a second after the first, movement artifacts due to breathing or position change do not occur. The high-energy image is made with the same machine settings as a standard film. The low-energy exposure yields poorer penetration and hence emphasizes bone shadows. A computer program "subtracts" the low-energy image from the high-energy one so as to provide clearer visualization of soft tissues.

The term **plain film** (not *"plane film"*) refers to a radiographic study performed without the use of contrast material. For each part of the body and each diagnostic purpose, standard procedures (positioning of the subject, machine voltage setting, exposure time) have been developed to yield the desired information with maximum speed and efficiency and a minimum of exposure to harmful radiation.

Chest X-ray (CXR)

The standard PA chest film is the most frequently performed of all plain radiographic examinations. For this study the patient stands facing the filmholder and the x-ray tube is aimed horizontally at the patient's back. The backs of the wrists are placed on the hips and the elbows rotated forward so as to move the scapulae laterally as far as possible, and the breath is held in full inspiration.

This single study can provide a great deal of critical diagnostic information. Solid tumors and abnormal accumulations of fluid (water density) are readily apparent when they encroach on lung tissue, which is largely filled with air (gas density). The heart and great vessels (aorta and venae cavae) appear sharply silhouetted against the background of air in lung tissue, so that abnormalities in their size and shape are also clearly evident.

Among the numerous indications for performing a chest x-ray are known or suspected disease affecting the respiratory, cardiovascular, or upper digestive system or other structures within or adjacent to the thorax; chest trauma; preoperatively in patients of uncertain cardiorespiratory status; postoperatively to assess success of surgery or look for complications; and for surveillance of workers exposed to certain airborne substances that can cause pulmonary fibrosis or malignancy.

In reading a chest film, the radiologist looks for changes in the density and contour of soft tissues (muscles of the neck and thorax, breasts); indications of deformity, disease, or trauma in bones (spine, ribs, scapulae, humeri); irregularities, thickening, or calcification of the pleural margins, or fluid in the pleural space; abnormalities of the diaphragmatic contour; and variations in the size, shape, and position of the heart, great vessels (aorta, pulmonary artery, superior and inferior venae cavae) and other structures in the mediastinum (the part of the thorax between the lungs). In a standard PA chest film the width of the cardiac shadow at its widest is normally less than half the width of the thorax at its widest. The comparison of these two widths (heart width divided by thoracic width), called the cardiothoracic ratio (CTR), is therefore normally less than 0.5.

The lungs are examined for areas of increased density (infiltrates, fibrosis, space-occupying lesions), cavitation, or atelectasis (collapse due either to blockage of a bronchus or to the presence of air in the pleural cavity). The air within the trachea and in the right and left main bronchi outlines these structures against the mediastinal soft tissues. Smaller branches of the respiratory tract, however, are visible only when surrounded by lung tissue containing not air but fluid, as in pneumonia (the so-called air bronchogram).

The normal "lung markings"—radiopaque tubular structures at the hila of the lungs, which branch and taper as they spread toward the periphery—are not bronchi but branches of the

right and left pulmonary arteries. Distortion or asymmetry of the pattern created by these vessels may indicate a space-occupying lesion within lung tissue, pneumothorax (air in the pleural space), or other abnormal condition.

A lateral chest film is often performed in conjunction with a PA film, or as a supplement to it when the initial study shows some abnormality. The lateral view shows substantially more of the lung bases than a PA view, and may reveal abnormalities concealed by the heart shadow in the PA view. A left lateral film (with the left side of the chest nearest to the film holder) is usually preferred because it provides a sharper image of the heart. Right and left oblique views of the chest may be obtained to clarify the diagnosis. A lateral film of the upper respiratory tract may be performed to assess the patency of the airway in cases of neck trauma.

A lordotic view is an anteroposterior chest film in which the x-ray beam is aimed slightly upward to improve visibility of the apices of the lungs, which are partly concealed by the clavicles in a PA film. Special positioning is used to assess the ribs and sternum for disease or injury. Films taken in both full inspiration and expiration are sometimes useful in detecting pneumothorax. Views made with the patient recumbent may show pleural fluid better than upright films.

Abdominal Films

Plain films of the abdomen are less valuable than chest films because most of the abdominal organs are of the same (water) density. Abdominal films are useful, however, in identifying disorders characterized by abnormal distribution of air or gas (distention of bowel due to obstruction, gas in the peritoneal cavity from a ruptured bowel), in confirming the presence and location of kidney stones and swallowed foreign bodies, and in identifying certain other disorders.

A plain film of the abdomen may be obtained as a screening examination, particularly in a patient with acute abdominal pain, to determine whether other studies are needed and to help in the selection of those studies. A plain film performed as a preliminary to contrast studies is called a scout film. Because such an examination is often done to screen for a stone in the urinary tract, it may also be called a KUB (kidneys, ureters, bladder) film.

A single abdominal film is ordinarily made with the patient lying supine (face up) and the film holder contained in a receptacle within the examining table. Although glass plates have not been used in diagnostic radiography for generations, the phrase *flat plate* lingers on as a term for such a flat abdominal film. When there is concern about the possibility of a ruptured bowel, with leakage of gas into the peritoneal cavity, several plain films may be made with the patient in different positions, usually flat, upright, and left lateral decubitus (that is, lying on the left side). For the latter examination, the film holder is placed vertically and the x-ray beam is directed horizontally across the table, hence the common term "cross-table view." Such a combination of films may be called an acute abdomen series or a free air study.

X-ray Pelvimetry

Radiographic examination of the pelvic bones was formerly a routine procedure in pregnant women whose pelvic dimensions were in doubt. This procedure is now seldom used because of concerns about the harmful effects on radiation on the fetus in early pregnancy and because of poor correlation between findings and outcomes. Clinical pelvimetry is discussed in Chapter 2.

Radiography of the Extremities

X-ray studies of the extremities are most often performed to assess the effects of injury (fracture, dislocation), to locate foreign bodies, or to diagnose disorders of bones or joints (congenital deformities, metabolic or circulatory disorders, benign and malignant tumors, rheumatoid arthritis, degenerative joint disease). A single x-ray view of an extremity may be of limited usefulness. Because all structures are superimposed in one composite two-dimensional image, a small fracture or zone of bone disease may escape detection. A metallic foreign body will probably be visible, but its exact location in the three-dimensional extremity cannot be determined from a two-dimensional study.

For most extremity studies, therefore, three exposures are made: anteroposterior (AP), lateral, and oblique. The term *anteroposterior* means that the x-rays are traveling from anterior to posterior. For an anteroposterior study of the wrist, the back (dorsum) of the subject's wrist is against the film holder, and the front (volar or palmar aspect) of the wrist is toward the x-ray tube. The lateral examination is made with the part rotated 90° from the AP position, and for an oblique view the positioning is approximately midway between AP and lateral. Two oblique views or other special positions may be appropriate for certain purposes. Specially shaped supports, sandbags, or other appliances may be used to keep certain parts (for example, the hand) properly positioned and immobile during the exposure.

In orthopedics, the measurement of distances and angles as shown in special radiographic projections is an important means of diagnosing congenital or acquired bone and joint problems and in planning surgery. A stress film is one in which mechanical stress is applied to one or more joints in an extremity while the exposure is being made. A stress film may show abnormal laxity of a joint, such as that due to a ligamentous tear, which would not be apparent on a standard view. Stress can be applied manually by the patient or by means of a strap, tape, or other appliance. In the examination of a shoulder to detect a tear of the acromioclavicular joint, films may be taken both with and without the subject holding a weight in the arm on the affected side.

Skull and Spine Films

X-rays of the axial skeleton (skull, spinal column, ribs, and sternum) may be performed in cases of injury or to diagnose bone or joint disease. However, specialized examinations (CT, MRI, angiography) have largely supplanted plain skull films in the assessment of brain disorders (hemorrhage, neoplasms), and are also more valuable than plain films in evaluating injury or disease of the vertebrae.

Special studies of the nasal bones, the bony orbit, and other facial bones may be performed to evaluate acute injury. Radiographic studies of the paranasal sinuses may show thickening of mucous membranes and an air-fluid level due to accumulation of secretions in a sinus whose ostium is blocked by swelling. However, such studies are both nonspecific and insensitive. Computed tomography (CT) is more accurate in the diagnosis of acute and chronic sinusitis, and shows nasal polyps better.

Mammography

Breast cancer is the most common malignancy in women, with about 182 000 new cases diagnosed annually in this country. This disease ranks second only to lung cancer as a cause of cancer deaths in women, with about 46 000 deaths yearly. A woman's lifetime risk of developing breast cancer is 8%; the risk increases with advancing age. Many other factors, including race, family history, and reproductive history, influence a woman's risk of developing breast cancer.

Mammography is the radiologic evaluation of the female breast, primarily to search for or evaluate abnormal masses that may be malignant. Most authorities currently recommend that every woman have a baseline mammogram by age 40 and annual mammograms after age 50. Examinations should start at an earlier age in women with a family history of early-onset breast cancer.

Special equipment and techniques have been devised to limit radiation exposure and enhance the diagnostic value of the procedure. The apparatus used to perform mammography includes, besides an adjustable x-ray source and a film holder, a compression paddle that serves to flatten

out the breast during the examination. By thinning the layer of tissue to be examined, compression permits a lower dose of radiation. In addition, the compression paddle steadies the patient and reduces the risk of movement during the exposure.

A screening mammogram is performed according to a standard protocol to evaluate the breasts of a woman who has no breast complaints or abnormal findings. In contrast, diagnostic mammography refers to a more specific and individualized radiographic study that is done to evaluate local breast pain or abnormal findings such

When Radiologists Saw Red

Before television technology became available to boost the clarity and contrast of fluoroscopic images, radiologists faced a difficult dilemma. If they used a voltage high enough to yield clean, sharp fluoroscopic images, they exposed themselves to dangerous, even life-threatening, cumulative doses of radiation. But at lower voltages the images appeared fuzzy and dull. Radiologists discovered that they could see low-voltage images much more clearly if, for several minutes before performing a fluoroscopic examination, they remained in the dark or covered their eyes with a blindfold. But although this period of dark adaptation sharpened the radiologists' perception of smudgy fluoroscopic images, it also wasted an enormous amount of time.

The solution eventually found was for the radiologist to wear a pair of red goggles instead of sitting idle in the dark. The goggles permitted reading, writing, eating, and the performance of other routine tasks, but blocked enough light that dark adaptation still occurred. Until the 1960s, many radiologists spent as much as one-third of their working days wearing red goggles.

as a palpable lump or nipple discharge or to follow up on an abnormal screening mammogram.

In screening mammography, an x-ray of each breast is made in two projections. For the mediolateral oblique view, the x-ray tube is positioned in front of the chest and aimed horizontally toward the breast to be examined, with the film holder placed laterally under the subject's raised arm. For the craniocaudal view, the film holder is placed horizontally under the breast and the x-ray beam is directed downward from above.

For interpretation, a film of the right breast is displayed side by side on a viewbox with the corresponding view of the left breast, as if they were mirror images. This facilitates comparison of the two breasts and serves to emphasize minor differences in their radiographic appearance. Digital mammography, permitting review of digital images on a high-resolution monitor, improves the accuracy of mammographic screening.

Mammographic findings that suggest cancer are ill-defined densities within breast tissue and microcalcifications (very small deposits of calcium), particularly those that are irregularly clustered or spiculated (appearing like small spikes or thorns). These findings are nonspecific. It is estimated that a woman having screening mammograms regularly throughout life has a 50% chance of eventually having a false-positive report (a mammogram that is suspicious for cancer in the absence of cancer).

Hence mammography is considered a screening procedure, and must be coordinated with other diagnostic measures such as physical examination, other imaging procedures (ultrasound, MRI, scintimammography, positron emission tomography), and biopsy of suspicious lesions. Mammography (rather than fluoroscopy) may be used to direct the placement of a needle or wire marker in a suspicious lesion in preparation for biopsy.

The reliability of mammography decreases as the density of breast tissue increases. Because younger women normally have denser breasts,

ultrasound examination may be preferred for them in the evaluation of breast masses. Ultrasound has the advantages that breast compression is unnecessary and there is no radiation exposure. Unlike routine mammography, however, ultrasonography requires considerable skill on the part of the examiner. Some authorities recommend that MRI be used for annual screening of women at high risk because it may detect tumors at an earlier stage than mammography.

Reporting of mammographic findings has been standardized by the Breast Imaging Reporting and Data System (BIRADS) in the following categories:

0	–	Incomplete examination
1	–	Negative
2	–	Benign abnormality noted
3	–	Probably benign findings; recommend repeat examination
4	–	Suspicious for malignancy; consider biopsy
5	–	Malignancy highly probable

Bone Densitometry

Osteoporosis, a common disorder of middle-aged and elderly women, is characterized by decreased mass and decreased mineral density of bone, with increased susceptibility to fractures. Bone mass declines with age and is influenced by sex, race, weight, and other factors. Osteoporosis is responsible for 50% of fractures occurring in women over age 50. Compression fractures of vertebrae and fractures of the wrist and hip (neck of the femur) due to falls are the most common. Assessment of bone density is currently recommended for all women over 65 and for younger women who are at increased risk of osteoporosis.

Because mineral density must be decreased by about one-third before any reduction is apparent in an x-ray image, standard radiography is an insensitive test for osteoporosis. Bone densitometry is an application of radiographic technology to osteoporosis screening. Most of the bone densitometry techniques in current use measure the extent to which a low dose of radiation is absorbed by bone. The subject sits or lies motionless with the body area under study placed between an x-ray source and a scanner. Skeletal areas examined include the wrist, lumbar spine, and hip. Besides producing an image of the area examined, the study yields a numerical score that can be used to measure the degree of osteoporosis and to quantify the risk of fracture.

The several methods used for bone densitometry include single-photon and dual-photon absorptiometry (SPA and DPA), single-energy and dual-energy x-ray absorptiometry (SXA and DEXA), and quantitative CT. An ultrasound procedure, which does not involve x-rays, is also available.

The interpretation of a bone densitometry study includes a comparison of the findings with established norms. The result of this comparison is reported as a T-score, which is based on comparison of the patient's bone mineral density with that of a healthy woman in her 30s. A Z-score, based on comparison of the patient's measurements with those of a person of the same sex and age, may also be calculated.

Exercises

Fill in the Blanks

1. A tremendous advancement over plain radiography is _____, in which a group of x-ray images are combined and analyzed by a computer so as to produce a series of cuts or sectional views. (Section IV)

2. High-frequency sound waves, far above the pitch audible to the human ear, and able to penetrate tissues and generate echoes that could be captured by suitable equipment and converted into visual images are known as _____. (Section IV)

3. _____ is the use of radioactive isotopes to create visual images of certain changes in living tissues. (Section IV)

4. A _____ dictates a report of findings observed during an examination and after review of films, with conclusions or radiographic diagnoses. (Section IV)

5. The term _____ refers to interpretation of radiographic findings, or the lack thereof, in the light of the patient's history and findings on physical examination and other diagnostic testing. (Section IV)

6. In _____, a continuous stream of x-rays passing through a part of the body is made to create an image on a television screen.

7. In contrast to conventional photography in which a positive image is printed on paper, an x-ray image is a _____ image on a sheet of film.

8. A structure or body area that allows x-rays to pass freely, resulting in a darker or black area on the film, is said to be _____.

9. A structure or object that blocks x-rays, resulting in less exposure of the film and a lighter or white area, is said to be _____.

10. A standard chest x-ray is taken with the front of the patient's chest against the filmholder and the x-ray source behind the patient. This is called a _____ view.

11. When the thoracic spine is the center of interest, the same part of the body is x-rayed with the patient's back nearest the film holder for a _____ view.

12. A _____ may be placed between the subject and the film to reduce soft-tissue scatter and the effects of lateral spreading (radiation).

13. The term _____ refers to a radiographic study performed without the use of contrast material.

Exercises

14. Lung collapse due either to blockage of a bronchus or to the presence of air in the pleural cavity is known as _____.

15. A _____ view is an anteroposterior chest film in which the x-ray beam is aimed slightly upward to improve visibility of the apices of the lungs, which are partly concealed by the clavicles in a PA film.

16. Chest films taken in both full inspiration and expiration are sometimes useful in detecting _____.

17. Smaller branches of the respiratory tract are visible only when surrounded by lung tissue containing not air but fluid, as in pneumonia—the so-called _____.

18. A plain film performed as a preliminary to contrast studies is called a _____.

19. An abdominal x-ray done to screen for a stone in the urinary tract may be called a _____ film.

20. _____, the old term for a supine abdominal film, lingers on although glass plates have not been used in diagnostic radiography for generations.

21. _____, _____, and _____ films may be made when there is concern about the possibility of a ruptured bowel, with leakage of gas into the peritoneal cavity.

22. A single x-ray view of an extremity may be of limited usefulness because _____.

23. For most extremity studies, therefore, three exposures are made: _____, _____, and _____.

24. A _____ may show abnormal laxity of a joint, such as that due to a ligamentous tear, which would not be apparent on a standard view.

25. _____ is the radiologic evaluation of the female breast, primarily to search for or evaluate abnormal masses that may be malignant.

26. A compression paddle that serves to flatten out the breast during mammography to _____ and _____.

27. Two projections used for screening mammography are _____ and _____.

28. Ill-defined densities within breast tissue and microcalcifications appearing like small spikes or thorns are said to be _____ or _____.

29. Standard radiography is an insensitive test for osteoporosis because _____

30. _____ is an x-ray study used to evaluate a patient for osteoporosis.

Exercises

Multiple Choice: Circle the letter of the best answer from the choices given.

1. A chest x-ray or other radiologic study may be performed as a screening procedure in a person without symptoms or suspected abnormalities for which of the following reasons? (Section IV)
    A. Routine health evaluations.
    B. Before certain types of surgery.
    C. In workers exposed to certain hazardous airborne substances.
    D. All of the above.
    E. A & C.

2. Standard x-ray procedures performed without contrast media include all of the following except
    A. Fluoroscopy.
    B. Mammography.
    C. Bone densitometry.
    D. Chest x-ray.
    E. Magnetic resonance imaging.

3. Which of the following units used to quantify absorbed radiation is a unit in the International System of Units?
    A. Roentgen.
    B. Rad.
    C. Joule.
    D. Rem.
    E. Sievert.

4. Radiopaque markers may be placed on the film for all of the following reasons except
    A. To distinguish right from left.
    B. To indicate which side is up.
    C. To indicate that the study was performed before or after a certain procedure.
    D. To indicate that the study was performed with or without weights or stress applied to an extremity.
    E. To show the exact site of a skin wound in a search for an imbedded foreign body.

5. The degree of density of bone, gallstones, urinary calculi, metallic foreign bodies including orthopedic hardware is said to be
    A. Metal density.
    B. Air density.
    C. Gas density.
    D. Liquid density.
    E. Fat density.

Exercises

6. The radiographic density of body fluids and most soft tissues other than fat is
   A. Metal density.
   B. Air density.
   C. Liquid density.
   D. Gas density.
   E. Fat density.

7. The most frequently performed of all plain radiographic examinations is the
   A. AP x-ray of the chest.
   B. PA and lateral chest x-ray.
   C. PA chest x-ray.
   D. Recumbent views of chest.
   E. Right and left oblique chest x-ray.

8. The normal "lung markings"—radiopaque tubular structures at the hila of the lungs, which branch and taper as they spread toward the periphery—are caused by
   A. The heart and great vessels.
   B. Calcifications of the pleural margins.
   C. Bronchioles, the smaller branches of the bronchi.
   D. Branches of the right and left pulmonary arteries.
   E. The mediastinal soft tissues.

9. For a left lateral decubitus film of the abdomen, the film holder is placed vertically and the x-ray beam is directed horizontally across the table, hence the common term _____.
   A. Cross-table view.
   B. Upright view.
   C. Supine view.
   D. PA view.
   E. AP view.

10. Flat, upright, and left lateral decubitus views of the abdomen taken when there is a concern about the possibility of a ruptured bowel may also be called
    A. Tomograms.
    B. Acute abdomen series.
    C. A free air study.
    D. Fluoroscopy.
    E. B & C.

Exercises

11. In an oblique view of the hand, the hand is positioned
    A. Perpendicular to the film.
    B. Approximately midway between AP and lateral.
    C. With the palm up and the back of the hand against the film.
    D. With the palm of the hand against the film.
    E. Vertical to the film.

12. The measurement of distances and angles as shown in special radiographic projections of an extremity is important
    A. In diagnosing congenital or acquired bone and joint problems and in planning surgery.
    B. In diagnosing abnormal laxity of a joint.
    C. In diagnosing tears of the ligaments.
    D. In assessing weight-bearing capacity of a joint.
    E. In identifying loose bodies in a joint.

13. In which view is the x-ray tube positioned in front of the chest and aimed horizontally toward the breast to be examined, with the film holder placed laterally under the subject's raised arm?
    A. Posteroanterior.
    B. Oblique.
    C. Cross-table.
    D. Mediolateral oblique.
    E. Craniocaudal.

14. In which view is the film holder placed horizontally under the breast and the x-ray beam is directed downward from above?
    A. Posteroanterior.
    B. Oblique.
    C. Cross-table.
    D. Mediolateral oblique.
    E. Craniocaudal.

15. Several methods used for bone densitometry include all of the following except
    A. Single-photon and dual-photon absorptiometry (SPA and DPA).
    B. Magnetic resonance imaging.
    C. Single-energy and dual-energy x-ray absorptiometry (SXA and DEXA).
    D. Quantitative CT.
    E. Ultrasound.

Exercises

Short Answers

1. Define or explain:

   a. cardiothoracic ratio _____
   _____

   b. contrast medium _____
   _____

   c. fluoroscopy _____
   _____

   d. osteoporosis _____
   _____

   e. radiopaque _____
   _____

   f. tomography _____
   _____

2. What might be some emergency indications for performing a chest x-ray?

   _____
   _____
   _____

3. List three radiographic studies mentioned in this chapter that have been supplanted by safer or more informative methods.

   a. _____
   b. _____
   c. _____

4. List several factors that might interfere with the quality or usefulness of an x-ray examination.

   _____
   _____
   _____
   _____

Exercises

5. What procedures are followed to reduce unnecessary exposure of patients and technicians to radiation during radiographic examinations?

_____

_____

_____

_____

_____

_____

6. Explain how the use of contrast material has helped to overcome the limitations of plain radiography.

_____

_____

_____

_____

7. List the radiographic views of the chest discussed in the text and the advantages of each.

_____

_____

_____

_____

8. Discuss the strengths and weaknesses of plain films of the abdomen.

_____

_____

_____

_____

Exercises

Activities for Application and Further Study

1. Summarize the three major categories of imaging discussed in the introduction to Section IV and the significance of each. (Section IV)

2. Search the Internet for images from the history of medicine. Try to find line drawings or paintings demonstrating normal and abnormal anatomy as well as disease states. Compare these to comparable photographic images. Summarize and share your findings with the class. (Section IV)

3. Explain what happens on a standard x-ray when two areas of different density overlap. Give an example. What happens when two areas of like density overlap? Give an example.

4. Find a sample report for a bone densitometry on the Internet. What is the numerical value for the Z score, the T score? Are they normal or abnormal? Were there any terms on the report not discussed in the text? List and define. Share your report with the class.

Contrast Radiography

11

Although a plain x-ray examination can often provide adequate diagnostic information about a bone injury, an aspirated or swallowed foreign body, or a pulmonary infiltrate, x-ray images of soft-tissue structures such as the brain and spinal cord and the circulatory, digestive, and genitourinary systems typically lack sufficient detail for diagnostic purposes because most of the structures represented in the image are of the same (water) density.

This deficiency has been very largely overcome by the use of contrast media in diagnostic radiography. A contrast medium (sometimes—but not in this book—called a dye) is a liquid or semisolid material, containing either a metallic salt or an iodide, that appears with metal density in a radiographic image. Introduced into a hollow structure such as the colon or the aorta, it imparts to an x-ray picture a solid, opaque image of that structure.

Contrast Radiography of the Central Nervous System

Encephalography (Ventriculography)

Radiographic examinations of the brain after replacement of some of the fluid in the ventricular system with air or gas (pneumoencephalography) or with iodine-based contrast medium, formerly widely used in the diagnosis of head trauma and intracranial hemorrhage and tumors, has been rendered obsolete by the superior sensitivity and greater safety of MRI and CT.

Myelography

A myelogram is a radiographic examination of the spinal cord after injection of a contrast agent into the subarachnoid space. The procedure is usually performed to identify abnormalities of the spinal cord and its nerve roots, particularly compression by a herniated disk, a tumor, arthritic osteophytes (spiky outgrowths of bone), or spinal

stenosis (narrowing of the spinal canal). After administration of local anesthetic, a needle is inserted under fluoroscopic guidance between two lumbar vertebrae, as in the diagnostic procedure of lumbar puncture and in spinal anesthesia, and a water-based or oil-based iodine agent is injected. The x-ray table is tilted in order to distribute the medium throughout the area under examination. In addition to fluoroscopy and spot films, computed tomography (CT, discussed in Chapter 12) may be performed. As after any lumbar puncture, headache is a common sequela of this procedure.

Contrast Radiography of the Respiratory Tract

Bronchography

In this procedure, which is intended to visualize the trachea, the right and left main bronchi, and segmental bronchi and their branches, an iodine-based contrast medium is instilled into the lower respiratory tract by means of a catheter introduced through a nostril and passed beyond the larynx and into the trachea. A more localized study may be performed in which the contrast medium is introduced into a specific bronchus by a bronchoscope under fluoroscopic or direct visual control. These procedures are used to investigate acute or chronic bronchial disease, particularly obstruction, bronchiectasis, and tumors. Contrast bronchography with iodine media has been largely supplanted by CT studies with inhaled xenon as a contrast medium.

Contrast Radiographic Studies of the Gastrointestinal Tract

The soft tissues of the digestive system are of so uniform a density that plain x-rays are of little use in identifying or characterizing disorders of this system. Only when air or gas outlines or distends a part of the gastrointestinal tract can it be distinguished from surrounding tissues. Hence virtually all radiographic studies of the esophagus, stomach, and small intestine require that the subject swallow a radiopaque contrast agent. For examinations of the colon, the contrast material is administered as an enema.

For many decades the standard contrast medium for gastrointestinal studies has been barium sulfate. Pure barium sulfate forms white or yellowish crystals and is odorless, tasteless, virtually insoluble, chemically inert, and nontoxic when consumed orally. Various concentrations of barium are used depending on the type of examination to be performed.

A hollow structure such as the stomach or the colon, when filled with barium, presents a uniform barrier to x-rays and appears in a film as a solid radiopaque mass. Hence anatomic variations due to tumors, ulceration, scarring, or external factors are visible only when they affect the outer margin of the image as seen in any given projection. For this reason, the patient must "roll like a log" to right and left on the x-ray table while the radiologist observes the barium image fluoroscopically and records spot films as appropriate. The radiologist may also apply pressure to the abdomen to distribute the barium throughout the lumen of the structure under examination.

The chief abnormalities that may be noted in a barium study are filling defects (areas where the barium fails to fill out the expected contour of the organ because of the presence of a tumor), ulcerations (breaks or erosions in the integrity of the mucosal lining), strictures (narrowing of the lumen due to scarring), distortion or displacement due to external factors (swelling, tumors, or hemorrhage outside the digestive tract), and disturbances in gastrointestinal motility (undue rapidity or slowness of peristaltic movement of barium through the tract).

The radiologist observes the part of the digestive system under study not only while it is filled with barium but also after most of the barium has passed through. Traces of barium remaining may show small ulcerations or other subtle abnormalities in the mucous membrane or in the outline of the structure. The sensitivity of this part of a barium study may be enhanced by performing an air-contrast (double-contrast) examination. For this procedure, air or gas is introduced into the digestive tract to distend its walls after most of the barium has passed through or, in the case of a barium enema, has been expelled from the colon. In an upper GI study, gas is generated by having the patient swallow crystals of baking soda (sodium bicarbonate). For double-contrast colon studies, air is injected with the enema apparatus.

Suspensions of barium sulfate used for upper gastrointestinal examinations have a thick, chalky consistency but seldom provoke nausea or vomiting. Barium sulfate administered by either oral or rectal route sometimes causes mild constipation for a day or two after the examination.

Barium Swallow

A barium swallow may be performed to evaluate gastrointestinal bleeding, pain or difficulty in swallowing, chest pain thought to be of esophageal origin, or as an adjunct to other diagnostic studies in disorders of the chest. The fasting patient, standing or seated, drinks a sufficient volume of barium solution to fill and outline the esophagus while the radiologist observes its passage fluoroscopically, taking spot films as appropriate. A contrast film of the esophagus may be called an *esophagram*, a word formed by abridgment of the older term *esophagogram*. (Avoid the incorrect spelling *esophogram*.)

Abnormalities that may be detected on barium swallow include ulcerations or strictures of the esophagus, perforation (evidenced by leakage of barium outside the lumen), esophageal varices (dilated veins due to obstruction of the hepatic portal circulation), tumors, foreign bodies, hiatal hernia (passage of part or all of the stomach into the thorax through an abnormally dilated opening in the diaphragm), and disorders of esophageal motility. Tumors and other abnormalities outside the esophagus may divert or distort the column of barium. After all of the barium has passed into the stomach, gastroesophageal reflux (backflow of stomach contents into the lower esophagus) may be demonstrated if the examiner applies pressure to the upper abdomen of the recumbent patient.

Upper GI (Gastrointestinal) Series, Small Bowel Study

When the diagnostic focus is not limited to the esophagus, the barium swallow examination is followed by observation of the passage of contrast medium into the stomach and duodenum, generally with the patient supine (lying face up) on the x-ray table. Barium examination of the stomach can show gastritis (inflammation of the gastric mucosa), gastric ulcer, and cancer of the stomach. Generally sufficient barium passes through the pylorus (the valvelike opening from the stomach into the small intestine) to permit visualization of the duodenum (first part of the small intestine) during the same session as the barium swallow. Examination of the duodenum may show an ulcer or obstruction (usually due to scarring from an old ulcer). Delay in appearance of barium in the duodenum indicates an abnormally prolonged gastric emptying time

Passage of barium through the small intestine normally takes 2-4 hours or longer. For a full upper GI examination with small-bowel follow-through, further fluoroscopic assessment and spot films are performed at intervals, ideally until some barium appears in the cecum (first part of the colon). Contrast studies of the small intestine may show evidence of abnormal intestinal transit time, a benign or malignant tumor, inflammatory bowel disease (Crohn disease), or bowel obstruction due to postoperative adhesions, volvulus (twisting of the bowel around itself), intussusception (slipping of a segment of intestine into the segment distal to it), or other causes.

Barium Enema

The standard radiographic examination of the large intestine involves introduction of barium solution into the rectum by means of an enema tube. In preparation for this examination, the colon must be emptied of stool by the use of laxatives, rectal suppositories, cleansing enemas, or some combination of these.

Indications for barium enema include unexplained lower abdominal pain, significant change in bowel habits, hematochezia (gross blood in stools), positive stool examination for occult blood, unexplained anemia or weight loss, and personal or family history of colonic polyps or cancer. The examination is contraindicated in acute abdominal pain or rectal bleeding of unknown origin, because in certain disorders distention of the colon with barium or injected air may rupture it. Recent bowel surgery and pregnancy are also relative contraindications. If an upper GI study has recently been performed, examination of the colon is postponed until barium remaining from the earlier examination has passed out of the body.

During the examination the radiologist instructs the patient to move from side to side on the x-ray table and applies pressure to the abdomen in order to fill all parts of the colon with barium. The procedure is not considered complete until some barium is seen in the distal ileum (the part of the small intestine that empties into the colon), indicating that the entire colon has been visualized. Failure of barium to fill the appendix may indicate either that the appendix is acutely inflamed or that it has been surgically removed. Barium enema examination can identify obstruction, diverticulosis (formation of outpouchings of the bowel wall, common with advancing age), benign or malignant tumors, or inflammatory bowel disease (ulcerative colitis). Findings must be coordinated with results of other studies, including endoscopy.

Cholangiography

One of the many biochemical functions of the liver is the production of bile, an excretory and digestive fluid containing bilirubin (a breakdown product of hemoglobin) and bile salts (chemical agents that aid in the digestion and absorption of fats in the small intestine). The biliary tract consists of the hepatic ducts, which collect newly formed bile from the liver tissue; the common bile duct, formed by the joining of the hepatic ducts, which carries bile to the duodenum; and the gallbladder, a pouch adjacent to the common bile duct in which bile is stored until needed.

Cholecystitis (inflammation of the gallbladder) and cholelithiasis (formation of gallstones) are relatively common disorders that often occur together. Plain radiography can show gallstones that contain calcium salts (not all of them do), but it cannot clearly indicate their position in the biliary tract. The tract itself cannot be seen in a plain x-ray study unless it contains air or gas.

Cholangiography is a radiographic study of the biliary tract with contrast material to identify the presence of inflammation, obstruction, stones, or other abnormality. In oral cholangiography, a contrast medium is administered orally. After this material is absorbed into the blood stream, the liver concentrates it and excretes it in the bile, so that it outlines the biliary ducts and gallbladder. This technique involves a delay of 12-15 hours between administration of contrast medium and its appearance in the gallbladder. Moreover, even a perfectly normal gallbladder often fails to visualize if liver function is abnormal or if absorption of the contrast medium is inadequate. Contrast medium that has been administered intravenously appears much more rapidly in the biliary tract, but reactions to injected medium are frequent. For these reasons, and because an ultrasound examination yields superior definition of the biliary tract and gallstones, oral and intravenous cholangiography have largely been abandoned.

However, cholangiographic methods in which contrast medium is injected directly into the biliary tract are of value in certain settings. Percutaneous cholangiography (introduction of contrast medium by means of a catheter placed through a skin puncture and threaded into the biliary tract under fluoroscopic control) can often provide a rapid diagnosis in acute biliary tract obstruction. In T-tube cholangiography, contrast medium is injected into the biliary tract through a T-tube, a temporary drain placed in the biliary tract after cholecystectomy (surgical removal of the gallbladder). The usual indication for this procedure is concern that some stones may remain in the biliary tract after surgery.

Imaging of the biliary tract after intravenous administration of a radionuclide (HIDA scan, discussed in Chapter 15) may be preferred to any of these contrast x-ray procedures. Cholecystokinin (CCK), a natural polypeptide hormone produced by the small intestinal mucosa, exerts various effects on the motility of the upper gastrointestinal tract and on its supply of digestive juices. Administered intravenously during the course of imaging studies of the biliary tract, it stimulates contraction of the gallbladder and increases bile flow as well as secretion of pancreatic and intestinal digestive juices.

Endoscopic Retrograde Cholangiopancreatography (ERCP)

This procedure, as its name indicates, is a radiographic study of the biliary and pancreatic ductal systems that involves injection of contrast medium in a retrograde direction (that is, against the normal flow of bile and pancreatic juice) by means of an endoscope passed through the mouth, esophagus, and stomach into the duodenum. The examination is performed in conjunction with other diagnostic methods (CT, ultrasound, nuclear scans) to identify stones, tumors, cysts, and other abnormalities causing obstruction to the outflow of bile or pancreatic juice.

Radiographic Studies of the Genitourinary System

Intravenous Pyelography (IVP)

The delineation of the urinary tract (renal pelves, ureters, bladder, and urethra) by means of a contrast agent can provide crucial information in cases of urinary obstruction, bleeding from the urinary tract, or abdominal trauma, and can identify and localize renal calculi as well as tumors or cysts both within the urinary tract and closely adjacent to it.

For this study a contrast agent is injected intravenously after performance of a scout film. Normally functioning kidneys extract this agent from the blood stream and excrete it into the urine, so that it outlines the entire urinary tract. Exposures of the lower abdomen and pelvis are made at standard intervals after administration of contrast medium. When the basic series has been completed, the patient is asked to void and another film is taken to assess residual urine in the bladder.

If the patient is slightly dehydrated for this study, the concentration of contrast medium will be higher and visualization of the urinary tract correspondingly sharper. Ideally the colon is emptied before the study. An interval of 2-3 days must elapse after a barium enema before this test is done, to allow contrast medium to be cleared from the bowel.

Retrograde Pyelography

In this procedure the upper urinary tract is visualized with contrast medium that has been injected directly into it, one ureter at a time, from below. With a cystoscope (see Chapter 8), a ureteral catheter is threaded under direct vision into the opening between one ureter and the bladder. An iodine-containing contrast medium is then injected in retrograde fashion (in the direction opposite that of the normal downward flow of urine through the ureter) under fluoroscopic monitoring and spot x-ray films are made.

Indications for retrograde pyelography include inconclusive findings on IVP and as an adjunct to cystoscopy in the evaluation of hematuria or in investigations for possible malignancy of the urinary tract. This procedure has the advantage that contrast medium appears immediately in full concentration in the ureter under examination, regardless of impairment in renal function. However, unlike an IVP this examination must usually be done under spinal or general anesthesia and requires placement of catheters by a urologist.

Voiding Cystourethrogram (VCUG)

This examination is performed in order to assess the anatomy of the bladder and urethra and, in particular, the function of the bladder during voiding. A contrast medium is instilled into the bladder by means of a urethral catheter. Spot films are recorded in various projections while the bladder is distended with medium. The catheter is then removed and further films are taken as the subject voids (empties the bladder). This procedure is used to diagnose structural disorders such as urethral stricture or obstruction due to prostatic disease, diverticula or neoplasms of the bladder, or disturbances in bladder function including irritable or neurogenic bladder and vesicoureteral reflux (backward leakage of urine into one or both distal ureters occurring with voiding, a predisposing factor for urinary tract infection).

In a variant of this procedure, the stress cystogram, the patient is not instructed to void while imaging studies are performed. Instead, the patient coughs, strains, or bears down as for a bowel movement, while trying to hold back the flow of urine. This test is done to detect stress incontinence (involuntary leakage of urine with increase of pressure in the abdominopelvic cavity, as from coughing or laughing) and to assess its severity.

Hysterosalpingography

This is a radiographic examination of the uterine cavity and uterine tubes by means of a contrast medium injected through the cervix. The principal indications for this procedure are infertility and habitual abortion (repeated miscarriage), but it may also be used to diagnose tumors and other disorders of the female genital tract.

A water-soluble iodine-containing contrast medium is injected through a catheter or cannula placed in the uterine cervix under direct vision through a vaginal speculum. A balloon-tipped injection catheter is usually used to prevent leakage of medium from the cervix during the injection. Filling of the uterine cavity and uterine tubes is monitored fluoroscopically and spot films are taken. The position of the patient on the x-ray table may need to be shifted in order to obtain adequate visualization of both tubes.

The procedure is not performed during pregnancy or menstruation. It is moderately painful but anesthesia is usually not required. Occasionally the injection of contrast medium under pressure corrects infertility by dilating a narrowed uterine tube without the need for other intervention.

Angiography

Angiography is the radiographic study of blood vessels (less often, lymph vessels) into which a radiopaque medium has been injected. Less than five years after the discovery of x-rays, anatomists made angiograms by injecting metallic mercury or solutions of lead or bismuth salts into the blood vessels of cadavers. Such substances were far too toxic to be used in living patients, and it was not until the 1920s that solutions of iodide salts came into use as contrast media in angiography. All media used for such studies today are iodide solutions.

Although these media are relatively safe, they can have unpleasant and even dangerous side-effects. The injection of iodide solution causes a local sensation of burning or flushing and often dizziness or nausea. In some patients, particularly those with pre-existing renal disease, dehydration, or congestive heart failure, iodide contrast media can cause transitory or permanent kidney damage.

Angiographic examinations are therefore contraindicated in patients with these conditions. Earlier iodide solutions used in angiography were ionic. Since about 1970, nonionic solutions have been available. Because these can be used at lower concentrations, they cause less discomfort and are theoretically less likely to impair renal function, but they are also much more expensive.

The principal reason for performing an angiographic examination is to detect malformation, narrowing (stenosis), blockage (occlusion), or injury of a blood vessel. In addition, angiography often enhances the diagnostic value of plain radiography by showing displacement of blood vessels or other changes of vascular pattern due to tumors, swelling, hemorrhage, or trauma. The injection of contrast medium may be made with the catheter so placed that an entire arterial system (for example, both renal arteries) is visualized (flush method), or the tip of the catheter may be directed into a specific vessel or branch for a more selective examination.

Angiography differs from most other contrast studies in two important respects: the structures that are to be outlined (blood vessels) are already full of fluid, and that fluid is in motion. Because injected contrast medium immediately becomes diluted by the blood, it must be highly concentrated in order to retain its potency as an opacifying agent. And because the medium is immediately swept along through the vessels by the flow of blood, an x-ray exposure must be made at the same instant as the injection.

In the early days of angiography, elaborate devices were employed to make a series of film exposures in rapid sequence so as to trace the flow of contrast medium through the vessels under study. Although rapid-sequence spot films may still be made in the course of an angiographic examination, the entire study is now also recorded videographically on tape. For ease of viewing and interpretation, angiographic images can be electronically enlarged to 2-3 times actual size without loss of fidelity.

In the angiography of some structures (brain, kidney) the passage of contrast medium can be observed and recorded radiographically not only through the arteries but also through the capillaries and the veins. In the capillary phase of such an angiogram, the entire organ appears diffusely opacified for a few seconds as the contrast medium filters through thousands of microscopic capillaries. Structural abnormalities such as cysts, solid tumors, or areas of hemorrhage or infarction may be particularly evident in such views. The venous phase of a cerebral or renal arteriogram is, in essence, a venogram (phlebogram), providing information about the structure and integrity of the venous drainage of the organ.

In some angiographic examinations, particularly those of the central nervous system and the abdominal aorta, two images at right angles to each other (an AP and a lateral view) may be obtained and recorded in rapid sequence during a single injection of medium. This biplane imaging lends a three-dimensional element to the interpretation of the study.

It is standard practice to expose and develop a plain film (scout film) of the area under study before performing angiography. The scout film gives basic structural information, confirms that the patient and the x-ray equipment are properly positioned for the desired examination, and may alert the radiologist or the technician to potential problems.

Angiographic images are viewed and recorded against a nonuniform background of bone and soft tissue that often obscures vascular details. In the 1960s an ingenious technique was introduced to "subtract" this unwanted background. This required making a positive "print" of the scout film with white light on a second piece of film, so that the densities of the first film were exactly reversed, white becoming black and black becoming white. This second film, when superimposed on an angiographic image (made after injection of contrast medium), served to mask everything that appeared in the scout film and to show only what was dif-ferent about the angiographic image—namely, the vessels as outlined by injected medium.

Nowadays masking is done by a computer in a technique known as digital subtraction angiography (DSA). The computer carries out this function so rapidly that the radiologist performing the examination sees the masked or subtracted version of the image in real time (that is, virtually at the time the medium is injected). DSA is particularly valuable in angiographic studies of the central nervous system.

Rapid injection of a small volume of carbon dioxide gas can be used in conjunction with digital subtraction angiography, particularly in persons who are allergic to iodinated media or who have impaired renal function. The injected gas acts as a negative contrast medium, allowing passage of more radiation through vessels filled with it. Carbon dioxide dissolves quickly in the blood and is then excreted by the lungs. Because of possible toxic effects on nerve tissue, this technique is not used in cerebral angiography.

The purposes for which angiographic studies are performed vary with the part of the circulatory system examined. Arteriography, which records the flow of contrast medium through some part of the arterial system, is by far the most important and widely used form of angiography. A major application of arteriography is in the evaluation of the chambers and valves of the heart, the coronary arteries, and the aorta and pulmonary arterial circulation. Arteriography is also extensively used to assess the circulation of the brain, the abdominal viscera, and the extremities. Venography (phlebography), the angiographic study of veins, and lymphography (lymphangiography), the study of lymphatic vessels, are less widely used but can yield information of crucial importance in certain settings.

Most angiographic procedures are "invasive," requiring injection of contrast medium through a flexible catheter of the appropriate caliber and shape that has been introduced into the circulatory system from outside the body. For some angiographic procedures, such as retinal angiography, contrast medium is injected intravenously. CT and MR angiography, which do not require catheter injection of contrast medium, are discussed in Chapters 12 and 14 respectively.

An angiographic catheter may be inserted into a peripheral vessel through a surgical incision, but more often it is introduced through a cannula or large-bore needle placed in the vessel via a skin puncture. For studies of the left ventricle, coronary arteries, aorta, and other centrally located arteries, the catheter is inserted through a peripheral artery and threaded "upstream" (against the flow of blood) under fluoroscopic monitoring. The vessel most often used for access to the central circulation is the right or left femoral artery, entered at the groin. Alternatively a brachial artery may be approached through the axilla. In translumbar aortography the catheter is placed in the abdominal aorta through a cutaneous puncture in the back. Before placement of the catheter the access site is scrubbed with surgical soap and a local anesthetic is injected. For some procedures, especially cerebral angiography, general anesthesia may be preferable.

Catheters are made of synthetic materials such as polyethylene and Teflon, and vary widely in caliber, length, shape, and in the number and placement of holes from which contrast medium is expelled. To improve rigidity and facilitate manipulation, a guidewire is placed inside the catheter. When it is necessary to change from one catheter to another during the course of a procedure such as coronary arteriography, a guidewire remains in place in the vessel while the first catheter is withdrawn and the second is threaded on it. Further information about vascular catheters is provided in Chapter 4.

Once the catheter has been placed, its outer end is attached to an apparatus for injecting contrast medium. The medium may be injected by a hand-actuated syringe, by a programmed power injector, or by intravenous drip, depending on the procedure. A second syringe or reservoir of saline solution is provided to flush the medium from the catheter between examinations. Both syringes, and sometimes also a manometer to measure pressure within the vessel, are attached to the catheter by means of a manifold or system of stopcocks. Injury to blood vessels by catheters, guidewires, and cannulas leads to the release of tissue factors that can cause thrombosis (clot formation) within the circulation. In order to prevent clotting, the saline solution contains the anticoagulant heparin.

Cerebral Angiography

Contrast examination of cerebral arteries is performed to identify and localize obstruction to blood flow and also to detect vascular anomalies such as aneurysm (abnormal local dilatation of an artery) and arteriovenous malformations. Because displacement of normal vascular patterns can indicate an intracranial tumor or a hematoma (local accumulation of blood due to hemorrhage) or other consequence of head trauma, cerebral angiography is often used in cases of head injury or as an adjunct to other studies in patients with unexplained severe headache, seizures, or other clues to the possible presence of a tumor. In addition, cerebral angiography is performed to provide vascular mapping before certain types of surgery, and it may also be done postoperatively to assess beneficial results of surgery or to look for complications.

Disorders of the blood supply of the brain are an important cause of disease and death. A stroke, also called a cerebral vascular accident (CVA) or brain attack, is any acute neurologic disorder resulting from impairment of cerebral blood supply and lasting for more than 24 hours. The type and severity of symptoms depend on the part of the brain affected and the extent of vascular compromise. The consequences of a stroke can vary from barely detectable neurologic impairment to rapid onset of coma followed by death. About 600,000 Americans experience strokes each year, and about 25% of these are fatal. Stroke ranks third as a cause of death in adults, following coronary artery disease and cancer.

The risk of stroke is greater in persons with hypertension, valvular heart disease, atrial fibrillation, elevated cholesterol, or diabetes mellitus and in cigarette smokers and persons who have had previous evidence of cerebral vascular disease or a family history of stroke. Most strokes are due to blockage of a major cerebral artery by thrombosis (less commonly, hemorrhage) at the site of atheromatous disease (inflammation and degeneration of the vessel wall, with deposits of cholesterol and often calcium). Another important cause is embolism—vascular obstruction by a clot that has become dislodged from its site of origin, usually the left atrium in a patient with atrial fibrillation, and has been carried by the blood stream until it reaches a vessel too small for it to pass through.

The treatment of stroke includes prompt intravenous administration of a thrombolytic agent—a drug that dissolves an obstructing clot. However, thrombolytic therapy is contraindicated when the stroke is due to hemorrhage rather than thrombosis, because hemorrhage may be worsened by this treatment. Cerebral angiography may therefore be used to rule out hemorrhage before administration of a thrombolytic agent. However, CT or MRI is often preferred to this more invasive procedure.

Four vessels arising from branches of the aortic arch provide most of the blood supply of the brain (see Fig.11.1). These are the right and left internal carotid arteries and the right and left vertebral arteries. The internal carotid arteries (branches of the common carotid arteries) pass upward from the thorax under cover of the muscles at the sides of the neck to enter the skull through the carotid foramina, each then dividing into an anterior and a middle cerebral artery. The vertebral arteries (branches of the subclavian arteries) pass upward alongside the cervical vertebrae to enter the skull through the foramen magnum along with the spinal cord. Here the vertebral arteries fuse to form the basilar artery, which passes forward beneath

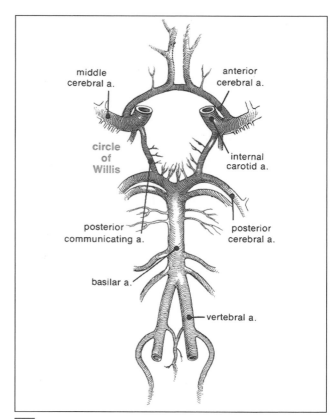

Fig. 11.1. Cerebral circulation

Reproduced with permission from *Melloni's Illustrated Medical Dictionary*, 4th ed. (2002)

the brain stem and redivides to form the right and left posterior cerebral arteries.

The terminal branches of these four vessels (the right and left anterior cerebral, the right and left middle cerebral, and the right and left posterior cerebral arteries) provide the principal blood supply to all parts of the brain. In addition, they all participate in the formation of the circle of Willis, an arterial ring lying beneath the brain and serving to maintain even flow.

Both anteroposterior and lateral projections are routinely made during cerebral angiography. A four-vessel study is an angiogram performed with the catheter in the aortic arch. Catheter access may be gained through a femoral or brachial artery. Manipulation of the catheter permits selective examination of individual arteries or their branches. Alternatively, contrast medium may be injected through a needle puncture of a common carotid artery. For bilateral examination this requires two punctures, and leaves the vertebrobasilar system unexamined. Carotid puncture is usually done under general anesthesia to minimize patient distress and to make it easier to keep the patient immobile during the examination.

Coronary Angiography

Heart attack (myocardial infarction) is the number one cause of death in both men and women in the United States. By far the majority of all heart attacks are caused by thrombosis (clot formation) in one or more coronary arteries affected by atherosclerosis.

Coronary angiography is currently the most precise diagnostic procedure available to confirm and localize narrowing of coronary arteries by disease and to estimate the extent to which blood flow is compromised. This examination is performed routinely in the assessment of patients with known or suspected coronary artery disease.

Modern techniques of coronary angiography have developed in parallel with the field of cardiac catheterization (discussed in Chapter 4), and both types of procedure are often performed during the same diagnostic session. Moreover, therapeutic procedures pertaining to interventional cardiology (percutaneous transluminal angioplasty, stent placement) may be undertaken immediately after angiography if one or more sites of significant vascular narrowing are identified. Continuous electrocardiographic monitoring of the patient is standard during coronary angiography.

The right and left coronary arteries, which supply blood to the myocardium (heart muscle), are the first branches of the aorta, arising immediately distal to the aortic valve (*see figure*). The right coronary artery (RCA) descends along the right side of the heart, dividing into a posterior descending and a marginal branch to supply the right atrium and right ventricle. The left coronary artery (LCA) divides in two just beyond its origin. The (left) anterior descending (LAD) branch passes downward along the sulcus or groove on the

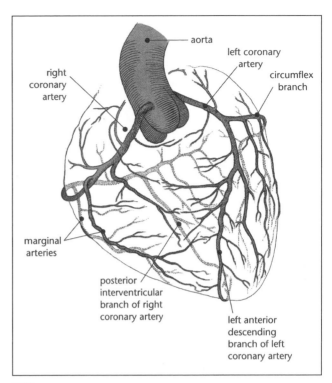

Fig. 11.2. Coronary circulation

Reproduced with permission from *Melloni's Illustrated Medical Dictionary*, 4th ed. (2002)

surface of the heart that corresponds to the anterior margin of the interventricular septum, and the circumflex branch winds posteriorly around the left side of the heart. These branches of the LCA supply the left atrium, the left ventricle, and most of the interventricular septum. The coronary arteries vary considerably in their branching patterns.

In coronary angiography, a catheter is introduced into a peripheral artery and advanced toward the heart under fluoroscopic guidance. The tip of the catheter is then manipulated into the origin of one of the two coronary arteries and contrast medium is injected. The positioning of the patient and of the radiographic equipment is arranged to provide optimum visibility of the vessels under study, and may be changed several times during the course of an examination. In about one-third of patients with coronary artery disease, angiography demonstrates significant stenosis in only a single vessel, most often the (left) anterior descending (LAD) artery.

Pulmonary Angiography

The principal reason for performing angiography of the pulmonary artery and its branches is to detect or confirm acute pulmonary embolism. A clot (thrombus) that has formed in a systemic vein and broken loose from its site of origin is called an embolus. Carried by the flow of blood to the vena cava and through the right atrium and right ventricle into the pulmonary artery, it can cause acute pulmonary hypertension followed by circulatory collapse and death.

The diagnosis of acute pulmonary embolism can generally be made with considerable probability by diagnostic measures other than pulmonary angiography. In certain cases, however, angiography may be required to confirm the diagnosis, to locate the embolus, or to assess the extent of vascular obstruction. This procedure can also be used to detect vascular abnormalities (congenital anomalies, aneurysm) and to enhance the sensitivity of chest radiography in evaluating tumors, emphysema, and other structural disorders that do not directly affect the blood vessels.

In order to visualize the pulmonary arterial circulation, contrast medium must be injected into the pulmonary artery by means of a catheter inserted in a peripheral vein and threaded "downstream" (in the same direction as normal venous blood flow) through the right atrium and right ventricle. Access via a femoral vein may be a poor choice in a patient with suspected or known thrombophlebitis in a lower extremity. In such cases a brachial vein or internal jugular vein approach may be preferred.

Aortography and Abdominal Visceral Angiography (Liver, Spleen, Pancreas)

Contrast imaging of the thoracic and abdominal aorta, with medium injected via a catheter introduced through a femoral or brachial artery, is indicated when other studies fail to provide adequate information about atherosclerotic lesions, aneurysms, or aortic dissection. By advancing the catheter under fluoroscopic monitoring, the radiologist can perform selective angiography of the liver, spleen, pancreas, or kidneys when indicated.

Indications for angiographic examination of the **liver** include investigations for cirrhosis, primary and metastatic tumors, and vascular anomalies. The liver has a dual blood supply consisting of the hepatic artery (derived from the celiac trunk, a major branch of the abdominal aorta) and the portal vein (which drains the spleen and digestive organs and delivers nutrients and other substances absorbed from the digestive tract to the liver for processing). In cirrhosis, obstruction to the flow of blood through the liver may cause portal hypertension, with severe disturbances of hepatic circulation. Angiographic examination of the portal vein can be performed by percutaneous catheterization of the vein.

Angiography of the **spleen** is used in the diagnosis of aneurysm of the splenic artery and acute or delayed hemorrhage after blunt abdominal trauma. Contrast study of the pancreatic circulation is seldom indicated, because other studies (CT and ultrasound) usually provide adequate information.

Renal Angiography

The renal arteries, which supply the kidneys, are the last major branches given off by the aorta before it divides to form the common iliac arteries. Examination of these vessels with contrast medium may be performed to identify renal artery stenosis (an important cause of secondary hypertension), thrombosis or embolism of a renal artery, or structural abnormality within a kidney due to congenital anomaly, trauma, or tumor. Renal angiography is also a standard part of the evaluation of a donor kidney for renal transplant.

For a general assessment of the renal vessels bilaterally, contrast medium is injected with a catheter whose tip lies in the abdominal aorta proximal to the origins of the renal arteries. A more selective examination can be performed by directing the catheter into the right or left renal artery. The capillary phase of renal angiography, sometimes called a nephrogram, is particularly valuable in detecting abnormalities in renal anatomy due to tumors, cysts, or infarction.

Peripheral Angiography

Radiographic examination of the arteries of the extremities with contrast medium is performed to identify and localize vascular obstruction due to atherosclerosis, malformations or aneurysms, the effects of trauma, and neoplasms. The site chosen for vascular access depends on the location of abnormal findings, known or presumed, and sometimes on the presence of concomitant disease.

A vasodilator (drug that dilates blood vessels) may be administered before the injection of contrast medium to enhance blood flow. For examinations of the lower extremity, exposures may be made on several pieces of film in a stepped sequence to follow the flow of contrast medium through the arteries from above downward.

Venography (Phlebography)

The principal reason for examining peripheral veins with contrast medium is to diagnose deep vein thrombosis (DVT; clotting of blood in deep veins of the pelvis or lower extremity, most often in the calf). The importance of this condition is that it poses a high risk of pulmonary embolism, in which clots become detached and travel through the right atrium and right ventricle to obstruct branches of the pulmonary artery. DVT may be accompanied by local pain and inflammation or may be "silent." The risk of this disorder is increased by sudden immobilization (as after surgery or severe injury), obesity, pregnancy, cigarette smoking, long-term use of oral contraceptives or estrogen replacement therapy, and certain coagulation disorders.

Before the performance of venography in the lower limb, tourniquets are applied just above the knee and just above the ankle to collapse the superficial veins, which are not involved in DVT. Because venography is an invasive procedure which may aggravate existing inflammation or thrombosis, other diagnostic measures such as Doppler ultrasonography and MRI may be preferred.

Lymphangiography

This is a radiographic examination of lymphatic channels, performed for the diagnosis of lymphomas (malignant tumors of lymphoid tissue) or of malignancies that have metastasized to lymph nodes. The procedure may also be used to help explain swelling of an extremity due to blockage of lymph channels (lymphedema).

Methylene blue, a nontoxic dye, is first injected subcutaneously between the fingers or toes of the limb under study. Over a period of several hours the lymphatic channels pick up the dye. Through a small skin incision, the examiner then inserts a fine-gauge needle into one of the channels outlined by dye. A suspension of radiopaque material in oil is pumped into the lymphatic circulation under pressure during a period of 1-2 hours. The flow of the medium is followed fluoroscopically and recorded in spot films.

Arthrography

Plain radiographic studies of the extremities are of limited usefulness in the examination of joints. Bones show clearly, cartilage almost as clearly, but soft tissues (ligaments and joint capsules, synovial membranes) are not well represented, nor are accumulations of fluid, blood, or pus within a joint space.

Arthrography is the radiographic examination of a joint into which a contrast medium has been injected. Indications for this procedure are unexplained pain, swelling, or dysfunction of a joint and investigation of complications following joint surgery. The joints most frequently examined by this technique are the temporomandibular (TMJ), shoulder, wrist, hip, knee, and ankle.

After administration of a local anesthetic, a needle is introduced into the joint space. Any fluid present is aspirated and preserved for laboratory study. Under fluoroscopic monitoring to assure that the needle is correctly placed, contrast material, air, or both are injected into the joint and spot films are taken in various projections. The examination is contraindicated in the presence of known or suspected infection within the joint.

Other Contrast Studies

Sialography or ptyalography (contrast study of a parotid gland duct) is performed to diagnose obstruction of the duct by calculus or tumor. If a scout film shows a calculus in the duct, the contrast study may be postponed or canceled. After injection of medium into the duct with a cannula inserted through the mouth, films are taken in various projections. The patient may be given lemon juice to stimulate salivary flow.

Dacryocystography is a contrast examination of the nasolacrimal duct, the passage that normally conducts tears from the eye to the nasal cavity. Contrast medium is injected into the lacrimal punctum (the opening of the duct near the inner canthus). The principal indication is epiphora (persistent overflow of tears due to obstruction of a nasolacrimal duct). CT is more often used than conventional radiography with this contrast procedure.

Galactography (ductogalactography), radiographic visualization of mammary gland ducts by means of contrast medium, may be performed in order to assess bleeding or discharge from a nipple or as an adjunct to mammography.

In **fistulography** (sinography), iodinated contrast medium is injected to permit radiographic mapping of a fistula or sinus tract. A fistula is an abnormal communication between one hollow organ or cavity and another, or between it and the skin. A sinus tract is an abnormal passage opening on the skin surface but ending blindly. Contrast studies help to determine the course and extent of fistulas and sinus tracts and to plan surgical excision. (Note: The term *fistulogram* is also used to refer to the radiographic examination, with injected contrast material, of an arteriovenous fistula such as is created for renal dialysis.)

Contrast Media

acetrizoate (Diaginol, Urokon)
diatrizoate (Angiografin, Hypaque, Renografin, Urografin, Urovison)
ethiodized oil (Ethiodol)
iodamide (Uromiro)
iodixanol (Visipaque)
iodized oil (Lipiodol Ultra Fluid)
iodophenylundecylic acid (iophendylate) (Pantopaque, Myodil).
ioglicate (Rayvist)
iohexol (Omnipaque)
iopamidol (Iopamiro, Isovue, Niopam, Solutrast)
iopentol (Imagopaque)
iopromide (Ultravist)
iothalamate (Conray)
iotrolan (Isovist)
ioversol (Optiray)
ioxaglate (Hexabrix)
ioxithalamate (Telebrix)
metrizamide (Amipaque)
metrizoate (Isopaque, Triosil)
propyliodone (Dionosil)

Exercises

Fill in the Blank

1. X-ray images of soft-tissue structures typically lack sufficient detail for diagnostic purposes because _____ _____.

2. A _____ is a liquid or semisolid material, containing either a metallic salt or an iodide, that appears with metal density in a radiographic image.

3. A _____ is a radiographic examination of the spinal cord after injection of a contrast agent into the subarachnoid space.

4. Spiky outgrowths of bone sometimes seen on a myelogram are called _____.

5. Narrowing of the spinal canal is known as _____.

6. _____ is a common sequela of myelography.

7. Only when _____ outlines or distends a part of the gastrointestinal tract can it be distinguished from surrounding tissues.

8. _____ is the contrast medium of choice for x-rays of the gastrointestinal system.

9. _____ in GI studies are areas where the barium fails to fill out the expected contour of the organ because of the presence of a tumor.

10. _____ are breaks or erosions in the integrity of the mucosal lining of the GI tract.

11. Narrowing of the lumen of the GI tract due to scarring is called a _____.

12. Distortion or displacement of the outline of gastrointestinal structures may be due to external factors such as _____, _____, or _____ outside the digestive tract.

13. Undue rapidity or slowness of peristaltic movement of barium through the tract are disturbances in gastrointestinal _____.

14. Air or gas is introduced into the digestive tract to distend its walls after most of the barium has passed through or, in the case of a barium enema, has been expelled from the colon in an x-ray procedure called an _____ or _____ examination.

15. A barium swallow may also be called an _____.

Exercises

16. Evidence of leakage of barium outside the esophageal lumen is an indication of _____.

17. Dilated veins due to obstruction of the hepatic portal circulation are _____.

18. Passage of part or all of the stomach into the thorax through an abnormally dilated opening in the diaphragm may be an indication of _____.

19. Backflow of stomach contents into the lower esophagus is evidence of _____.

20. An upper GI series generally refers to a contrast x-ray examination of the _____.

21. A small bowel study is a contrast examination of the _____.

22. The _____ is the valvelike opening from the stomach into the small intestine.

23. _____ is twisting of the bowel around itself.

24. Slipping of a segment of intestine into the segment distal to it is _____.

25. The medical term for gross blood in stools is _____.

26. Barium enema is contraindicated in acute abdominal pain or rectal bleeding of unknown origin because in certain disorders _____.

27. _____ is a condition characterized by the formation of outpouchings of the bowel wall, common with advancing age.

28. Inflammatory bowel disease includes _____ and _____.

29. _____ is a radiographic study of the biliary tract with contrast material to identify the presence of inflammation, obstruction, stones, or other abnormality.

30. _____ is performed by the introduction of contrast medium by means of a catheter placed through a skin puncture and threaded into the biliary tract under fluoroscopic control.

31. _____, administered intravenously during the course of imaging studies of the biliary tract, stimulates contraction of the gallbladder and increases bile flow as well as secretion of pancreatic and intestinal digestive juices.

32. _____ is backward leakage of urine into one or both distal ureters occurring with voiding, a predisposing factor for urinary tract infection.

Exercises

33. _____ is involuntary leakage of urine with increase of pressure in the abdominopelvic cavity, as from coughing or laughing.

34. _____ is radiographic examination of the uterine cavity and uterine tubes by means of a contrast medium injected through the cervix.

35. _____ is the radiographic study of blood vessels (less often, lymph vessels) into which a radiopaque medium has been injected.

36. The vessel most often used for access to the central circulation is the _____, entered at the groin.

37. When it is necessary to change from one catheter to another during the course of a procedure such as coronary arteriography, a _____ remains in place in the vessel while the first catheter is withdrawn and the second is threaded on it.

38. _____ is inflammation and degeneration of the vessel wall, with deposits of cholesterol and often calcium.

39. In about one-third of patients with coronary artery disease, angiography demonstrates significant stenosis in only a single vessel, most often the _____ artery.

40. _____ is clotting of blood in deep veins of the pelvis or lower extremity, most often in the calf.

41. The angiographic procedure used to diagnose DVT is known as _____ or _____.

42. _____ or _____ (contrast study of a parotid gland duct) is performed to diagnose obstruction of the duct by calculus or tumor.

43. _____ is a contrast examination of the nasolacrimal duct, the passage that normally conducts tears from the eye to the nasal cavity.

44. _____ is the radiographic visualization of mammary gland ducts by means of contrast medium.

45. In _____, iodinated contrast medium is injected to permit radiographic mapping of a fistula or sinus tract.

Exercises

Multiple Choice: Circle the letter of the best answer from the choices given.

1. Structures which typically lack sufficient detail on plain x-rays for diagnostic purposes include all the following except
   A. Brain and spinal cord.
   B. Circulatory.
   C. Vertebrae.
   D. Digestive.
   E. Genitourinary system.

2. The limitations of plain x-rays in diagnosing soft tissue structures is overcome with the use of
   A. Arthroscopy.
   B. PA and lateral views.
   C. Oblique views.
   D. Contrast media.
   E. Tangential views.

3. A procedure usually performed to identify abnormalities of the spinal cord and its nerve roots, particularly compression by a herniated disk, a tumor, arthritic osteophytes, or spinal stenosis is
   A. A bronchogram.
   B. A myelogram.
   C. An encephalogram.
   D. A ventriculogram.
   E. A pneumoencephalogram.

4. On a study of the GI tract, contrast medium is distributed throughout the area being studied by
   A. Tilting the table the patient is lying on.
   B. Having the patient roll from side to side.
   C. Instilling the contrast medium under pressure.
   D. Having the patient walk around the examining room.
   E. None of the above.

5. Abnormalities that may be detected on barium swallow include all of the following except
   A. Ulcerations, strictures, or perforations of the esophagus.
   B. Disorders of esophageal motility.
   C. Esophageal varices.
   D. Gastroesophageal reflux.
   E. Gastritis.

Exercises

6. After all of the barium has passed into the stomach, the examiner may apply pressure to the upper abdomen of the recumbent patient in an effort to demonstrate
    A. Gastroesophageal reflux.
    B. Esophageal varices.
    C. Hiatal hernia.
    D. Perforation of the lumen.
    E. Ulceration of the lumen.

7. Delay in appearance of barium in the duodenum indicates
    A. The presence of a hiatal hernia.
    B. Perforation of the lining of the stomach.
    C. Gastroesophageal reflux.
    D. An abnormally prolonged gastric emptying time.
    E. Inflammation of the gastric mucosa.

8. Fluoroscopic assessment and spot films performed at intervals, ideally until some barium appears in the cecum is necessary in order to perform
    A. A full colonoscopic examination.
    B. A full upper GI examination with small-bowel follow-through.
    C. An air contrast upper GI study.
    D. A double contrast barium enema.
    E. A gastric emptying study.

9. A barium enema may be contraindicated or delayed in all of the following cases except
    A. Acute abdominal pain.
    B. Recent bowel surgery.
    C. Pregnancy.
    D. Recent upper GI study.
    E. Gross blood in the stools.

10. A barium enema is not considered complete until
    A. Barium passes through the pylorus.
    B. Barium is seen in the distal ileum.
    C. Barium enters the appendix.
    D. Barium is seen in the duodenum.
    E. Barium fills the gastric pouch.

Exercises

11. The usual indication for a T-tube cholangiogram is
    A. The rapid diagnosis in acute biliary tract obstruction.
    B. To identify the presence of inflammation.
    C. Concern that some stones may remain in the biliary tract after surgery.
    D. To evaluate the function of the liver.
    E. To determine patency of the common duct.

12. A radiographic study in which contrast is introduced by means of an endoscope passed through the mouth, esophagus, and stomach into the duodenum to evaluate the biliary tract is the
    A. Endoscopic retrograde cholangiopancreatography.
    B. Upper GI series with small bowel follow-through.
    C. Lower gastrointestinal series.
    D. Intravenous cholecystogram.
    E. Oral cholecystogram.

13. The entire urinary tract can be evaluated by exposures of the lower abdomen and pelvis made at standard intervals after IV administration of contrast medium in which of the following procedures?
    A. Retrograde pyelogram.
    B. Voiding cystourethrogram.
    C. Intravenous cholangiogram.
    D. Intravenous pyelogram.
    E. Stress cystogram.

14. The upper urinary tract can be studied by introducing an iodine-containing contrast medium by means of a catheter threaded under direct vision into the opening between the ureter and bladder in which of the following procedures?
    A. Retrograde pyelogram.
    B. Voiding cystourethrogram.
    C. Intravenous cholangiogram.
    D. Intravenous pyelogram.
    E. Stress cystogram.

15. An examination performed to assess the anatomy of the bladder and urethra and, in particular, the function of the bladder during voiding is the
    A. Voiding cystourethrogram.
    B. Intravenous cholangiogram.
    C. Intravenous pyelogram.
    D. Stress cystogram.
    E. Retrograde pyelogram.

Exercises

16. In which of the following procedures is the patient instructed to cough, strain, or bear down as for a bowel movement, while trying to hold back the flow of urine?
    A. Voiding cystourethrogram.
    B. Hysterosalpingogram.
    C. Intravenous pyelogram.
    D. Stress cystogram.
    E. Retrograde pyelogram.

17. A computer technique which masks everything that appeared in the scout film and shows only what was different about the angiographic image is known as
    A. Lymphangiography.
    B. Digital subtraction angiography.
    C. Cerebral angiography.
    D. Arteriography.
    E. Venography.

18. Angiographic study of the brain and its arteries is known as
    A. Carotid angiogram.
    B. Renal angiogram.
    C. Cerebral angiogram.
    D. Coronary angiogram.
    E. Pulmonary angiogram.

19. Angiographic study of the vessels of the heart is known as
    A. Carotid angiogram.
    B. Abdominal aortogram.
    C. Cerebral angiogram.
    D. Coronary angiogram.
    E. Renal angiogram.

20. Angiographic study of the artery going to the lungs is known as
    A. Pulmonary angiogram.
    B. Abdominal aortogram.
    C. Cerebral angiogram.
    D. Carotid angiogram.
    E. Renal angiogram.

Exercises

21. An angiographic study used to evaluate the arteries of the extremities is
    A. Renal angiogram.
    B. Pulmonary angiogram.
    C. Peripheral angiogram.
    D. Coronary angiogram.
    E. Abdominal aortogram.

22. An angiographic study used to evaluate the circulatory system of the kidneys is
    A. Renal angiogram.
    B. Pulmonary angiogram.
    C. Peripheral angiogram.
    D. Coronary angiogram.
    E. Abdominal aortogram.

23. Which of the following angiographic procedures is used to evaluate the mammary ducts?
    A. Venography, phlebography.
    B. Sialography, ptyalography.
    C. Dacryocystography.
    D. Galactography.
    E. Fistulography.

24. Which of the following angiographic procedures is used to evaluate an abnormal communication between one hollow organ or cavity and another?
    A. Venography, phlebography.
    B. Sialography, ptyalography.
    C. Dacryocystography.
    D. Galactography.
    E. Fistulography.

25. Which of the following studies is used to diagnose obstruction of the parotid gland duct by calculus or tumor?
    A. Venography, phlebography.
    B. Sialography, ptyalography.
    C. Dacryocystography.
    D. Galactography.
    E. Fistulography.

Exercises

Short Answers

1. Define or explain:

   a. barium sulfate _____

   _____

   b. biplane imaging _____

   _____

   c. cholecystokinin _____

   _____

   d. double contrast study _____

   _____

   e. embolus _____

   _____

   f. IVP _____

   _____

   g. scout film _____

   _____

   h. sialography _____

   _____

   i. T-tube cholangiogram _____

   _____

2. Why is a scout film routinely made before the injection of contrast medium?

   _____

   _____

   _____

   _____

3. List some examinations discussed in this chapter that might be done as emergency procedures.

   _____

   _____

   _____

Exercises

4. List some examinations discussed in this chapter that have been largely supplanted by safer or more informative examinations.

_____

_____

_____

_____

5. What are some possible adverse consequences or complications of angiography?

_____

_____

_____

_____

6. Describe the limitations of contrast studies of the gastrointestinal tract.

_____

_____

_____

_____

7. What are the advantages of cholangiography over plain radiography in diagnosing disorders of the biliary tract and gallbladder?

_____

_____

_____

_____

8. What advantage does the retrograde pyelogram have over an intravenous pyelogram? What disadvantage?

_____

_____

_____

_____

Exercises

9. Angiography differs from most other contrast studies in two important respects. What are they?

_____

_____

_____

_____

10. Distinguish among arteriography, venography, and lymphangiography.

_____

_____

_____

_____

_____

_____

_____

_____

Activities for Application and Further Study

1. Discuss the various approaches for the introduction of contrast material in angiographic procedures. Which, if any, of these might be considered "invasive"?

2. List the primary arteries supplying the heart musculature and the portion of the heart each supplies. Disease of which artery might be most critical for survival? Support your answer.

3. From the list of contrast media in the box at the end of the chapter, identify one or two used for each of the following procedures: cerebral angiography, coronary angiography, renal angiography, and peripheral angiography.

Computed Tomography 12

LEARNING OBJECTIVES

Upon completion of this chapter, the student should be able to

- Explain how computed tomography differs from standard diagnostic radiography;

- List some advantages and applications of computed tomography;

- Discuss the use of contrast media in CT.

Computed tomography (CT), also called computed axial tomography (CAT), is an application of computer technology to diagnostic radiology. Instead of exposing a sheet of photographic film after passing through the subject, the x-rays are detected and recorded by one or more scintillation counters (devices that detect and measure radiation). The x-ray source and scintillation counter are mounted on a frame or gantry, allowing them to rotate 360° around the subject and "cut" across any selected plane. A series of exposures are made according to a predetermined protocol that has been programmed into the equipment. Data on the amount of x-ray that penetrates the subject at each exposure are collected, digitized, stored, and analyzed by a computer that generates a cross-sectional image or profile corresponding to the plane cut by the x-ray beam.

A CT examination suite contains, besides the x-ray source, scintillation counters, and table, a work station including a control console where the examination is programmed and a microcomputer that processes data and generates images. The operations performed by the computer are divided into an acquisition phase (collection of data) and a reconstruction phase (analysis of data and assembly of CT images). Images are displayed

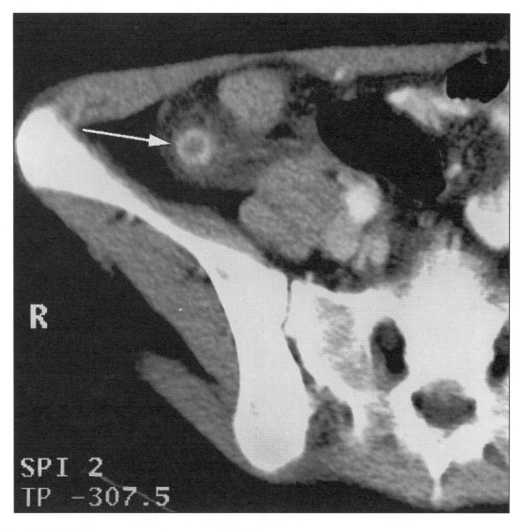

Fig. 12.1. Axial CT scan, acute appendicitis.
Minimally distended appendix with an enhancing wall (arrow). Copyright-protected material used with permission of the author, Brian Mullan, M.D., Univ. of Iowa's *Currents Magazine*, and Virtual Hospital, www.vh.org.

on a screen and recorded on film besides being stored digitally.

A CT examination results in a series of images or slices showing the anatomy of the subject at right angles to the x-ray beam, exactly as if the body were actually being sliced into cross-sections. For viewing, CT images are always oriented as if the subject were lying supine (face up) and the observer were looking at the sections from the subject's feet. The thickness of each slice and the distance between slices are determined by computer settings. An examination can result in sample slices at regular intervals or in a sequence of contiguous images without intervals of unexamined tissue between them.

In conventional CT, the x-ray source moves from one position to another in stepwise fashion around the patient and exposures are made individually. In helical (or spiral) CT (see Fig.12.1) the x-ray tube emits radiation continuously as it rotates through a predetermined arc while the table supporting the subject moves at a constant speed at a right angle to this arc to yield a series of cuts. Helical CT is more expensive, but it provides significant technical advantages. In a conventional CT examination, breathing movements and random shifts in the patient's position between slices can introduce artifacts. Because it produces a series of images more quickly, helical CT allows an entire organ or body region (for example, the liver or the thorax) to be scanned during a single session.

The information acquired during a CT examination is stored as raw digital data. By manipulating these data, the radiographer can enhance the visibility of certain tissues or structures as they appear in an image, while suppressing others.

A digital image consists of thousands of very small square pixels (picture elements). For each pixel, a number (in Hounsfield units; see box) indicates the amount of radiation that was absorbed by the tissue at the point in the image that is represented by that pixel. The denser the tissue, the higher the number. Bone, of maximum

Hounsfield Unit

The Hounsfield unit was named after the British electrical engineer Sir Godfrey Newbold Hounsfield, born in 1919, who developed the first clinically useful CT machine. This unit was conceived as a means of standardizing the measurement of linear attenuation values for various tissues. Water was assigned a value of zero and air a value of -1000. Each Hounsfield unit therefore represents a difference of 0.1% (that is, one thousandth) of the full range of attenuation values between these two substances.

The use of Hounsfield units permits comparison of imaging data obtained from various CT scanners having different x-ray beam characteristics. It also facilitates the establishment of reference windows as explained in the text. Godfrey Hounsfield shared the 1979 Nobel Prize in Medicine or Physiology with an American, Allan MacLeod Cormack, his fellow pioneer in the development of CT technology.

density, is arbitrarily assigned a Hounsfield number of 1000, while air (gas), of minimum density, has a value of -1000.

As in a conventional radiographic image (negative), areas with very high numbers appear white on a CT monitor or on x-ray film, and those with very low numbers appear black. Structures intermediate in density appear in various shades of gray depending on their Hounsfield numbers.

Instead of creating an image in which the various shades composing the gray scale are spread out evenly from -1000 to 1000, the radiographer can limit the range of densities to be displayed. A *window* is a limited range of densities chosen to enhance minor contrasts within tissues of that range. For example, a window ranging from -200 to 300 might be chosen to emphasize subtle contrasts in the densities of mediastinal soft tissues in a CT examination of the thorax. The window width in this case is 500 (the algebraic difference between -200 and +300). The window level, which is automatically the midpoint of the range, is 50.

Tissues whose densities are reflected by Hounsfield numbers within the range represented by the window will appear in the image in various shades of gray. Moreover, the whole range of shades of gray will be distributed only among tissues within that range. Structures whose Hounsfield values are close to the window level will appear in a shade of gray exactly intermediate between black and white. Any structure having a Hounsfield number above the top figure of the window will appear completely white and any structure having a number below the bottom figure will appear completely black. The data from a single scan can be processed repeatedly with different windows to accentuate different features of the part examined.

By more sophisticated programming of the CT computer, it is possible to perform multiplanar reconstructions (projections of anatomy in planes other than at a right angle to the x-ray beam) and even three-dimensional imaging (sometimes called virtual endoscopy because the images generated are similar to what could be seen by actual inspection with an endoscope).

Computed tomography has replaced conventional x-ray studies for many applications because it permits finer discrimination between tissue densities. Contiguous soft-tissue structures whose borders or silhouettes are not represented in an x-ray image can often be clearly distinguished in a CT scan. Hence CT provides superior visualization of enlarged or displaced organs and of soft-tissue masses (cysts, neoplasms, hemorrhage), and is particularly valuable in diagnostic screening of the head, thorax, abdomen, and pelvis. In addition, it is more sensitive than con-

ventional radiology in detecting variations in calcification and bone density and in identifying subtle fractures.

CT examinations of the head are useful in identifying and localizing hemorrhage both after acute trauma (to identify epidural or subdural hematoma) and in stroke (to rule out hemorrhage before administration of a thrombolytic agent). In the diagnosis of pulmonary embolism, CT is approximately as accurate as a ventilation-perfusion scan (discussed in Chapter 15). Studies of the respiratory tract with helical CT and multiplanar imaging have application in the diagnosis of bronchial disease and asthma and in screening high-risk populations (e.g., smokers over 60) for lung cancer. In acute abdominal pain, CT is valuable in diagnosing such disorders as ureteral calculus, bowel obstruction, and appendicitis. It can also detect deep vein thrombosis (DVT) in the pelvis or a lower extremity.

As with conventional radiography, the sensitivity of some computed tomography studies can be enhanced by administration of a contrast medium during the examination.

Barium may be given orally or rectally in studies of the gastrointestinal tract. In CT angiography, an iodide contrast medium is infused intravenously rather than being introduced into an artery by catheter. After making a circuit through the heart and lungs, the medium appears in the arterial supply of the structures being studied in sufficient concentration to render those vessels and structures visible. This technique has the advantage of not requiring placement of an arterial catheter.

Another contrast medium used with CT is xenon, a colorless, odorless, and chemically inert elemental gas. Inhalation of a mixture of xenon and oxygen results in excellent demarcation of respiratory passages on CT scanning. Inhaled xenon is absorbed into the circulation and rapidly diffused throughout the body, enhancing the visibility of soft tissues such as abdominal viscera. Because it readily passes the blood-brain barrier, xenon studies are valuable in the evaluation of regional cerebral blood flow. Administration of xenon by inhalation is safe, provided that an adequate concentration of oxygen is combined with it. Xenon studies are very expensive.

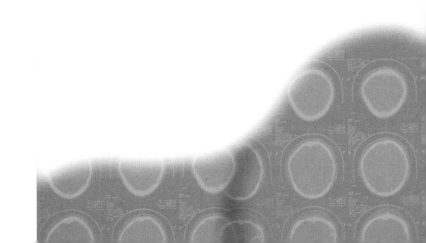

Exercises

Fill in the Blanks

1. The _____ phase of computed tomography consists of the collection of data and a _____ phase consists of the analysis of data and assembly of CT images.

2. Projections of anatomy in planes other than at a right angle to the x-ray beam are called _____.

3. Inhalation of a mixture of _____ and oxygen results in excellent demarcation of respiratory passages on CT scanning.

4. For viewing, CT images are always oriented as if the subject were lying _____ and the observer were looking at the sections _____.

5. The advantage of _____ is that using them permits comparison of imaging data obtained from various CT scanners having different x-ray beam characteristics.

Multiple Choice: Circle the letter of the best answer from the choices given.

1. Which of the following contrast media is administered by inhalation?
   A. Barium sulfate.
   B. Xenon.
   C. Diatrizoate.
   D. Iothalamate.
   E. Metrizamide.

2. _____ generates a cross-sectional image or profile corresponding to the plane cut by the x-ray beam.
   A. Conventional computed tomography.
   B. Plain radiography.
   C. Contrast-enhanced radiography.
   D. Helical computed tomography.
   E. Angiography.

3. On a CT study, a Hounsfield unit of 1000 would indicate the density of which of the following?
   A. Gas.
   B. Air.
   C. Bone.
   D. Solid organs.
   E. Hollow organs.

Exercises

4. Mediastinal soft tissue densities might be represented by a Hounsfield unit of which of the following?
   A. -1000 to 1000.
   B. 500
   C. -1000
   D. 1000
   E. -200 to 300

Short Answers

1. Define or explain:

   a. scintillation counter _____

   _____

   b. virtual endoscopy _____

   _____

   c. xenon _____

   _____

2. List some types of examination for which CT scanning is superior to conventional radiography.

   _____

   _____

   _____

   _____

   _____

3. What are some advantages of CT angiography over conventional angiography?

   _____

   _____

   _____

   _____

   _____

Exercises

4. In what ways does helical CT differ from the more conventional procedure?

_____

_____

_____

_____

_____

5. What might be the advantage of producing contiguous CT images of a body area?

_____

_____

_____

_____

6. Why would a radiographer choose to limit the range of densities to be displayed? Give examples.

_____

_____

_____

_____

Activities for Application and Further Study

1. List and define 10 terms related to computerized tomography.

   a. _____

   _____

   b. _____

   _____

   c. _____

   _____

   d. _____

   _____

   e. _____

   _____

Exercises

f. _____

_____

g. _____

_____

h. _____

_____

i. _____

_____

j. _____

_____

Ultrasonography

13

LEARNING OBJECTIVES

Upon completion of this chapter, the student should be able to

- State the basic principles of diagnostic ultrasonography;

- List advantages and disadvantages of this method;

- Describe the application of the Doppler principle to ultrasonography;

- Explain the use of ultrasound in obstetrics and cardiology.

Chapter Outline

Ultrasonography

Obstetrical Ultrasound

Echocardiography

Ultrasonography

Ultrasonography (or sonography) is a means of visualizing internal structures by observing the effects they have on a beam of sound waves. The term ultrasound refers to the fact that the sound waves used for this procedure have a higher frequency (pitch) than the human ear can detect. The upper limit of human hearing is about 20 000 Hz (hertz, or cycles per second). Diagnostic ultrasonography uses frequencies between 1 and 10 million Hz (1-10 MHz). Ultrasound technology is also used therapeutically in the treatment of acute or chronic soft-tissue pain and to shatter urinary calculi (lithotripsy).

Ultrasound waves pass through air, gas, and fluid without being reflected. However, they bounce back from rigid structures such as bone and gallstones, creating an echo that can be detected by a receiver. Solid organs such as the liver and kidney partially reflect ultrasound waves in predictable patterns. Waves are also reflected from the interface between two structures having different acoustic properties, such as fluid and the structure that contains it (e.g., cyst, urinary bladder).

Ultrasound waves for diagnostic sonography are generated by a piezoelectric crystal or ceramic chip, which emits vibrations when stimulated by electricity. A device that converts one type of energy into another in this fashion is called a transducer. The same crystal also acts as a receiver, detecting echoes and converting them back into electrical signals. Although it emits bursts of ultrasound at a rate of 1000 per second, a transducer actually functions as a receiver most (99.9%) of the time.

The transducer used in ultrasonographic examinations is contained in a hand-held scanning head or probe, which the examiner places on the surface of the patient's body. A gel is applied to the skin surface to reduce friction and ensure even contact. During the examination the patient feels only the pressure and movement of the scanning head.

The echoes detected by the receiver and transformed by it into electrical data are processed by a computer and converted to an image on a television screen. In analyzing sonographic data, the computer uses the strength of each echo to determine the acoustical impedance (resistance to the passage of sound waves) of the structure that generated it, and the echo time (delay in return of echo after emission of the sound wave) to determine the distance between the transducer and the structure. The images produced are in gray-scale. That is, each pixel ("picture element," smallest discrete component of the image) appears in a shade of gray whose darkness or lightness is in proportion to the intensity of the signal represented. Sonographic images can be printed on film or paper or recorded on videotape.

A tissue or organ that reflects ultrasound strongly is said to be hyperechoic, or to display high echogenicity, while a tissue that reflects ultrasound weakly is said to be hypoechoic and to display low echogenicity. Because water and other fluids do not reflect at all, they are said to be anechoic or sonolucent (by analogy with *translucent* and *radiolucent*). A highly echogenic structure, such as a bone, prevents sound waves from generating images of tissues behind it, a phenomenon known as acoustic shadowing.

A-mode sonography, using a solitary transducer, yields only information about the size or position of a given target, such as a mass or organ. In B-mode sonography, a scanner containing as many as 100 transducers, each "viewing" the subject from a slightly different angle, permits the generation of a two-dimensional image.

Rapid processing of signals can convert a succession of B-mode scans into a sequence of images that, like the images on motion picture film, flow together to give the observer an illusion of motion. This is called M-mode (for "motion") or real-time scanning. By this technique movement (for example, the beating of the heart) is perceived as it occurs. In addition, moving the scanner rapidly back and forth over the area under study generates a series of images, each "seen" from a slightly different angle, which lend a three-dimensional element to visual interpretation. (By the application of technology similar to that used in computed tomography, two-dimensional B-mode sonographic images can also be combined to produce three-dimensional images.)

Since its development in the 1950s, ultrasonography has become a standard imaging technique, replacing x-ray and other diagnostic methods for many applications. Because no harmful radiation is involved, it is particularly useful during pregnancy and in the examination of children. However, the sensitivity and accuracy of a sonographic examination depend on the skill and experience of the examiner to a greater extent than with conventional radiography, CT, or MRI.

Certain areas cannot be adequately evaluated by ultrasound. Because the scanning head must come into contact with the body surface, examination may not be feasible in cases of open wounds or dressings. The skull blocks sound waves from penetrating the brain, and gas within the digestive tract scatters waves. Hence for abdominal and pelvic sonography, a full bladder is helpful because it displaces bowel and creates a readily observable reference point. Sonohysterography is a variation on the standard pelvic ultrasound examination in which saline solution (not a contrast agent) is injected into the uterine cavity by a catheter inserted through the cervix. This procedure distends the cavity, providing clearer sonographic definition of polyps, fibroids, or other abnormalities.

Ultrasonography is widely used in the diagnosis of acute or chronic pain, masses, and trauma of the abdomen or pelvis. Because it can determine the size of masses and distinguish between cysts and solid tumors, it is a standard procedure in evaluating masses or swellings in the thyroid gland, liver, pancreas, spleen, kidney, and prostate. Because it shows gallstones and urinary calculi clearly, it is particularly useful in obstructive disease of the biliary and urinary tracts. It can also be used to guide the performance of a biopsy, particularly of the prostate, or (during surgery) the placement of a needle in a cyst or other lesion.

The Doppler effect (*see box*) can be applied to ultrasonography to detect the motion of blood in blood vessels and through the heart. In pulsed-wave Doppler sonography, this is achieved by the use of programmed pulses and sophisticated analysis of data. Continuous-wave or "bedside" Doppler sonography is performed with a self-contained hand-held device that uses two crystals simultaneously, one to send and one to receive. The ultrasonic signals detected are converted to audible sounds, whose pitch provides information about blood flow through the artery or vein under study. For arterial studies a blood pressure cuff is applied to control flow during the examination.

What Is the Doppler Effect?

The Doppler principle, first formulated by the Austrian mathematician Christian Doppler (1803-1853), refers to the change in the observed frequency of sound waves (or other waves) when the distance between the source of the waves and the observer is changing. If, while driving, you pass a ringing bell or honking horn that is stationary, the pitch (musical note) seems to drop suddenly at the moment you pass the source of sound. The reason is that, as you approach the source of the sound, the waves reach you slightly sooner than if you were standing still, so that, for you, their frequency is higher. As you move away from the source of sound, the waves reach you slightly later than if you were standing still, so that their observed frequency is lower. This principle is used by highway patrol radar to measure the speed of an approaching vehicle, by weather radar to track storms, and in astronomy to observe the motion of stars.

Duplex Doppler sonography combines standard ultrasound imaging with computer analysis of Doppler data to graph the speed and direction of blood flow through the vessels under study. A further refinement is the use of color to indicate the direction of blood flow. In color Doppler sonography, each pixel containing information on blood flow is color-coded according to the direction and velocity of blood flow, blue indicating flow away from the transducer and red indicating flow toward the transducer.

Obstetrical Ultrasonography

Ultrasonography is a routine part of prenatal care. Ordinarily an obstetrical sonogram is performed at 18 to 20 weeks' gestation. An examination may be performed earlier to confirm the presence of pregnancy or, in cases of vaginal bleeding, to assess fetal viability and rule out ectopic pregnancy. (A fetal heartbeat can normally be observed on sonography by the seventh week of gestation.) Other specific indications for diagnostic sonography during pregnancy include diagnosis of multiple pregnancy, fetal malformation, or polyhydramnios (excessive amniotic fluid) and localization of the placenta (in cases of placenta previa or before amniocentesis). Transvaginal sonography, with the scanning head placed inside the vagina, yields superior detail in certain circumstances.

Sonography permits accurate determination of fetal size and calculation of gestational age. Early in pregnancy the crown-rump length is most useful in calculating age. Later the biparietal diameter (transverse width of skull) correlates most closely with age. In the third trimester, the circumference of the fetal abdomen may be measured as a means of estimating fetal size and weight.

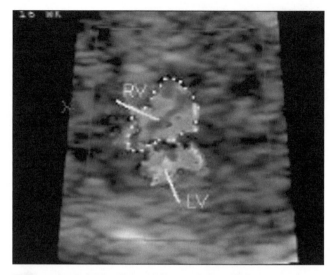

Fig. 13.1. Color Doppler ultrasound of fetal heart. Credit: Greggory R. DeVore, M.D., http.//www.fetalecho.com

Echocardiography

Echocardiography is the application of ultrasonography to the examination of the heart. An echocardiogram, performed with a scanning head applied to the anterior and lateral chest wall, gives information about the size of the cardiac chambers (atria and ventricles), the thickness and motion of chamber walls, and the condition of the pericardium and great vessels. The addition of Doppler imaging shows the direction and velocity of blood flow, assesses valve function, and permits calculation of the ventricular ejection fraction (the proportion of the blood present in the left ventricle at the end of diastole that is ejected during systole, usually expressed as a percent rather than a fraction). An electrocardiogram tracing is recorded simultaneously with the echocardiogram.

Echocardiography is a standard procedure in the evaluation of congenital and acquired valvular disease, including mitral valve prolapse, and in congestive heart failure and other disorders characterized by inadequate pumping action of the heart. A general reduction in ventricular wall motion is called hypokinesis; a more localized reduction of motion is called asyneresis. An ejection fraction less than 40% suggests cardiac failure.

Exercises

Fill in the Blanks

1. _____ is a means of visualizing internal structures by observing the effects they have on a beam of sound waves.

2. The term ultrasound refers to the fact that the _____ used for this procedure have a higher _____ than the human ear can detect.

3. Therapeutic uses of ultrasound technology include _____ and _____.

4. A device that converts one type of energy into another is called a _____.

5. The term _____ refers to resistance to the passage of sound waves.

6. The term _____ refers to the delay in return of echo after emission of the sound wave.

7. Sonographic images produced are in gray-scale; that is, each pixel appears darker or lighter in proportion to the _____ of the signal represented.

8. A tissue or organ that reflects ultrasound strongly is said to display _____.

9. A tissue that reflects ultrasound weakly is said to be _____.

10. Images sequenced like the images on motion picture film that flow together to give the observer an illusion of motion are known as M-mode sonography or _____.

11. M-mode sonography is useful for imaging the _____.

12. Because the scanning head must come into contact with the body surface, examination may not be feasible in cases of _____.

13. For abdominal and pelvic sonography, a full bladder is helpful because _____.

14. _____ is a variation on the standard pelvic ultrasound examination in which saline solution is injected into the uterine cavity by a catheter inserted through the cervix, providing clearer definition of polyps, fibroids, or other abnormalities.

15. The _____ is most useful in calculating age early in a pregnancy.

16. The term *biparietal diameter* refers to the _____ and is useful for determining fetal _____ later in pregnancy.

Exercises

17. In the third trimester, the circumference of the fetal abdomen may be measured as a means of _____.

18. The _____ is the proportion of the blood present in the left ventricle at the end of diastole that is ejected during systole.

19. _____ is a general reduction in ventricular wall motion.

20. A more localized reduction of motion is called _____.

21. An _____ of less than 40% suggests cardiac failure.

Multiple Choice: Circle the letter of the best answer from the choices given.

1. In analyzing sonographic data, the computer uses the strength of each echo to determine the _____ of the structure that generated it.
    A. Echo time.
    B. Acoustical impedance.
    C. Transducer signal.
    D. Piezoelectric crystal.
    E. Pixellated elements.

2. In analyzing sonographic data, the computer uses the _____ to determine the distance between the transducer and the structure.
    A. Acoustical impedance.
    B. Transducer signal.
    C. Piezoelectric crystal.
    D. Pixellated elements.
    E. Echo time.

3. A tissue or organ that reflects ultrasound strongly is said to be
    A. Piezoelectric.
    B. Pixellated.
    C. Hyperechoic.
    D. Hypoechoic.
    E. Anechoic.

Exercises

4. A tissue that reflects ultrasound weakly is said to
    A. Display low echogenicity.
    B. Display high echogenicity.
    C. Display lots of pixels.
    D. Block most ultrasound signals.
    E. Display no echoes.

5. Water and other fluids that do not reflect at all are said to be
    A. Piezoelectric.
    B. Pixellated.
    C. Hyperechoic.
    D. Hypoechoic.
    E. Anechoic.

6. A phenomenon known as acoustic shadowing is caused by sound waves bouncing off a highly echogenic structure such as
    A. Water.
    B. Soft tissue.
    C. Bone.
    D. Brain.
    E. Heart.

7. A type of sonography that uses a solitary transducer and yields only information about the size or position of a given target, such as a mass or organ, is
    A. B-mode sonography.
    B. A-mode sonography.
    C. M-mode sonography.
    D. Ultrasonography.
    E. Pulsed-wave Doppler sonography.

8. The type of sonography in which a scanner containing as many as 100 transducers, each "viewing" the subject from a slightly different angle, permits the generation of a two-dimensional image is
    A. B-mode sonography.
    B. A-mode sonography.
    C. M-mode sonography.
    D. Ultrasonography.
    E. Pulsed-wave Doppler sonography.

Exercises

9. Converting a succession of B-mode scans into a sequence of images by rapid processing of signals so that the images flow together to give the observer an illusion of motion, like that of motion picture film, is
   A. Pulsed-wave Doppler sonography.
   B. B-mode sonography.
   C. A-mode sonography.
   D. Ultrasonography.
   E. M-mode sonography.

10. The detection of the motion of blood in blood vessels and through the heart is possible by means of a special type of sonography known as
    A. Pulsed-wave Doppler sonography.
    B. B-mode sonography.
    C. A-mode sonography.
    D. Ultrasonography.
    E. M-mode sonography.

11. A type of sonography that combines standard ultrasound imaging with computer analysis of Doppler data to graph the speed and direction of blood flow through the vessels under study is
    A. Color Doppler sonography.
    B. Duplex Doppler sonography.
    C. Pulsed-wave Doppler sonography.
    D. A-mode sonography.
    E. M-mode sonography.

12. In _____, each pixel containing information on blood flow is color-coded according to the direction and velocity of blood flow, blue indicating flow away from the transducer and red indicating flow toward the transducer.
    A. Color Doppler sonography.
    B. Duplex Doppler sonography.
    C. Pulsed-wave Doppler sonography.
    D. A-mode sonography.
    E. M-mode sonography.

13. All of the following types of sonography are used to image the heart and circulation except
    A. Color Doppler sonography.
    B. Duplex Doppler sonography.
    C. Pulsed-wave Doppler sonography.
    D. A-mode sonography.
    E. M-mode sonography.

Exercises

14. Specific indications for diagnostic sonography during pregnancy include all of the following except
    A. Diagnosis of multiple pregnancy.
    B. Diagnosis of fetal malformation.
    C. Polyhydramnios (excessive amniotic fluid).
    D. Localization of the placenta.
    E. Determining the sex of the fetus.

15. Sonography permits accurate determination of fetal size and/or calculation of gestational age by
    A. Measuring the crown-rump length.
    B. Measuring the circumference of the fetal abdomen.
    C. Measuring the biparietal diameter.
    D. All of the above.
    E. None of the above.

16. An ordinary echocardiogram is used for all of the following except
    A.   To determine the size of the cardiac chambers and the thickness and motion of chamber walls.
    B. To calculate the ventricular ejection fraction.
    C. To assess the condition of the pericardium and great vessels.
    D. To evaluate for mitral valve prolapse.
    E. To diagnose congestive heart failure.

17. With the addition of Doppler imaging, an echocardiogram can be used
    A. To calculate the ventricular ejection fraction.
    B. To determine the size of the cardiac chambers and the thickness and motion of chamber walls.
    C. To assess the condition of the pericardium and great vessels.
    D. To evaluate for mitral valve prolapse.
    E. To diagnose congestive heart failure.

18. Congestive heart failure is evident on Doppler echocardiogram when
    A. Hypokinesis is evident.
    B. Asyneresis is evident.
    C. The ejection fraction is less than 40%.
    D. The mitral valve is prolapsed.
    E. Blood flow velocity is indeterminable.

Exercises

Short Answers

1. Define or explain:
   a. acoustic shadowing _____
   _____

   b. Doppler effect _____
   _____

   c. pixel _____
   _____

   d. polyhydramnios _____
   _____

   e. sonolucent _____
   _____

2. List some body areas for which ultrasonography is superior to conventional x-ray.
   _____
   _____
   _____
   _____

3. Ultrasonography is used in neurosurgery to aid the placement of instruments or localization of structures in the brain. It is not used, however, for routine examinations of the brain or spinal cord. Why not?
   _____
   _____
   _____
   _____

4. What are some indications for performing obstetric ultrasonography before 18 weeks' gestation?
   _____
   _____
   _____
   _____

Exercises

5. What types of ultrasound examination might be performed in an emergency situation?

_____

_____

_____

_____

6. Describe how ultrasound works.

_____

_____

_____

_____

_____

_____

_____

_____

Activities for Application and Further Study

1. Bring to class (or find on the Internet) examples of obstetrical ultrasound images. Compare with others brought in by class members (or those found on the Internet). Identify the ages of the fetuses. What are the prominent features of the fetus at the ages represented by the images collected? Summarize in writing.

2. Find images of the Internet of the following studies of the heart:
   Color Doppler sonography.
   Duplex Doppler sonography.
   Pulsed-wave Doppler sonography.
   M-mode sonography.
   Summarize the differences in appearance as well as diagnostic capabilities.

Magnetic Resonance Imaging

14

Magnetic resonance imaging is a method of visualizing internal structures electronically rather than with x-rays. Although this technique yields cuts or cross-sectional images similar to those of computed tomography, it is based on entirely different physical principles.

As with x-ray and ultrasound, MRI detects and records differences in the physical properties of contiguous or adjacent tissues—for example, bone as contrasted with muscle, or normal liver as contrasted with a cyst. But whereas an x-ray examination detects varying resistance of tissues to penetration by x-rays, and ultrasonography detects varying resistance to penetration by sound waves, MRI detects varying concentrations or densities of hydrogen atoms (protons) in tissues.

A magnet attracts not only iron atoms but also any other atoms that, like iron, have an unequal number of protons and neutrons in their nuclei. The degree to which such an atom responds to magnetic attraction depends on its nuclear structure and is expressed as a physical constant called **spin**.

The simplest of all atoms is that of hydrogen, which, with but a single proton in its nucleus, possesses spin and responds to magnetic attraction. If the human body is placed in a static magnetic field of sufficient strength, then a significant number of its hydrogen atoms align themselves with the field like trillions of infinitesimal compass needles.

In an MRI examination, the patient is placed inside a static magnetic field generated by a large, powerful magnet. A pulse of radio waves (excitation pulse) is then used to create, for a brief period, a second magnetic field at a right angle to the static field. While this second field is acting on the body, the hydrogen ions (protons) change their orientation, and when the second field is turned off, they go back to their previous orientation to the static magnetic field.

As the protons return to their previous orientation, they give off a stream of radiofrequency energy or "signal," which can be detected by a suitably placed receiving coil. The intensity of the signal given off by any tissue is proportional to the hydrogen ion concentration (or proton density) of that tissue. Muscle emits a very high signal, bone a very low one, air or gas almost none.

The time it takes for the protons to return to their former orientation after an excitation pulse is called the spin-lattice relaxation time, abbreviated as T1 (the Greek letter *tau*). This time interval, a fraction of a second, is directly proportional to the hydrogen ion density or proton density (PD) of the sample. The greater the proton density of the tissue examined, the greater the delay in returning to the previous orientation, and the longer the T1.

When the excitation pulse is applied, the protons in the sample respond together, or in phase, as they take up their new orientation. After the excitation pulse ceases, but before all the protons have come back to their former orientation to the static magnetic field, they tend to get out of phase with each other, as adjacent molecules collide. Once the protons go out of phase, a signal can no longer be detected by the receiving coil. The time it takes for the protons to go out of phase is called the spin-spin relaxation time, or T2. Obviously T2 is always shorter than T1.

Because both T1 and T2 vary in proportion to the proton density of the sample, they can be used by a computer to generate an image of the sample. However, direct measurement of T1 is not possible, since the signal is lost as soon as the protons go out of phase. There are also technical obstacles to the precise measurement of T2. Some of these obstacles are eliminated by the **spin echo technique**, in which the excitation pulse is followed, after a brief interval, by a second and stronger pulse. This results in the generation of an echo signal, from which T2 can be determined. The time that elapses between the first pulse and the appearance of the echo is called the **echo time** (TE).

In order to obtain cross-sectional images, it is necessary to modify the magnetic resonance system by adding yet a third magnetic field. This **gradient magnetic field**, created by a separate coil, introduces a positional element into the signals detected by the receiver. A computer decodes and analyzes the signals, generating two-dimensional cross-sectional images of the subject in much the same way that CT images are produced (*see Fig. 14.1*). The series of images or slices generated are displayed on a screen and recorded on film. As with CT, images are oriented as if the subject were supine and the observer were at the subject's feet.

The intensity of the signal emitted by various tissues, and the contrast between various tissues, can be adjusted by manipulating the strength, direction, and duration of pulses. In practice, a number of different pulses and time intervals are used in predetermined series called pulse sequences, and the resulting spin echo signals are averaged. Repetition time (TR) is the interval between one pulse sequence and the next.

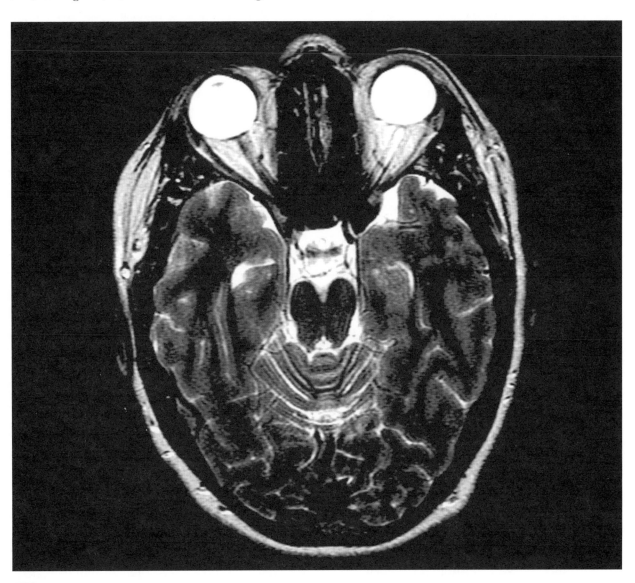

Fig. 14.1. MRI of head. Reference: J. Hornak, http://www.cis.rit.edu

An image generated with a pulse sequence using a relatively short TR (0.6 seconds or less) is called a T1 weighted image, because it reflects the T1 of the specimen to a greater extent than the T2. An image generated with a longer TR (2.0 seconds or more) is called a T2 weighted image. Differential weighting of MRI images is carried out because T1 and T2, although they are both related to proton density, reflect somewhat different properties of tissues.

In a T1 weighted image, water and watery fluids (urine, cerebrospinal fluid) appear dark because their intensity with this technique is low; they are therefore said to be hypointense. Fat, fresh hemorrhage, slowly moving blood, and fluids with high protein content such as mucus appear bright (are hyperintense) with T1 weighting. In contrast, water is hyperintense in a T2 weighted image and soft tissues including muscle and fat yield a low signal. Regardless of weighting, bone, calcifications, and air or gas are always hypointense, appearing dark in an MR image.

With an inversion recovery pulse sequence, the first excitation pulse is aimed directly opposite to the field (that is, at an angle of 180° to it) and the second pulse is delivered at a 90° angle to it. A STIR (short T1 inversion recovery) sequence is particularly useful in suppressing the signal emitted by fat (which has a shorter T1) while retaining the signals characteristic of soft tissue (intermediate T1) and water (long T1) proton densities. A FLAIR (fluid-attenuated inversion-recovery) sequence generates T2-weighted images with no appreciable signal from fluid, making it valuable in detecting lesions in the subarachnoid space and ventricular system of the brain.

MRI has largely replaced conventional radiography for applications in which it provides superior discrimination among tissue densities. In the examination of the central nervous system, MRI shows the plaques of demyelination characteristic of multiple sclerosis. Although CT is preferred for distinguishing between ischemic and hemorrhagic strokes and in identifying subarachnoid hemorrhage, MRI is a more sensitive indicator of early ischemia and infarction, and of lesions in the posterior cranial fossa (brain stem and cerebellum).

MRI is also valuable in determining the location, size, and shape of tumors, particularly in the brain and liver, and in the diagnosis of bone and joint disorders (internal derangements, ligamentous tears, spinal cord compression due to disk herniation or spinal stenosis). MRI may detect tumors at an earlier stage than mammography, and has been recommended by some authorities for annual surveillance of women at high risk.

Because the apparatus generates a strong magnetic field, jewelry, watches, and other metal objects must be removed before the examination. MRI is contraindicated for patients with ferrous metal prostheses or implanted cardiac pacemakers. For the duration of the examination, which may take more than an hour, the patient lies motionless on a narrow table within the cylindrical magnet. Some patients become claustrophobic in these circumstances or may find it difficult to remain still. MRI examination is often not feasible in the critically ill or injured patient, who may require supportive care and frequent assessment.

Magnetic resonance imaging does not expose the patient to ionizing radiation. Although no adverse effects on the fetus have been documented, the American College of Obstetricians and Gynecologists and the National Radiological Protection Board have advised against the use of MRI during the first trimester of pregnancy.

Contrast agents, such as barium and iodides, that are used in radiology are not effective in improving the clarity of MRI images. However, the metallic element gadolinium possesses physical properties that render it particularly suitable as a contrast agent in MRI examinations. Although biologically inert, it enhances the MRI signal of any tissue or area in which it accumulates by shortening the T1 of adjacent protons.

Intravenously administered gadolinium is quickly distributed throughout the circulation, showing blood vessels, highly vascular tissues, and zones of hemorrhage with great clarity. MRI angiography with intravenous gadolinium is useful in rapid diagnosis of aortic aneurysm and renal artery stenosis. This contrast medium can also be used in procedures such as arthrography. Injected gadolinium is cleared from the body in 3-6 hours. Unlike iodide contrast media, it is not toxic to the kidneys, and allergic and other side-effects are rare.

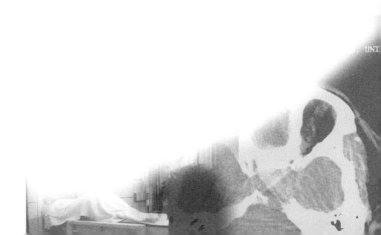

Exercises

Fill in the Blanks

1. Magnetic resonance imaging is similar to computed tomography in that it _____.

2. An MRI magnet attracts not only iron atoms but also any other atoms that, like iron, have _____ and neutrons in their nuclei.

3. _____ is a physical constant which is an expression of the degree to which such an atom, depending on its nuclear structure, responds to magnetic attraction.

4. T2 is always _____ than T1.

5. Cross-sectional images are obtained in an MRI scan by adding a third magnetic field called the _____.

6. In practice, a number of different pulses and time intervals are used in predetermined series called _____.

7. Images that appear bright on an MRI are said to appear _____.

8. Images that appear dark on an MRI are said to appear _____.

9. A _____ is particularly useful in suppressing the signal emitted by fat (which has a shorter T1) while retaining the signals characteristic of soft tissue (intermediate T1) and water (long T1) proton densities.

10. A _____ generates T2-weighted images with no appreciable signal from fluid, making it valuable in detecting lesions in the subarachnoid space and ventricular system of the brain.

11. _____ enhances the MRI signal of any tissue or area in which it accumulates by shortening the T1 of adjacent protons.

Multiple Choice: Circle the letter of the best answer from the choices given.

1. The degree to which such an atom responds to magnetic attraction depends on its nuclear structure and is expressed as a physical constant called
   A. Excitation pulse.
   B. Spin.
   C. Echo time (TE).
   D. Spin-lattice relaxation time (T1).
   E. Spin echo technique.

Exercises

2. The time it takes for the protons to return to their former orientation after an excitation pulse is called the
   A. Spin-lattice relaxation time (T1).
   B. Echo time (TE).
   C. Spin-spin relaxation time (T2).
   D. Spin.
   E. Repetition time (TR).

3. The time it takes for the protons to go out of phase is called the
   A. Spin-lattice relaxation time (T1).
   B. Repetition time (TR).
   C. Spin-spin relaxation time (T2).
   D. Spin.
   E. Echo time (TE).

4. Following the excitation pulse, after a brief interval, by a second and stronger pulse is called the
   A. Pulse sequence.
   B. Excitation pulse.
   D. Spin.
   E. Spin echo technique.

5. The time that elapses between the first pulse and the appearance of the echo is called the
   A. Repetition time (TR).
   B. Spin.
   C. Echo time (TE).
   D. Spin-lattice relaxation time (T1).
   E. Spin echo technique.

6. The interval between one pulse sequence and the next is known as the
   A. Repetition time (TR).
   B. Spin.
   C. Echo time (TE).
   D. Spin-lattice relaxation time (T1).
   E. Spin echo technique.

7. An image generated with a pulse sequence using a relatively short TR (0.6 seconds or less) is called
   A. Spin image.
   B. A T2 weighted image.
   C. Gradient image.
   D. A T1 weighted image.
   E. Spin echo image.

Exercises

8. An image generated with a longer TR (2.0 seconds or more) is called
   A. Spin image.
   B. A T2 weighted image.
   C. Gradient image.
   D. A T1 weighted image.
   E. Spin echo image.

9. An intravenously administered imaging agent that is quickly distributed throughout the circulation, showing blood vessels, highly vascular tissues, and zones of hemorrhage with great clarity, and thus useful in MRI angiography in rapid diagnosis of aortic aneurysm and renal artery stenosis, is known as
   A. Barium.
   B. Ultravist.
   C. Visipaque.
   D. Gadolinium.
   E. Angiografin.

Short Answers

1. Define or explain:
   a. gadolinium _____
   _____

   b. pulse sequence _____
   _____

2. List some types of examination for which MRI is preferred to conventional radiography.
   _____
   _____
   _____
   _____

3. In what circumstances might MRI examination not be feasible?
   _____
   _____
   _____
   _____

Exercises

4. What types of examination mentioned in this chapter might be performed in an emergency situation?

    _____

    _____

    _____

    _____

5. List some differences between a T1 weighted image and a T2 weighted image.

    _____

    _____

    _____

    _____

6. How does MRI differ from standard x-rays and ultrasonography?

    _____

    _____

    _____

    _____

7. Summarize how MRI images are made.

    _____

    _____

    _____

    _____

Activities for Application and Further Study

1. Find on the Internet photos of both traditional and open MRI machines. Survey your classmates, friends, and family members to find out how many, if any, would have problems being placed in a traditional MRI. Is there a difference in cost between closed and open MRI? If so, would that make a difference to those you survey?

2. Find on the Internet examples of normal and abnormal brain MRI images. Can you see the abnormalities? Can you label the lobes of the brain and other structures based on the MRI images?

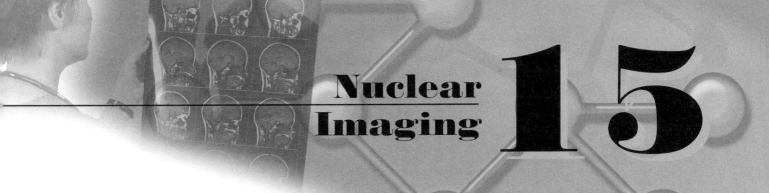

Nuclear Imaging 15

Nuclear medicine applies the principles of nuclear physics to both the diagnosis and treatment of disease. Diagnostic procedures in which radioactive substances are used can be divided into those that create visual images and those that do not. Nuclear imaging techniques are discussed in this section and other types of radiodiagnostic procedures are discussed in Chapters 20 and 24.

The basis of all nuclear diagnosis is the introduction into the body, by ingestion, injection, inhalation, or some other route, of a radioactive tracer—a substance that has been tagged or labeled by having a radioactive isotope incorporated into its chemical structure (*see box*). After an interval the distribution or concentration of the tracer is assessed or measured in some way. In nuclear imaging, that assessment results in a picture or graphic representation of the distribution of the tracer. The term radiopharmaceutical is sometimes applied to radioactive tracers used in diagnostic procedures, although strictly speaking it refers only to radioisotopes that are administered for therapeutic purposes, such as radioactive iodine used to suppress hyperactive thyroid tissue in Graves disease.

Unlike other imaging techniques, nuclear imaging appraises the function of the structures under study rather than their anatomy (size, shape, position). The significance of increased or decreased uptake of a radiotracer depends on the tissue under study and the biochemical nature of the substance into which the radioisotope has been incorporated.

For example, radioactive iodine is used to study the function of the thyroid gland, which normally extracts iodine from the circulation. If administration of radioactive iodine is followed after an interval by the finding of an even distribution of radioactivity throughout the thyroid gland, the conclusion is that the gland is functioning normally. A "hot" zone (an area of increased uptake of radioisotope) corresponding to the position of a nodule in the thyroid gland suggests that the nodule consists of hyperactive thyroid tissue. A "cold" nodule is more likely to represent a malignant tumor, which is unable to concentrate iodine like normal thyroid tissue.

Technetium (*see box on p. 212*) is the most widely used radioisotope in nuclear imaging. In a HIDA (hepatobiliary iminodiacetic acid) scan, intravenously administered technetium Tc 99m N(2,6-dimethylphenylcarboylmethyl) iminodiacetic acid outlines the biliary tract, showing obstruction by stones or tumor. This procedure is often preferred to x-ray studies with injected contrast media. Scanning of the scrotum after intravenous administration of technetium Tc 99m pertechnetate can identify acute reduction of blood supply to a testicle when testicular pain and swelling are due to torsion (twisting) of the spermatic cord. Injected white blood cells labeled with technetium Tc 99m HMPAO (hexamethylpropyleneamine oxime) cluster at sites of inflammation, such as an abscess, the intestinal wall in Crohn disease, or the bone marrow in acute osteomyelitis, permitting localization of these sites and distinguishing them from other pathologic processes.

Standard scanning procedures have been devised for many tissues and organs, including the brain, heart, lungs, liver, and kidneys. For each of these examinations the choice of radiotracer, the route of administration, the interval between administration and scanning, and the details of the scanning procedure depend on the metabolism of the organ or tissue in question and the type of information to be determined by the procedure.

The dosage of a radioisotopic tracer is measured in millicuries (mCi) (*see box on p. 212*). The amount of radiation absorbed by the patient in standard nuclear imaging studies is small and not harmful, and tracers are normally cleared from the body within a few hours or days. These studies are, however, contraindicated in women who are or may be pregnant, because of the sensitivity of the fetus to even small amounts of

What Is a Radioisotope?

All of the substances known to chemistry consist of a relatively small number (108 at latest count) of constituent elements. An element may be defined as a substance that cannot be broken down into a simpler substance. Examples are oxygen, carbon, iron, and sulfur. The physical and chemical properties of an element depend on the structure of its atoms, all of which are identical, or nearly so.

An atom is a submicroscopic particle of matter consisting of a nucleus and one or more electrons orbiting around it, as the moon rotates around the earth and the earth around the sun. The nucleus is made up of protons and neutrons. (Exception: The nucleus of a hydrogen atom contains one proton and no neutrons.) Protons have a positive electric charge and electrons have a negative electric charge. Imbalances and changes in these charges are responsible for chemical reactions such as oxidation and reduction.

All atoms of a given element have the same number of protons in their nuclei, and that number is the atomic number of the element. For example, the atomic number of hydrogen is 1; that of carbon, 6; that of sulfur, 16, and so on. However, not all atoms of a given element have the same number of neutrons in their nuclei.

The mass (that is, the weight) of an atom depends on the number of protons and neutrons in its nucleus. (In computations of mass, electrons are left out of account.) The mass number (formerly, "atomic weight") of an element is the weight of the particles composing its nucleus. The mass number is an arbitrary value based on the relative weight of various atoms. Originally the weight of a hydrogen atom was taken as having a mass number of 1.0. Nowadays, however, mass numbers are based on 12.0 as the mass number of carbon.

Atoms of a given element that vary in the number of neutrons in their nuclei, and hence in their mass numbers, are called **isotopes** of that element. An element as it occurs in nature is often a mixture of several isotopes. For such an element, the mass number given in reference works (e.g., chlorine, 35.45; iron, 55.85) is the average of the mass numbers of the various isotopes as they occur in nature. Hence the mass number of an element (unlike its atomic number) is often not an integer (whole number).

The mass number of any given isotope, however, is always a whole number. By convention, the mass number is shown as a superscript number before the symbol of the element (^{32}P, an isotope of phosphorus with a mass number of 32; ^{14}C, an isotope of carbon with a mass number of 14). Alternatively the mass number may follow the symbol of the element, without a hyphen: P 32, C 14.

Some isotopes of certain elements (and all isotopes of elements with atomic numbers above 89) are unstable, undergoing a steady nuclear decay accompanied by a discharge of energy in various forms (alpha and beta particles, gamma rays, positrons). This discharge of energy, called radioactivity, was discovered in 1896 by the French physicist Antoine Henri Becquerel (1852-1908).

Like x-rays, radioactivity causes certain chemical substances to break up into ions (hence "ionizing radiation") and can have harmful effects on living tissue. In addition to radioisotopes that occur in nature, some have been produced artificially by bombarding stable isotopes with a proton beam generated by a cyclotron.

The rate of nuclear decay of any given isotope is constant. One way of quantifying the rate is to determine its half-life, the time required for one-half of a sample of the isotope to undergo radioactive decay. The half-life of ^{214}Po (polonium) is 164 μ (microseconds) (0.000164 seconds); that of ^{14}C (carbon 14, used to date archaeologic objects derived from formerly living materials) is 5730 years; that of ^{87}Rb (rubidium) is 4.9×10^{10} years, which is millions of times longer than the highest estimates for the age of the universe.

What Is Technetium?

The radioisotope that is most widely used for nuclear imaging is technetium 99m (Tc 99m), whose atomic number is 43. Technetium is a radioactive metallic element that appears in the spectra of some stars but can be found in only minute quantities on Earth in its natural state. It was the first element to be synthetically produced, as reflected by its name (from Greek *tekhnetos* 'synthetic'). It is produced abundantly, as a waste product of nuclear reactors, by the decay of zirconium 99 (Zr 99). It can also be made by bombarding molybdenum 99 (Mo 99), another nuclear waste product, with deuterium nuclei (two-proton nuclei of H 2, also called heavy hydrogen). The isotope of technetium used in medicine is technetium 99m (the *m* stands for *metastable*), which has a half-life of about 6 hours.

radiation. Another contraindication is recent administration of a radiopharmaceutical, such as radioactive iodine for the treatment of Graves disease, or recent performance of another nuclear diagnostic procedure.

Radiation can be detected and measured in various ways. Like x-rays, radiation exposes photographic film that has been protected from light. A Geiger counter measures radiation by recording its ionizing effect on argon gas. A scintillation counter (from Latin *scintilla* 'spark') contains materials that fluoresce (emit light) when struck by radiation, similar to the coating on a television screen or computer monitor. This fluorescence can be used to expose photographic film or can be converted to an electrical signal.

The earliest nuclear imaging methods employed a rectilinear scanner. This is a scintillation counter that detects radiation from a single

narrow source, the radiation passing through a collimator (a fine slit) to reach the detecting crystal. In order to create an image, such a scanner must track back and forth across the area under study—for instance, the thyroid gland—stopping and starting at predetermined intervals. Radiation detected during each rest is recorded as a darker or lighter spot on light-sensitive paper. In this way a picture is gradually formed, in which darker spots represent zones of higher iodine concentration and lighter spots represent zones of poor iodine uptake.

As with radiography, the application of computer technology to nuclear imaging has greatly broadened its diagnostic potential and permitted the generation of two-dimensional (tomographic) and three-dimensional images. Nowadays most imaging studies are performed with a gamma camera. This is a scintillation counter with many collimators and a complex electronic program that analyzes radiation from many sources at once and fuses the data into a two-dimensional image. This image can be displayed on a television monitor, recorded photographically, and stored digitally.

In multiple-gated acquisition (MUGA) scanning, computer analysis of radionuclide emissions

What Is a Millicurie?

One millicurie (1 mCi) is one thousandth of a curie (0.001 Ci), and a curie is defined as that quantity of a radioisotope that decays at a rate of 3.7×10^{10} disintegrations per second. The curie is named for Marie Curie (1867-1934), born Maria Sklodowska, who received a Nobel Prize for Physics in 1903 in recognition of her isolation of radium, and a Nobel Prize for Chemistry in 1911 in recognition of her further work on radiation.

from the heart results in a composite scan assembled from a series of successive images, all taken at the same point in the cardiac cycle to eliminate blurring due to motion. Comparison of ventricular volumes at the end of diastole and at the end of systole permits calculation of the ejection fraction.

The radioactive tracer used in positron emission tomography (PET) is a man-made isotope whose nuclear decay results in the release of subatomic particles called positrons. Scintillation data are collected simultaneously by a ring of counters surrounding the subject. In a manner analogous to computed tomography (CT), these data are then used to construct a two-dimensional, color-coded image to reflect concentration density.

The glucose analogue 2-(fluorine-18)fluoro-2-deoxy-d-glucose (FDG) is used in positron emission tomography to locate zones of heightened energy metabolism. PET scanning provides valuable information about brain function in Alzheimer and other dementias, parkinsonism, epilepsy, brain tumors, and stroke. This technique is also used to assess coronary blood flow and to study solitary pulmonary nodules and other masses. PET is expensive and can only be performed where there is ready access to a cyclotron (nuclear accelerator) to generate the needed radioisotopes.

Single-photon emission computed tomography (SPECT) is another form of nuclear imaging using computer software to generate two- and three-dimensional images (*see box*). The incorporation of single-photon technology into nuclear imaging greatly improves the contrast and resolution of the images produced. SPECT has found particular application in providing information about regional blood flow, in assessing disorders of the heart and lungs, and in the evaluation of head injuries, seizure disorders, stroke, brain tumors, and dementia.

What Is a Photon?

Electromagnetic radiation, including light, x-rays, and gamma rays, behaves sometimes as a wave motion and sometimes as a stream of particles. Modern physics allows for the possibility that either of these concepts is valid, and even for the possibility that they both are.

A quantum is the smallest discrete unit or particle of anything, including energy, that can exist independently. In the context of a particle theory of radiation, a photon is a quantum of electromagnetic energy, assumed to have zero mass and no electrical charge. A single-photon emission detector is just what its name says—a device that is capable of detecting and recording photons one at a time, instead of responding to bursts or parcels of varying numbers of photons. By way of analogy, a turnstile at an amusement park counts individual visitors, whereas counting shuttle bus arrivals would yield only an approximate estimate of the number of visitors per day.

Ventilation-Perfusion Scan

In this procedure two scans of the lungs are performed in succession with different radionuclides administered by different routes. First a ventilation scan with inhaled radioactive xenon gas is done to show which parts of the lungs are filled with inspired gas and which, if any, are not. After all of the xenon has been washed out of the respiratory tract with ordinary air, technetium Tc 99m macroaggregated albumin is administered intravenously. A second lung scan is then performed to assess the perfusion (circulatory distribution) of radionuclide through lung tissue.

A ventilation-perfusion scan is done when acute pulmonary embolism is suspected, and its rationale is as follows. Pulmonary embolism is blockage of a branch of the pulmonary artery by a clot that has traveled from elsewhere in the circulation, usually from a vein in a lower limb. Although such blockage may be evident on a simple perfusion scan, an abnormal scan can also result if a zone of lung tissue has poor circulation because of pre-existing disease. Hence a ventilation scan is also done, so that any areas of lung tissue with chronic impairment of circulation can be identified. A ventilation-perfusion mismatch—an area with normal ventilation but blocked perfusion—probably represents a zone of acute pulmonary artery blockage due to embolism.

The incorrect expression V/Q scan is sometimes applied to this procedure by confusion with a different type of pulmonary study involving blood gas analysis.

Bone Scintigraphy (Bone Scan)

The isotopic tracer technetium Tc 99m methylene diphosphonate (MDP), administered intravenously, binds to apatite (the crystalline calcium compound of which bone largely consists). The tracer is taken up in higher amounts by areas of bone in which there is heightened osteoblastic activity (new bone formation). This technique is useful in detecting osteomyelitis (infection of bone marrow), primary and metastatic tumors of bone, and subtle fractures missed by x-ray studies (including stress fractures, vertebral fractures due to sports injuries, and pathologic fractures due to osteoporosis or corticosteroid therapy). It may also be used to screen a child with unexplained evidence of trauma for abuse. Findings on technetium bone scanning are somewhat nonspecific, and must be interpreted in the light of the patient's history and physical findings and the results of other tests. Other radioisotopic tracers (gallium, technetium-labeled WBCs) may be useful in distinguishing changes due to infection from those due to trauma or metabolic bone disease.

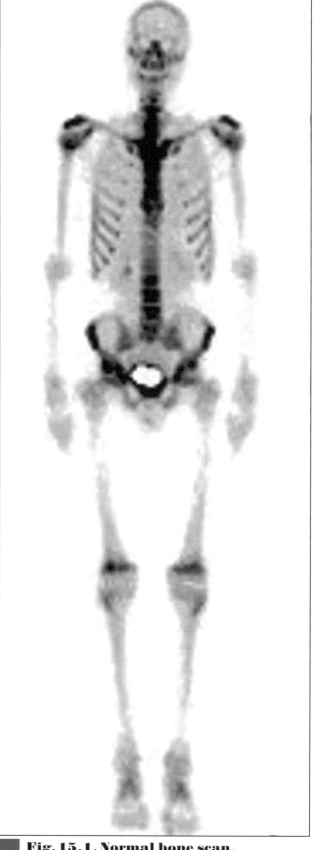

Fig. 15.1. Normal bone scan.

Copyright Imaginis Corporation: http://imaginis.com/cancer/cancer_medicalimaging.asp

Radionuclides Used in Diagnostic Imaging

fluorine F 18   Half-life: 1.9 hr
  fluorine F 18 2-(fluorine-18) fluoro-2-deoxy-
  d-glucose (FDG)

gallium Ga 67   Half-life: 78 hr
  gallium Ga 67 citrate (Neoscan, Hepatolite)
  gallium Ga 67 citrate-labeled white blood
  cells

indium In 111   Half-life: 2.8 days
  indium In 111 capromab pendetide
    (Prosta-Scint)
  indium In 111 labeled platelets
  indium In 111 labeled white blood cells
  indium In 111 oxime
  indium In 111 oxyquinoline
  indium In 111 pentetate disodium
    (In 111 DTPA)
  indium In 111 pentreotide (Octreoscan)
  indium In 111 satumomab pendetide
    (OncoScint CR/OV)
  indium In 113m Half-life: 1.6 hr
  indium In 113m colloid

iodine I 123   Half-life: 13.2 hr
  iodine I 123 sodium iodohippurate
    (Nephroflow)
  iodine I 123 iofetamine (Spectamine)

iodine I 125   Half-life: 60.1 days
  iodine I 125 albumin (Jeanatope)
  iodine I 125 human serum albumin
    (I 125 RISA, IHSA, Isojex)
  iodine I 125 iothalamate (Glofil)

iodine I 131   Half-life: 8 days
  iodine I 131 albumin (Megatope)
  iodine I 131 albumin aggregate
    (Albumotope L S)
  iodine I 131 iodomethylnorcholesterol
    (I 131 NP-59)

iodine I 131 metaiodobenzylguanidine
  (I 131 mIBG)
iodine I 131 sodium iodide (I 131 NaI)
iodine I 131 sodium iodohippurate
  (Hippuran, Hipputope)

technetium Tc 99m   Half-life: 6 hr
  technetium Tc 99m albumin aggregate
    (Lungaggregate, Macrotec, MPI MAA,
    Pulmolite, TechneScan MAA)
  technetium Tc 99m albumin colloid
    (Microlite)
  technetium Tc 99m apcitide (Acutect)
  technetium Tc 99m arcitumomab
    (CEA-Scan)
  technetium Tc 99m biciromab
  technetium Tc 99m bicisate (Neurolite)
  technetium Tc 99m depreotide (Neotect)
  technetium Tc 99m disofenin (diisopropyl
    IDA, Tc 99m DISIDA, Hepatolite)
  technetium Tc 99m ethyl cysteinate dimer
    (Tc 99m ECD)
  technetium Tc 99m etidronate (hydroxy-
    ethilidene diphosphonate, Tc 99m
    HEDSPA, Tc 99m EHDP, Osteoscan)
  technetium Tc 99m exametazine (hexam-
    ethylpropyleneamine oxime, HMPAO,
    Ceretec)
  technetium Tc 99m ferpentetate
  technetium Tc 99m furifosmin
  technetium Tc 99m gluceptate (Tc 99m
    glucoheptonate, Tc 99m GH,
    Glucoscan)
  technetium Tc 99m human albumin
    microspheres (Tc 99m HAM)
  technetium Tc 99m human serum albumin
    (Tc 99m HSA)
  technetium Tc 99m labeled red blood cells
    (Tc 99m RBC, RBC-Scan, Ultratag)
  technetium Tc 99m labeled white blood cells
    (Tc 99m WBC)
  technetium Tc 99m lidofenin HIDA
    (TechneScan HIDA)

technetium Tc 99m macroaggregated
albumin

technetium Tc 99m mebrofenin (trimethyl-
bromo-IDA, Choletec)

technetium Tc 99m medronate (methylene
diphosphonate, MDP, Amerscam
MDP, Osteolite)

technetium Tc 99m mertiatide (mercapto-
acetyltriglycine, Tc 99m MAG,
TechneScan MAG3)

technetium Tc 99m micisate (Neurolite)

technetium Tc 99m (N (2,6-dimethyl-
phenylcarboylmethyl) iminodiacetic
acid, Technescan)

technetium Tc 99m oxidronate
(Tc 99m HDP, Osteoscan HDP)

technetium Tc 99m pamidronate
(aminohydroxypropane diphosphonate)

technetium Tc 99m pentetate (diethylene-
triamine pentaacetic acid, Tc 99m
DTPA)

technetium Tc 99m pentetreotide
(Octreo-Scan)

technetium Tc 99m pyrophosphate
(Tc 99m PYP, AN-Pyrotec, Phosphotec,
Pyrolite, TechneScan PYP)

technetium Tc 99m satumomab pendetide
(Onco-Scint CR/OV)

technetium Tc 99m sestamibi (methyloxy-
isobutyl isonitrile, Tc 99m MIBI,
Cardiolite)

technetium Tc 99m siboroxime

technetium Tc 99m sodium medronate
(methylene diphosphonate,
Tc 99m MDP)

technetium Tc 99m sodium pertechnetate

technetium Tc 99m succimer
(dimercaptosuccinic acid,
Tc 99m DMSA)

technetium Tc 99m sulfur colloid
(Tc 99m SC)

technetium Tc 99m teboroxime (CardioTec)

technetium Tc 99m tetrofosmin (Myoview)

thallium Tl 201 Half-life: 73 hr
thallium Tl 201 sodium chloride
thallium Tl 201thallous chloride

xenon Xe 127 Half-life: 36.4 days
xenon Xe 127

xenon Xe 133 Half-life: 5.3 days
xenon Xe 133

Exercises

Fill in the Blanks

1. Some isotopes of certain elements (and all isotopes of elements with atomic numbers above 89) are unstable, undergoing a steady nuclear decay accompanied by a discharge of energy in various forms; this discharge of energy is known as _____.

2. One way of quantifying the rate of nuclear decay of any given isotope is to determine its _____, the time required for _____ of a sample of the isotope to undergo radioactive decay.

3. Strictly speaking, the term _____ refers only to radioisotopes that are administered for therapeutic purposes.

4. The basis of all nuclear diagnosis is the introduction into the body, by ingestion, injection, inhalation, or some other route, of a _____—a substance that has been tagged or labeled by having a radioactive isotope incorporated into its chemical structure.

5. _____ is the most widely used radioisotope in nuclear imaging.

6. The dosage of a radioisotopic tracer is measured in _____.

7. A _____ measures radiation by recording its ionizing effect on argon gas.

8. A _____ is defined as that quantity of a radioisotope that decays at a rate of 3.7×10^{10} disintegrations per second.

9. In _____ scanning, computer analysis of radionuclide emissions from the heart results in a composite scan assembled from a series of successive images, all taken at the same point in the cardiac cycle to eliminate blurring due to motion.

10. The radioactive tracer used in _____ is a man-made isotope whose nuclear decay results in the release of subatomic particles called positrons.

11. The abbreviation PET stands for _____.

12. The abbreviation SPECT stands for _____.

13. The _____ scan is done with inhaled radioactive xenon gas to show which parts of the lungs are filled with inspired gas and which, if any, are not.

14. A second lung scan is performed with IV technetium Tc 99m macroaggregated albumin to assess the _____ (circulatory distribution) of radionuclide through lung tissue.

Exercises

15. _____ is blockage of a branch of the pulmonary artery by a clot that has traveled from elsewhere in the circulation, usually from a vein in a lower limb.

16. The isotopic tracer technetium Tc 99m methylene diphosphonate (MDP), administered intravenously, binds to _____ (the crystalline calcium compound of which bone largely consists).

17. The term _____ activity refers to new bone formation.

18. The term _____ refers to infection of bone marrow.

Multiple Choice: Circle the letter of the best answer from the choices given.

1. An area of increased uptake of radioisotope corresponding to the position of a nodule in the thyroid gland suggesting that the nodule consists of hyperactive thyroid tissue is referred to as
   A. Radioactivity.
   B. A hot zone.
   C. A cold nodule.
   D. A radioisotope.
   E. A tracer.

2. _____ is more likely to represent a malignant tumor, which is unable to concentrate iodine like normal thyroid tissue.
   A. Radioactivity.
   B. A hot zone.
   C. A cold nodule.
   D. A radioisotope.
   E. A tracer.

3. A device that contains materials that fluoresce (emit light) when struck by radiation, which fluorescence can be used to expose photographic film or can be converted to an electrical signal, is the
   A. Geiger counter
   B. Gamma camera.
   C. Rectilinear scanner.
   D. Collimator.
   E. Scintillation counter.

Exercises

4. A fine slit through which the radiation passes to reach the detecting crystal is a
   A. Geiger counter
   B. Gamma camera.
   C. Rectilinear scanner.
   D. Collimator.
   E. Scintillation counter.

5. Most imaging studies are performed with a _____, a scintillation counter with many collimators and a complex electronic program that analyzes radiation from many sources at once and fuses the data into a two-dimensional image.
   A. Geiger counter
   B. Gamma camera.
   C. Radiopharmaceutical.
   D. Collimator.
   E. Rectilinear scanner.

6. A nuclear imaging procedure used to determine the ejection fraction of the ventricles of the heart is the
   A. MUGA scan.
   B. HIDA scan.
   C. PET scan.
   D. SPECT scan.
   E. Ventilation-perfusion scan.

7. The imaging agent of choice used in positron emission tomography (PET) to locate zones of heightened energy metabolism is
   A. Gallium Ga 67.
   B. Indium In 111.
   C. Technetium Tc 99m.
   D. Glucose analogue 2-(fluorine-18)fluoro-2-deoxy-d-glucose (FDG).
   E. Iodine I 123.

8. A nuclear imaging procedure used to outline the biliary tract, showing obstruction by stones or tumor is the
   A. MUGA scan.
   B. Ventilation-perfusion scan.
   C. PET scan.
   D. SPECT scan.
   E. HIDA scan.

Exercises

9. A nuclear imaging procedure used when acute pulmonary embolism is suspected is the
   A. MUGA scan.
   B. HIDA scan.
   C. PET scan.
   D. SPECT scan.
   E. Ventilation-perfusion scan.

Short Answers

1. Define or explain:
   a. HIDA scan _____
   _____

   b. isotope _____
   _____

   c. photon _____
   _____

   d. ventilation-perfusion scan _____
   _____

2. What is the essential difference between nuclear imaging and all other standard imaging techniques?
   _____
   _____
   _____
   _____

3. List some situations in which nuclear imaging is standard.
   _____
   _____
   _____
   _____

Exercises

4. List some circumstances in which nuclear imaging would not be feasible.

    _____

    _____

    _____

    _____

5. List some nuclear imaging procedures that might be performed in emergency situations.

    _____

    _____

    _____

    _____

6. How is the mass number of an isotope represented?

    _____

    _____

7. Why is a simple perfusion scan often not adequate to diagnosed acute pulmonary embolism?

    _____

    _____

    _____

    _____

Activities for Application and Further Study

1. The isotope ^{14}C (carbon 14) is used to date archaeologic objects derived from formerly living materials. Using a pharmaceutical reference book (or the Internet), find a medical diagnostic use for carbon 14.

2. Until recently, PET scanning was primarily a research procedure. Why do you think this was the case? Support your answer.

3. Find on the Internet color images of MUGA, HIDA, PET, and SPECT scans. What differences do you see in the images? Can you identify the structures being studied?

Anatomic Pathology

Pathology is the branch of medicine that studies the structural and functional changes produced in the living body by injury or disease. The application of pathologic information to medical practice occurs at several levels.

First, pathology is one of the basic sciences, along with anatomy, biochemistry, physiology, and pharmacology, learned during the preclinical years of medical school. Knowledge of the effects of specific diseases on the structure and function of specific organs and tissues governs, to a great extent, a physician's approach to the evaluation, diagnosis, and treatment of patients.

Second, in an effort to learn the nature, cause, and extent of disease in a particular patient, and also to assess the effects of treatment, the physician may subject various tissues, fluids, or other materials removed from the patient's body to pathologic examination. Tests of blood and urine are part of any thorough diagnostic evaluation. Organs and tissues removed during surgical procedures are routinely submitted to a pathologist for gross and microscopic study. The information obtained from this study helps to confirm the preoperative diagnosis and, in cases of malignancy, to determine the extent of disease and the adequacy of surgical removal.

A third application of pathology to practical medicine occurs when an autopsy is performed to discover the cause of the patient's death and to correlate the medical history with postmortem findings. Besides providing data for official certification of the cause of death, autopsy findings may have great legal importance—for example, in a case of suspected homicide. In addition, information about the cause of death and the precise nature of the patient's disease contributes to the unending learning process of the treating physician and of other health professionals who attend the autopsy as an educational experience.

Under ordinary circumstances, autopsies and pathologic examinations of tissue specimens are performed by pathologists—physicians with postdoctoral training and certification by the American Board of Pathology. The pathologist's examination of specimens is not limited to naked-eye inspection but also includes microscopic examination and perhaps chemical or other testing. For this reason, pathology is a laboratory-based specialty, and the majority of pathologists perform at least a part of their professional activities in hospitals.

The practice of pathology is divided into three principal branches. Anatomic pathology is concerned with the gross and microscopic changes brought about in living human tissues by disease. Clinical pathology refers to the laboratory examination of bodily fluids and waste products such as blood, spinal fluid, urine, and feces. Forensic pathology involves the application of knowledge comprised by the other two branches to certain issues in both civil and criminal law. The practice of forensic pathology is largely confined to official settings. The standard pathology residency lasts four years, the training time being variously divided between anatomic and clinical pathology. Pathologists who serve as medical examiners, coroners, or forensic consultants usually have additional training in forensic pathology.

Much of the day-by-day work in clinical pathology is done by medical technologists. These are specially trained nonphysicians who, under the supervision of a pathologist, perform routine laboratory examinations of blood, urine, and other fluids, and prepare tissue specimens for microscopic examination by a pathologist. Clinical pathology is discussed in Chapters 19-24.

Normal Anatomy and Histology

16

Gross and Microscopic Anatomy: General Concepts

The essence of anatomic pathology practice is observing and interpreting changes or variations from the normal or expected appearance of tissues. Hence the pathologist must be intimately familiar with the gross and microscopic features of normal, healthy tissue, and pathology reports typically contain many references to such features. This chapter provides a concise survey of gross and microscopic anatomy, with emphasis on terminology.

For purposes of description and discussion, the human body is divided into several systems, each having a general biological function. For example, the function of the digestive system is to take in nutrients and dispose of associated wastes. Each system is composed of organs. An organ is defined as an anatomically differentiated and isolated structure with a specific function. Each of the organs that compose the digestive system—esophagus, stomach, small and large intestines, salivary glands, liver, gallbladder, pancreas—has its specific role in the overall process of digestion.

Organs are composed of tissues, each of which, when subjected to microscopic examination, is found to have a characteristic and more or less homogeneous composition. The stomach, for example, consists of three concentric layers, each containing a different type of tissue. The innermost layer is a lining of mucous membrane; the intermediate layer is a sheath of muscle; and the outermost layer is a coating of connective tissue.

A tissue is made up of cells. The cell is the smallest and simplest independent unit of living matter. Although all cells have certain features in common, many are highly specialized in structure and function. The cells of the lining of the stomach, for example, can be divided into undifferentiated columnar epithelial cells, which serve mainly as structural units or building blocks; chief cells, which produce the digestive enzyme pepsin; parietal cells, which produce hydrochloric acid; and goblet cells, which produce mucus.

This division and classification of bodily structures is not absolute. For example, the pancreas belongs to the digestive system because it produces digestive enzymes, but it also belongs to the endocrine system because it secretes insulin, glucagon, and other hormones. Some regard the skin and even the blood as organs; others would call the skin a tissue and the blood simply a body fluid. But for practical purposes, the breakdown into systems, organs, tissues, and cells works well.

Solid and Hollow Viscera

The term **viscus** (plural, **viscera**) refers to any of the organs in the thoracic and abdominal cavities. Viscera can conveniently be classed as either solid or hollow organs, each class having its own basic structural plan. It is usual to divide the tissues composing a solid organ such as the liver or the kidney into **parenchyma**, the specialized cells that are unique to the organ and that enable it to perform its function, and **stroma**, the supporting framework of connective tissue. The stroma is also called interstitial tissue. Typically a solid organ is encased in a more or less dense capsule of connective tissue, from which **septa** (walls, divisions) or **trabeculae** (bands, strands) or both extend into the substance of the organ, dividing the parenchyma into small but grossly visible lobules. The more intimate interweaving of parenchyma and stroma is appreciable only on microscopic study.

Besides the partitioning of tissue into lobules, an organ may have several major structural divisions or lobes. The thyroid gland and the left lung have two, the right lung three, the liver four. The term **hilum** refers to a notch or cleft in the contour of an organ, where arteries, veins, ducts, or other structures enter or leave. For example, a ureter, a renal artery, and a renal vein are attached at the hilum of each kidney. The extremities of a vertically positioned organ may be referred to as **poles**—thus, the upper (or superior) pole of the kidney, the lower (or inferior) pole of the testis.

Inspection of the cut surface of certain organs, such as the kidney and the adrenal gland, reveals two grossly distinguishable zones, an outer **cortex** and an inner **medulla**. The difference in appearance between the two zones results from differences in cell type, in the proportion between parenchyma and stroma, and in the orientation of parenchymal elements.

The hollow interior of a tubular structure such as the aorta, the trachea, and the colon is called its **lumen**. Most hollow and tubular organs are made up of layers of different kinds of tissue. Typically there is a lining of epithelium with its basement membrane and lamina propria; then a layer of smooth muscle, often subdivided into an inner layer with fibers running circumferentially and an outer layer with fibers running longitudinally; and finally an outer coat of connective tissue. The terms **tunica** and **lamina** are used as well as English **coat** and **layer** to designate these structural divisions. In medical parlance the mucous lining of a tubular or hollow structure is often called simply the **mucosa** (for **tunica mucosa**); the muscular layer, the **muscularis** (for **tunica muscularis**); the outer layer, the **fibrosa** (for **tunica fibrosa**) in the case of an organ whose covering blends in with surrounding structures, and the **serosa** (for **tunica serosa**) in the case of an organ covered by a serous membrane.

Membranes, Blood Vessels

A **fascia** is a sheet or layer of connective tissue that binds or invests an organ or body region. Subcutaneous fascia of variable thickness is present under the skin over the entire body surface. Muscles and groups of muscles are typically covered and separated by a layer of fascia.

Peritoneum is a continuous serous membrane that covers the entire inner surface of the abdominal cavity and all the organs it contains. The parts of this membrane that cover the walls of the abdominal cavity are called **parietal** peritoneum, and the parts covering the organs are called **visceral** peritoneum. In similar fashion, the parietal and visceral **pleura** respectively line the thoracic cavity and cover the lungs. The parietal and visceral **pericardium** respectively line the pericardium and cover the heart.

Some notion of the circulation of blood through tissues is necessary for an understanding of many basic concepts in pathology. Virtually every tissue in the body except mature cartilage and the central nervous system is filled with a meshwork of microscopic blood vessels, the capillaries, which deliver oxygen and nutrients and remove carbon dioxide and other wastes. Arteries carry oxygenated blood from the left ventricle of the heart to the tissues and organs of the body. The arteries keep branching repeatedly until the branches are of microscopic size. These arterioles branch further to become capillaries, whose walls are composed of a single layer of very thin epithelial cells (endothelium). Capillaries do not pass straight through tissue but branch repeatedly and join other capillaries to form a network. This arrangement of numerous connections among adjacent vessels is called an anastomosis. The flow of blood through a capillary bed is regulated by arterioles, which act as valves by virtue of the smooth-muscle fibers in their walls. For example, capillary flow in the skin is reduced by exposure to cold, increased by exposure to heat.

The joining together of many capillaries forms a venule, and the joining together of many venules forms a vein. Veins carry blood back to the heart to be reoxygenated in the lungs. A major artery is usually accompanied along its course by a vein that drains the structure supplied by the artery, and often by a nerve as well. The combination of an artery, one or more veins, and a nerve is called a **neurovascular bundle**. The vascular supply of a solid viscus usually enters at its hilum. Hollow and tubular organs in the abdominal cavity receive their blood supply through a fold of tissue that also anchors the organ to the body wall. For the small intestine this fold is called the mesentery. By extension, the prefix **mes(o)-** is used to name attachments of other organs: mesoappendix, mesocolon.

Sections and Directions

Certain terms in descriptive anatomy refer to imaginary cuts made through the body or through an organ in various planes. In pathology, such terms are sometimes used in this figurative sense and sometimes refer to actual cuts made through an organ or body part with a knife or microtome. A sagittal section divides a structure into right and left segments; a coronal section, into upper and lower segments; a frontal section, into front and rear segments. A cross (or transverse) section divides an elongated structure at right angles to its long axis (length). A longitudinal section divides an elongated structure parallel to its length.

The following terms are used extensively in discussing anatomic relationships:

anterior—front, toward the front of the body.

caudal—lower in the body.

cranial—higher in the body.

distal—further away from the center of the body or some other point of reference. (The thumb is distal to the wrist.)

dorsal—pertaining to or in the direction of the back.

inferior—lower, downward.

lateral—further away from the midline of the body. (The lungs are lateral to the heart.)

medial—nearer to the midline of the body. (The nipple is medial to the axilla.)

posterior—rear, toward the back.

proximal—nearer to the center of the body or some other point of reference. (The wrist is proximal to the thumb.)

superior—upper, upward.

ventral—pertaining to or in the direction of the front surface of the body.

Microscopic Anatomy and Histology

The Cell

The cell is both the structural and the functional unit of all living things, plant and animal. Each cell is isolated from its surroundings by an enclosing membrane. Each cell, given the proper environment and nutrients, is capable of carrying on all the vital functions proper to it, independently of other cells. Generally speaking, the function or action of a tissue is simply the aggregate of the functions or actions of its cells. The term **protoplasm** is used as a generic designation for all living material, without regard to its organization into cells or tissues.

It is convenient to start by discussing an ideal or typical cell, and then to consider how various types of cells are modified in structure for specific functions. Within each cell is a fluid called **cytoplasm**, which is a colloidal suspension of proteins, amino acids, carbohydrates, and electrolytes in water. The cell membrane is neither an impermeable barrier nor a biologically inert one. It allows water and substances of low molecular weight such as sodium, calcium, glucose, and amino acids to pass into and out of the cell. Only in special circumstances, however, can it be traversed by more complex substances such as enzymes and nucleoproteins. Moreover, the cell membrane actively "pumps" certain substances in and others out. This accounts for the higher concentration of potassium in a living cell than in its immediate environment, and the lower concentration of sodium.

The most conspicuous internal feature of a cell is generally its **nucleus**, a dense and roughly spherical mass of protein, DNA, and RNA, which controls such cellular functions as energy metabolism and protein synthesis. The nucleus also contains the genetic coding that determines what kind of cell this is, and that will be passed on to any daughter cells formed from it. Although all cells in the human body contain in their nuclei the genetic coding received from parental sperm and oocyte, only spermatozoa and oocytes have the capacity to transmit this genetic material to a new individual. The nucleolus is a sharply defined body containing RNA that is often visible within the nucleus.

The growth of any tissue or organ comes about mainly through an increase in the number of its cells. An adult has more cells, not larger cells, than a child. In cell multiplication, one cell divides into two identical daughter cells, each of which is endowed with a full complement of genetic material, and nothing except these daughter cells remains of the parent cell. As a preliminary to cell division, the nucleus undergoes a splitting of its genetic material into two equal portions. In this process, which is called mitosis, the normally tangled chromatin material composing the nucleus separates into clearly distinguishable bands of DNA called chromosomes.

The appearance of these "mitotic figures" in a high proportion of the cells of a tissue indicates that the tissue is actively growing or developing. Most cells retain throughout life their ability to undergo mitosis and cell division when this is necessary for growth, the repair of injury, or the replacement of dead or diseased cells. Nerve cells of the central nervous system, by exception, lose their ability to reproduce even before fetal development is complete.

Other structural elements besides the nucleus can be seen in the cytoplasm of some cells. These, collectively known as organelles or organoids, include mitochondria, microsomes, the central body or centrosome, and the Golgi apparatus. Much of the ultrastructure of the cell can be seen only by electron microscopy, and is therefore not germane to routine pathology work. However, standard histologic preparations often show cytoplasmic granules that are characteristic of certain cells. In addition, the cytoplasm of some cells may contain pigment, fat globules, or minute bubbles of air or gas called vacuoles.

While many cells are strictly limited by their genetic makeup to a single form and function,

others have the capacity to undergo marked changes in type and structure to meet the evolving needs of the tissues in which they reside. Some cells are capable of traveling or migrating through tissue in response to various chemical stimuli. For example, neutrophils in great numbers can move from the blood through capillary walls and into injured or diseased tissue as part of an inflammatory response. Cells that are actively motile in a fluid medium are said to show ameboid movement—that is, movement like that of the amebas, one-celled animal organisms. In ameboid movement an extrusion of the cell called a pseudopod is first put forward, and then the rest of the cell "flows" into it.

In most tissues, cells are arranged in sheets, strands, clusters, tubules, sacs, or other characteristic patterns depending on their function. These groups of cells are held together by bands or bridges of protein between their membranes. The term syncytium refers to a complex of originally distinct cells that have fused to form a continuous mass of protoplasm with many nuclei but no intervening cell membranes. Cells are surrounded by or immersed in an intercellular fluid similar in composition to cytoplasm. This serves as a medium for the diffusion of nutrients, oxygen, and wastes in appropriate directions.

Many tissues contain large proportions of noncellular material. For example, connective tissue consists largely of fibers formed by cells but structurally distinct from them. In some tissues, such as the outer (cornified) layers of the skin, cells that have lost their nuclei and ceased to live remain for a time as essential structural elements.

All of the cells of the body have developed from a single fertilized oocyte. This development involves not only a vast increase in the number of cells but also their differentiation into many structural and functional types. As we proceed to a discussion of the various types of cells found in the human body, the reader is urged to keep in mind that cell descriptions are based primarily on the appearance of dead cells that have been chemically preserved, dehydrated, and hardened, sliced into transparent sections, and artificially colored. An appearance or finding that results from the technique used to prepare a slide, rather than from any natural or pathologic process, is called an **artifact.** Vacuolation, shrinkage, and distortion of cells are often artifactual rather than pathologic in origin.

Most tissues do not take up chemical stains evenly. Nuclear material, which is slightly acidic, attracts basic (alkaline) stains such as hematoxylin. Cytoplasm and non-nuclear material attract acidic stains such as eosin. Many cells and tissue components are identified by and named for their staining properties: eosinophil 'attracting eosin,' basophil 'attracting basic stains,' chromophobe 'repelling (literally, 'fearing') color,' argentaffin 'having an affinity for silver stains,' and so on.

Tissues

The tissues of the body can be divided into a relatively small number of types on the basis of characteristic cells, structural organization, similarity of function, and common embryonic origin. For most purposes, a classification into five tissue types—epithelium, connective tissue, muscle, nerve, and hemolymphatic—is sufficiently specific.

Epithelium

Most of the surfaces in the body, including skin and mucous membranes, the linings of hollow and tubular organs in the digestive, respiratory, and urogenital systems, and the linings of the chest and abdominal cavities, consist of a tissue called epithelium. Epithelial tissue is made up almost entirely of cells, with very little intercellular material. Epithelial cells show a marked capacity for regeneration, and in some epithelial tissues, such as the lining of the digestive tract, the turnover under normal conditions is very rapid.

Epithelial cells vary considerably in shape and arrangement, depending on whether their princi-

pal function is to contain, to conduct, or to protect (*see Fig. 16.1*). Epithelial cells are classified according to shape as squamous (flat, scalelike), cuboidal, or columnar. Simple epithelium consists of but a single layer of cells; in stratified epithelium there are several layers. The term **pseudostratified** is applied to certain simple columnar epithelial surfaces where variation in the positions of nuclei creates the illusion of several layers.

The free surface of an epithelial cell may show modifications of various kinds. For example, the pseudostratified columnar epithelium lining the trachea and bronchi is equipped with whiplike cilia that, by their beating motion, keep the mucus film moving upward toward the pharynx. The brush border of certain cells in the kidney, the striated border of certain cells in the intestine, and the microvilli of cells in several areas are further examples of surface modifications. Underlying a zone of epithelium and separating it from deeper structures is a distinct layer of connective tissue called the basement membrane.

Some specialized epithelial cells have secretory capabilities. A secretory cell is one that produces a chemical substance whose functions are performed outside the cell. Such cells secrete mucus, digestive enzymes, and hormones. Secretory epithelium is known as glandular tissue, and any structure that is differentiated to produce a secretion may be called a gland.

Most glandular cells are cuboidal or columnar in shape. Some contain distinctive cytoplasmic granules representing stored secretions or their chemical precursors. A gland may consist of a single cell, such as the goblet cell, which releases its secretion of mucus directly into the interior of the trachea, stomach, or intestine. Or a group of secretory cells may be arranged in a cup- or flask-shaped acinus or alveolus. A number of these acini (alveoli) may be disposed around a single duct, which carries away their secretion, and a number of such ducts may unite to form a larger duct.

Throughout the respiratory and digestive tracts are found numerous alveolar glands whose

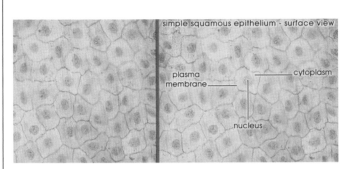

surface view, simple squamous epithelium

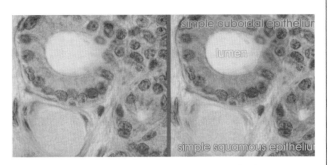

simple cuboidal epithelium, kidney tubules in cross section

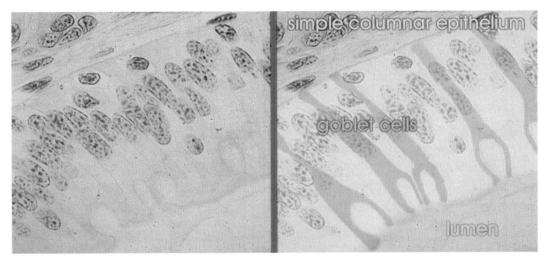

simple columnar epithelium (intestinal lining)

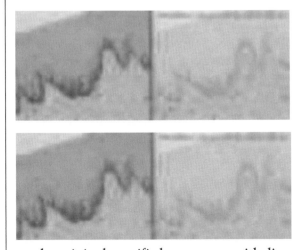

nonkeratinized stratified squamous epithelium

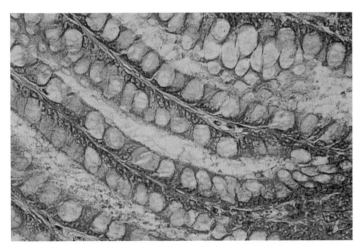

tubular glands lined with simple cuboidal epithelium, colon—intestinal glands

Fig. 16.1. Types of epithelium. Images created by P. Gregory, Biology Laboratory Specialist at Tyler Junior College, http://science.tjc.edu/images/histology/epithelium.htm; tubular glands from Betsy Ott, Tyler Junior College, Tyler, TX.

secretions lubricate the lining surfaces. Serous glands produce a thin, watery secretion, while mucous glands produce a thicker secretion containing the protein mucin. Some gland alveoli contain cells of both serous and mucous types. Glandular structures with ducts (such as the salivary glands and the mammary glands) are called exocrine. Glands that release their secretions directly into the circulation (such as the thyroid and adrenal glands) are called endocrine or ductless glands, and their secretions are called hormones.

Certain terms and concepts regarding epithelium need clarification here. The epithelial lining found in most internal organs and ducts is known as mucous membrane (membrana mucosa) or simply mucosa. A mucous membrane may consist of squamous, cuboidal, or columnar cells. Beneath its basement membrane is a loose connective tissue layer called the lamina propria. Most mucous membranes are supplied with mucous glands that keep the surface lubricated. The mucosa of much of the urinary tract, however, despite its name, contains no mucous glands.

The type of epithelium that lines the pericardium, thorax, and abdomen and covers the organs they contain is called a serous membrane or serosa. Here, again, the term is misleading, for serosal surfaces do not contain serous glands. They are lubricated by a watery fluid filtered from the blood. The type of epithelium found in serosal surfaces is called mesothelium, and the type lining blood vessels is called endothelium. Both mesothelium and endothelium consist of very thin, flat, polygonal cells, but the terms refer to the location of the epithelium in each case rather than to its structural characteristics.

Connective Tissue

The term **connective tissue** includes bone, cartilage, tendons, ligaments, the dermis or true skin, subcutaneous fat, and many other supporting and investing structures. Connective tissues are, so to speak, the timbers, nails, bricks, and mortar of

the body. While varying greatly in composition, all connective tissues have certain features in common. They contain a higher proportion of noncellular material than other tissues, chiefly because bundles and networks of fibers provide more strength, cohesion, and durability than aggregations of living cells. The cells and fibers of connective tissue are embedded in a homogeneous, nonfibrous, gel-like material called ground substance, which is distinct from the intercellular fluid also present.

Connective-tissue cells are relatively few in type. The **fibroblast** (or fibrocyte) is a large flat cell with several branches or processes that extend through the surrounding tissue and may touch the processes of other fibroblasts. The function of the fibroblast is to produce fibers. In mature, healthy connective tissue, the fibroblasts are few and not especially active. In tissue that is growing or undergoing repair, fibroblasts are more numerous and more active.

Histiocytes (also called macrophages) are large cells of irregular shape, with small nuclei. They are at least functionally related to certain other cells found throughout the body and known generically as phagocytes. All of these cells have the property of surrounding and engulfing or "swallowing" foreign material, bacteria or other invading microorganisms, and degenerating or diseased tissue elements, which they then break down and remove.

Small, round, or oval **plasma cells,** which differentiate from B lymphocytes in bone marrow and produce antibodies, are found sparsely distributed in most connective tissues. **Mast cells** are large oval cells that produce and store complex chemical substances, including histamine and heparin, for release as needed. Certain tissues contain highly specialized pigment cells which produce and store the pigment responsible for the color of the skin and the iris of the eye. Bone and cartilage also contain specialized cells that will be described shortly.

Each connective-tissue fiber is actually a bundle of fibrils. Although fibrils do not branch, fibers do branch and interconnect. Connective-tissue fibers are divided on the basis of their physical characteristics into collagenous, elastic, and reticular. **Collagenous** fibers are larger in caliber and tougher than the other types. **Elastic** fibers are thinner and, as their name implies, more elastic. They show a greater tendency to form webs or lattices. **Reticular** fibers are still more delicate and still more apt to form fine networks. They have an affinity for silver stains but do not show well in routine histologic preparations. Reticular cells, found typically in association with networks of reticular fibers, are probably modified fibroblasts but may be more closely related to histiocytes.

Connective tissue can be divided on the basis of its structural organization into six distinct types. **Loose** (or areolar) **connective tissue** consists of freely woven meshes of fibers with many open spaces filled by ground substance and intercellular fluid. This type of tissue is found in the subcutaneous fascia and in the stroma or structural framework of solid organs such as the liver, kidney, and pancreas. **Dense connective tissue** (also called regular connective tissue), which shows a more compact arrangement of fibers in sheets or cords, occurs in ligaments, tendons, and the dermis. **Reticular connective tissue**, consisting of reticular fibers and reticular cells, forms the framework of lymphoid organs (spleen and lymph nodes) and of bone marrow.

Adipose or fatty **tissue** consists mostly of specialized cells packed tightly in a sparse fibrous matrix. Each cell contains a large fat globule, which displaces the cytoplasm and pushes the nucleus against one side of the cell. Fatty tissue serves as a shock absorber and thermal insulator. It is distributed in variable amounts in the subcutaneous tissue and forms cushioning layers around certain organs such as the kidney and the eye.

Cartilage has a highly condensed but elastic ground substance that lends it both toughness and flexibility. Dense aggregations of fibers are embedded in this ground substance. Relatively rare cartilage cells or chondrocytes are also seen, each occupying a hollow space or lacuna in the cartilage. Chondrocytes have large nuclei and their cytoplasm contains fine granules and fat droplets. They are active in the formation and growth of cartilage but relatively inert in mature tissue. Regeneration of damaged cartilage occurs only to a limited extent.

Three types of cartilage are identified. **Hyaline cartilage**, by far the most abundant, contains collagenous fibers. It is found in the nose, larynx, trachea, and bronchi, and as a covering for the joint surfaces of bones. **Elastic cartilage** (also called yellow cartilage from its gross appearance) contains elastic fibers. It occurs in the external ear and the epiglottis. **Fibrous cartilage** (or fibrocartilage) features an extremely dense aggregation of collagenous fibers that make it particularly tough. It is found in the intervertebral disks.

Bone derives its unique rigidity from its calcium content. It is formed by the deposition of minute crystals of calcium salts either in a connective-tissue matrix (intramembranous bone, as in the cranial vault) or by replacement of hyaline cartilage (intracartilaginous or enchondral bone, as in the long bones of the extremities). The microscopic structural unit of bone is the osteon or haversian system, consisting of ten or more thin layers called lamellae arranged concentrically around a haversian canal. These haversian canals branch and intersect to serve as passages for blood vessels and nerves. Osteocytes, the characteristic cells of bone, appear in lacunae from which radiate numerous fine channels or canaliculi to accommodate the delicate processes extending from the cells. Osteoblasts are cuboidal cells with eccentric nuclei and basophilic cytoplasmic granules, which appear in developing, growing, healing, or regenerating bone. In areas where damaged or diseased bone is being broken down, multinucleated giant cells called osteoclasts are often found. These apparently arise by transformation and fusion of osteoblasts.

Muscle

The third major tissue type is muscle. All muscle tissue consists of bundles or sheets of long, narrow cells arranged in parallel and having the capacity to shorten under appropriate electrochemical stimulation. The collective effect of the simultaneous shortening of many thousands of muscle cells is a contraction of the muscle as a whole. Muscle tissue is divided into three distinct types.

Smooth muscle (so called by contrast with striped muscle, to be discussed shortly) consists of long, spindle-shaped cells usually found tightly packed together in sheets. Smooth muscle is also called involuntary muscle because it responds only to stimuli from the autonomic nervous system and is not under voluntary control. Smooth muscle forms part of the walls of tubular and hollow organs, including most of the structures in the respiratory, digestive, and urinary tracts, and of blood vessels other than capillaries. Smooth muscle also appears in the skin (where it is responsible for making hairs stand on end), the iris, and the spleen.

Skeletal, striped, or voluntary **muscle** is the type found in the large muscle masses of the trunk and extremities, which hold the body erect and serve for locomotion and other voluntary activities. Each of the voluntary muscles is made up of long cylindrical strands or fibers, which are bunched into groups called fasciculi. Muscle fibers, unlike those of connective tissue, are composed of living cells, several hundred cells sometimes combining to form a single fiber. The term striped refers to the fine, regular cross striations that are characteristic of skeletal-muscle fibers. This banded or striped appearance results from the arrangement in alternating layers of two proteins, actin and myosin, which are involved in muscle contraction. Changes in the bulk of a skeletal muscle due to exercise or wasting reflect changes in the size of muscle fibers, not changes in their numbers. Each muscle fiber is covered by a membrane called a sarcolemma. The small amount of delicate connective tissue between fibers is known as endomysium.

Cardiac muscle, found only in the heart, makes up nearly the whole of that organ. In microscopic appearance it closely resembles skeletal muscle. A unique feature of cardiac muscle is the presence of intercalated disks, which are irregular transverse bands lying at the junctions of two cells.

Nerve

Nervous tissue is the most highly specialized type of tissue in the body, and nerve cells show the most extreme differentiation of structure. The unique property of all nerve cells is to conduct electrochemical impulses. Each nerve cell, or neuron, consists of a cell body (or perikaryon) with one or more processes extending from it. These processes, which function like the wires or terminals of an electrical device, are divided into two types. Dendrites, relatively short and extensively branching, generally conduct impulses toward the cell body, while axons, long and less branched, generally carry impulses away from the cell body. The axon of a spinal cord cell may be more than 50 cm long. Most neurons have relatively large nuclei with prominent nucleoli. In addition, the cytoplasm of neurons contains a coarsely granular basophilic material rich in DNA, which is called Nissl substance.

The nervous system is a complex network of neurons, vastly more intricate in its circuitry than any possible computer. Particularly in the central nervous system—the brain and spinal cord—neurons are densely packed together in intimate physical and electrical association. The point where the process of one neuron makes electrochemical contact with the process or body of another neuron is called a synapse. A nerve fiber is simply the axon of a nerve cell. Typically these fibers or axons are grouped together, in bundles of hundreds or thousands, to form the nerve tracts within the central nervous system as well as the peripheral nerves extending from it to all parts of the body. White matter is nerve tissue in the central nervous system that consists principally of fibers (axons), and gray matter is nerve tissue consisting principally of cell bodies. A ganglion is a mass of nerve cell bodies adjacent to a peripheral nerve.

In peripheral nerves, each axon is covered by a fine membrane, the neurilemma or sheath of Schwann, which consists of delicate Schwann cells wrapped around the axon. In addition, some axons carry a coating of fatty material called myelin inside the neurilemma. This myelin (or medullary) sheath shows constrictions, the nodes of Ranvier, at intervals along its course where two Schwann cells adjoin. Neurons vary greatly in the type and arrangement of their processes, depending on their function. As noted earlier, nerve cells do not normally undergo mitosis after fetal development is complete, nor can one kind of nerve cell mutate or metamorphose into another type. However, as the central nervous system matures, nerve cell processes extend, become more numerous and more complex, and establish an increasing number of connections with other neurons.

Axons within the central nervous system lack a neurilemma, but other non-nerve cells are present to serve a supporting function. These are known collectively as neuroglia or simply glia. Neuroglia is seen with difficulty in standard histologic preparations. Glial cells are classified as astrocytes (astroglia), star-shaped cells with many processes, found particularly in the gray matter of the brain and spinal cord; oligodendroglia, smaller cells with fewer processes, found in both gray and white matter; microglia, very small cells resembling fibroblasts in appearance and having phagocytic functions; and ependyma, a columnar epithelium-like tissue lining the cavities of the brain and spinal cord.

Hemolymphatic System

The final class of bodily tissues comprises a group of cells that are found in both the circulating blood and in certain tissues and organs, particularly the bone marrow, the spleen, and the lymph nodes. These may be collectively designated hemolymphatic cells.

Blood consists of a fluid called **plasma** in which various cells or "formed elements" are suspended. Plasma, which is mostly water, contains electrolytes (sodium, potassium, calcium, chloride, bicarbonate), proteins (albumin, globulins), nutrients (glucose, lipids, amino acids), wastes (urea, creatinine), and dissolved gases (oxygen, carbon dioxide). Blood clots when fibrinogen (one of the globulins) is activated to form fibrin. Plasma from which the fibrin has been removed is called serum.

The formed elements of the blood (red blood cells, white blood cells, and platelets) are the subject matter of hematology. Accordingly, they are discussed in Chapter 19.

Lymphoid tissue is not a separate tissue type. It consists simply of large numbers of lymphocytes (small white blood cells with relatively large nuclei, essential components of the immune system) in a meshwork of reticular connective tissue. Lymphocytes develop in this tissue by differentiation from reticular cells. Loose aggregations of lymphoid tissue are found in the intestinal wall and other parts of the body. More highly organized masses of lymphoid tissue occur in the spleen, thymus, lymph nodes, and tonsils.

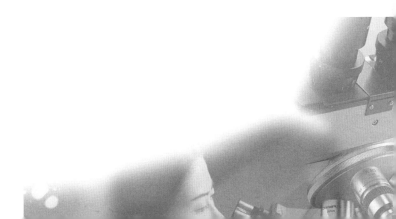

Exercises

Fill in the Blanks

1. _____ is the branch of medicine that studies the structural and functional changes produced in the living body by injury or disease. (Section introduction)

2. _____ are physicians with special postdoctoral training and certification who perform pathologic examinations of tissue specimens and autopsies. (Section introduction)

3. The practice of pathology is divided into three principal branches: _____ is concerned with the gross and microscopic changes brought about in living human tissues by disease; _____ refers to the laboratory examination of bodily fluids and waste products such as blood, spinal fluid, urine, and feces; _____ involves the application of knowledge comprised by the other two branches to certain issues in both civil and criminal law. (Section introduction)

4. _____ are specially trained nonphysicians who, under the supervision of a pathologist, perform routine laboratory examinations of blood, urine, and other fluids, and prepare tissue specimens for microscopic examination by a pathologist. (Section introduction)

5. The human body is divided into several _____, each having a general biological function, and further divided into _____, defined as an anatomically differentiated and isolated structures with a specific function, which are composed of different types of _____, in turn composed of _____, the smallest and simplest independent unit of living matter.

6. The term _____ (plural, _____) refers to any of the organs in the thoracic and abdominal cavities.

7. A solid organ is typically encased in a more or less dense capsule of connective tissue, from which _____ (walls, divisions) or _____ (bands, strands) or both extend into the substance of the organ.

8. Inspection of the cut surface of certain organs, such as the kidney and the adrenal gland, reveals two grossly distinguishable zones, an outer _____ and an inner _____.

9. In medical parlance the mucous lining of a tubular or hollow structure is often called simply the _____ (for _____).

10. In the case of a tubular or hollow organ whose covering blends in with surrounding structures, the outer layer is known as the _____ (for _____).

11. In the case of a tubular or hollow organ covered by a serous membrane, the outer layer is known as the _____ (for _____).

Exercises

12. The parietal and visceral _____ respectively line the pericardium and cover the heart.

13. Virtually every tissue in the body except _____ and the _____ is filled with a meshwork of microscopic blood vessels, the capillaries, which deliver oxygen and nutrients and remove carbon dioxide and other wastes.

14. Arteries branch repeatedly into smaller structures known as _____, which branch into microscopic structures known as _____.

15. The walls of capillaries are composed of a single layer of very thin _____ cells, a structure known as the _____.

16. The joining together of many capillaries forms a _____, and the joining together of many of these forms a _____.

17. Only _____ and _____ have the capacity to transmit genetic coding received from parental sperm and egg to a new individual.

18. As a preliminary to cell division, the nucleus undergoes a splitting of its genetic material into two equal portions, a process called _____.

19. _____ are cells that can move from the blood through capillary walls and into injured or diseased tissue as part of an inflammatory response.

20. An appearance or finding that results from the technique used to prepare a slide, rather than from any natural or pathologic process, is called an _____.

21. Eosinophils, basophils, chromophobes, and argentaffin cells are examples of cells named for their _____.

22. _____ cells are flat and scalelike.

23. The term _____ epithelium refers to epithelium composed of several layers of cells.

24. Underlying a zone of epithelium and separating it from deeper structures is a distinct layer of connective tissue called the _____.

25. A group of secretory cells arranged in a cup- or flask-shaped manner is referred to as an _____ or _____.

26. Glandular structures with ducts (such as the salivary glands and the mammary glands) are called _____.

Exercises

27. Glands that release their secretions directly into the circulation (such as the thyroid and adrenal glands) are called _____ or ductless glands, and their secretions are called _____.

28. The type of epithelium found in serosal surfaces is called _____, and the type lining blood vessels is called _____.

29. The _____ (or _____) is a large flat cell with several branches or processes that extend through surrounding connective tissue and may touch the processes of other cells of the same type.

30. Connective-tissue fibers are divided on the basis of their physical characteristics into _____ fibers, which are larger in caliber and tougher than the other types, _____ fibers, which are thinner and show a greater tendency to form webs or lattices, and _____ fibers, which are still more delicate and still more apt to form fine networks.

31. _____ forms part of the walls of tubular and hollow organs, including most of the structures in the respiratory, digestive, and urinary tracts, and of blood vessels other than capillaries.

32. Three names for the type of muscle that holds the body erect and serves for locomotion and other intentional activities are _____, _____, and _____.

33. A unique feature of _____ muscle is the presence of intercalated disks, which are irregular transverse bands lying at the junctions of two cells.

34. Structures in the nerve cells known as _____, relatively short and extensively branching, generally conduct impulses toward the cell body, while _____, long and less branched, generally carry impulses away from the cell body.

35. Another name for a nerve cell is a _____.

36. _____ are non-nerve cells that serve a supporting function to the axons within the central nervous system.

37. Substances such as electrolytes (sodium, potassium, calcium, chloride, bicarbonate), proteins (albumin, globulins), nutrients (glucose, lipids, amino acids), wastes (urea, creatinine), and dissolved gases (oxygen, carbon dioxide) are found in a component of blood known as _____.

38. _____ consists simply of large numbers of small white blood cells with relatively large nuclei, essential components of the immune system, in a meshwork of reticular connective tissue.

Exercises

Multiple Choice: Circle the letter of the best answer from the choices given.

1.　The cells of the lining of the stomach that serve mainly as structural units or building blocks are
　　A.　Chief cells.
　　B.　Goblet cells.
　　C.　Undifferentiated columnar epithelial cells.
　　D.　Parietal cells.
　　E.　Enucleated cells.

2. The cells of the lining of the stomach that produce the digestive enzyme pepsin are
　　A.　Enucleated cells.
　　B.　Parietal cells.
　　C.　Goblet cells.
　　D.　Undifferentiated columnar epithelial cells.
　　E.　Chief cells.

3.　The cells of the lining of the stomach that produce hydrochloric acid are
　　A.　Parietal cells.
　　B.　Undifferentiated columnar epithelial cells.
　　C.　Chief cells.
　　D.　Enucleated cells.
　　E.　Goblet cells.

4.　The cells of the lining of the stomach that produce mucus are
　　A.　Chief cells.
　　B.　Enucleated cells.
　　C.　Parietal cells.
　　D.　Goblet cells.
　　E.　Undifferentiated columnar epithelial cells.

5.　The specialized cells that are unique to an organ such as the kidney or liver and that enable it to perform its function are known as
　　A.　Hilum.
　　B.　Parenchyma.
　　C.　Interstitial tissue.
　　D.　Stroma.
　　E.　Trabeculae.

Exercises

6. A notch or cleft in the contour of an organ, where arteries, veins, ducts, or other structures enter or leave is known as the
   A. Parenchyma.
   B. Hilum.
   C. Lobe.
   D. Pole.
   E. Stroma.

7. The hollow interior of a tubular structure such as the aorta, the trachea, and the colon is called its
   A. Mucosa.
   B. Stroma.
   C. Lumen.
   D. Tunica.
   E. Lamina.

8. The fascia is defined as
   A. The upper and lower extremities of a vertically positioned organ.
   B. A notch or cleft in the contour of an organ, where arteries, veins, ducts, or other structures enter or leave.
   C. A continuous serous membrane that covers the entire inner surface of the abdominal cavity and all the organs it contains.
   D. A lining of epithelium with its basement membrane and lamina propria.
   E. A sheet or layer of connective tissue that binds or invests an organ or body region.

9. A continuous serous membrane that covers the entire inner surface of the abdominal cavity and all the organs it contains is known as the
   A. Pleura.
   B. Visceral peritoneum.
   C. Peritoneum.
   D. Visceral pleura.
   E. Pericardium.

10. A continuous serous membrane that covers the entire inner surface of the thoracic cavity is known as the
    A. Visceral pleura.
    B. Parietal pleura.
    C. Pericardium.
    D. Visceral peritoneum.
    E. Peritoneum.

Exercises

11. The small intestine receives its blood supply through a fold of tissue, which also anchors it to the body wall, called the
    A. Peritoneum.
    B. Pleura.
    C. Hilum.
    D. Mesentery
    E. Neurovascular bundle.

12. A _____ section divides a structure into upper and lower segments.
    A. Coronal.
    B. Cross.
    C. Frontal.
    D. Longitudinal.
    E. Sagittal.

13. A _____ section divides an elongated structure at right angles to its long axis (length).
    A. Coronal.
    B. Cross.
    C. Frontal.
    D. Longitudinal.
    E. Sagittal.

14. A _____ section divides a structure into right and left segments.
    A. Coronal.
    B. Cross.
    C. Frontal.
    D. Longitudinal.
    E. Sagittal.

15. A _____ section divides a structure into anterior and posterior segments.
    A. Coronal.
    B. Cross.
    C. Frontal.
    D. Longitudinal.
    E. Sagittal.

16. A _____ section divides an elongated structure parallel to its length.
    A. Coronal.
    B. Cross.
    C. Frontal.
    D. Longitudinal.
    E. Sagittal.

Exercises

17. The cell contains a colloidal suspension of proteins, amino acids, carbohydrates, and electrolytes in water known as the
    A. Protoplasm.
    B. Membrane.
    C. Cytoplasm.
    D. Chromosomes.
    E. DNA.

18. A dense and roughly spherical mass of protein, DNA, and RNA, which controls such cellular functions as energy metabolism and protein synthesis, found in the cell is its
    A. Cytoplasm.
    B. Protoplasm.
    C. Chromosomes.
    D. Organelle.
    E. Nucleus.

19. A complex of originally distinct cells that have fused to form a continuous mass of protoplasm with many nuclei but no intervening cell membranes is known as
    A. A syncytium.
    B. A sheet.
    C. A strand.
    D. Stroma.
    E. Epithelium.

20. Tissue made up almost entirely of cells, with very little intercellular material, covering most surfaces of the body, including skin and mucous membranes, the linings of hollow and tubular organs in the digestive, respiratory, and urogenital systems, and the linings of the chest and abdominal cavities can be classified as
    A. Connective tissue.
    B. Epithelial tissue.
    C. Hemolymphatic tissue.
    D. Muscle tissue.
    E. Nerve tissue.

21. Glands contain a specialized type of epithelial cell known as a _____ that produces a chemical substance (such as mucus, digestive enzymes, and hormones) whose functions are performed outside the cell.
    A. Fibroblasts.
    B. Secretory cells.
    C. Histiocytes.
    D. Macrophages.
    E. Plasma cells.

Exercises

22. The term _____ includes bone, cartilage, tendons, ligaments, the dermis or true skin, subcutaneous fat, and many other supporting and investing structures.
    A. Connective tissue.
    B. Epithelial tissue.
    C. Hemolymphatic tissue.
    D. Muscle tissue.
    E. Nerve tissue.

23. Cells which surround and engulf or "swallow" foreign material, bacteria or other invading microorganisms, and degenerating or diseased tissue elements, which they then break down and remove, may be called all of the following except
    A. Histiocytes.
    B. Macrophages.
    C. Phagocytes.
    D. Plasma cells.
    E. Microglia.

24. Large oval cells that produce and store complex chemical substances, including histamine and heparin, for release as needed are called
    A. Histiocytes.
    B. Schwann cells.
    C. Phagocytes.
    D. Plasma cells.
    E. Mast cells.

25. _____ consists of bundles or sheets of long, narrow cells arranged in parallel and having the capacity to shorten under appropriate electrochemical stimulation.
    A. Connective tissue.
    B. Epithelial tissue.
    C. Hemolymphatic tissue.
    D. Muscle tissue.
    E. Nerve tissue.

26. _____ is the most highly specialized type of tissue in the body; its cells exhibit the unique property of conducting electrochemical impulses and show the most extreme differentiation of structure.
    A. Nerve tissue.
    B. Muscle tissue.
    C. Hemolymphatic tissue.
    D. Epithelial tissue.
    E. Connective tissue.

Exercises

27. The point where the process of one neuron makes electrochemical contact with the process or body of another neuron is called
    A. An axon.
    B. The neurilemma.
    C. A synapse.
    D. A ganglion.
    E. A dendrite.

28. Star-shaped glial cells with many processes, found particularly in the gray matter of the brain and spinal cord are called
    A. Astrocytes (astroglia).
    B. Ependyma.
    C. Microglia.
    D. Oligodendroglia.
    E. Schwann cells.

29. Smaller glial cells with fewer processes, found in both gray and white matter are called
    A. Astrocytes (astroglia).
    B. Ependyma.
    C. Microglia.
    D. Oligodendroglia.
    E. Schwann cells.

30. _____ consist of very small glial cells resembling fibroblasts in appearance and having phagocytic functions.
    A. Astrocytes (astroglia).
    B. Ependyma.
    C. Microglia.
    D. Oligodendroglia.
    E. Schwann cells.

31. Glial cells forming a columnar epithelium-like tissue lining the cavities of the brain and spinal cord are classified as
    A. Astrocytes (astroglia).
    B. Ependyma.
    C. Microglia.
    D. Oligodendroglia.
    E. Schwann cells.

Exercises

32. Tissue that comprises a group of cells found in both the circulating blood and in certain tissues and organs, particularly the bone marrow, the spleen, and the lymph nodes is the
    A. Nerve tissue.
    B. Muscle tissue.
    C. Hemolymphatic tissue.
    D. Epithelial tissue.
    E. Connective tissue.

33. Highly organized masses of lymphoid tissue occur in all of the following structures except the
    A. Spleen.
    B. Thymus.
    C. Lymph nodes.
    D. Tonsils.
    E. Bone marrow.

Short Answers

1. Define pathology. Name and define its three principal branches.

    _____

    _____

    _____

    _____

    _____

    _____

2. Define or explain:
    a. cortex _____

    _____

    b. medulla _____

    _____

    c. organ _____

    _____

    d. parenchyma _____

    _____

    e. stroma _____

    _____

Exercises

3. Describe the basic structural features of a cell.

_____

_____

_____

_____

_____

_____

_____

_____

4. What are mitotic figures?

_____

_____

_____

_____

5. What is the general term for the type of tissue that forms coverings and lining membranes?

_____

_____

_____

_____

6. In what kind of structure is endothelium found?

_____

_____

_____

_____

Exercises

7. What basic type of tissue contains the highest proportion of noncellular material?

    _____

    _____

    _____

    _____

8. What is the function of fibroblasts?

    _____

    _____

    _____

    _____

9. In what type of tissue are haversian systems found?

    _____

    _____

    _____

    _____

10. State two important differences between smooth and skeletal muscle.

    a. _____

       _____

       _____

    b. _____

       _____

       _____

11. What type of cell has processes called axons and dendrites?

    _____

    _____

    _____

    _____

Exercises

12. What English words are roughly synonymous with Latin *tunica* and *lamina*?

_____

_____

13. What is the difference between visceral and parietal peritoneum?

_____

_____

_____

_____

14. What structures are typically found in a neurovascular bundle?

_____

_____

_____

_____

15. Connective tissue can be divided on the basis of its structural organization into six distinct types. List and give examples of each type.

a. _____

b. _____

c. _____

d. _____

e. _____

f. _____

16. List and give a brief, one-sentence definition for each of the five tissue types discussed in this chapter.

a. _____

_____

b. _____

_____

c. _____

_____

Exercises

d. _____

_____

e. _____

_____

Activities for Application and Further Study

1. The application of pathologic information to medical practice occurs at several levels. Summarize the three levels of application discussed in your text and give examples. (Section V)

2. Why is important to note the appearance of normal, healthy tissue in a pathology report?

3. Using the directional terms list from the text (the one beginning with *anterior*), structure 12 statements illustrating your understanding of each term. For example, "the thumb is distal to the wrist." Do not use the examples from the text.

Procedures and Practices in Anatomic Pathology

17

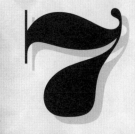

LEARNING OBJECTIVES

Upon completion of this chapter, the student should be able to

- Describe the gross examination of tissue specimens;

- Outline the procedure for preparing stained sections of tissue for microscopic examination;

- Discuss the basic techniques and diagnostic roles of cytologic studies, biopsies, and autopsies.

This chapter surveys the range of basic procedures performed in anatomic pathology: the gross and microscopic examination of tissue specimens obtained by biopsy or at autopsy and of cells obtained by scraping or washing.

Gross Examination of Tissue

The materials examined by an anatomic pathologist fall into two major classes: specimens taken from living patients and autopsy specimens. At autopsy it is feasible to remove vital organs such as the heart and the liver in their entirety and subject them to thorough, destructive dissection. Specimens from living patients are necessarily limited in type and volume. Such specimens are either tissues or organs removed during surgical operations or samples of material (biopsy specimens) removed from the living body for the purpose of examination.

Whereas the pathologist obtains and selects autopsy material for examination, specimens from the living patient are generally obtained by other physicians and submitted for study to the pathologist. Virtually all tissue specimens, regardless of how and by whom they are obtained, are subjected to certain routine procedures. As soon as possible after being removed from the body, the specimen is placed in a glass, plastic, fiberglass, or aluminum bottle, jar, or bucket containing a fluid called a fixative. The fixative has several purposes: to arrest the process of decomposition that begins almost at once in devitalized tissue, to kill bacteria and fungi in or on the specimen, and to begin hardening the tissue to facilitate preparation for microscopic study.

The most commonly used fixative is a 10% aqueous solution of formalin. Because formalin is made by bubbling formaldehyde gas through water, it is often called simply "formaldehyde." Formalin is inexpensive and highly suitable for most purposes. However, several other fixatives are available and may be preferred for special applications. The following list includes most of the fixatives in general use as well as certain chemicals that are included in the formulas of several fixatives.

Histologic Fixatives

absolute alcohol
acetic acid
acetone
Altmann solution
Bouin solution
buffered formalin
Carnoy solution
Carson solution
chlorpalladium
chromic acid
Delafield solution
Flemming solution
formaldehyde
formalin
formalin-alcohol
formalin-ammonium bromide
formol-Müller solution
FU-48 Zenker solution
Gendre solution
glacial acetic acid
glutaraldehyde
Helly Zenker-formalin solution
Jores solution
Kaiserling solution
Maximow solution
Millonig phosphate-buffered formalin
Müller solution
neutral (buffered) formalin
osmic acid
osmium tetroxide
picric acid
potassium bichromate (or dichromate)
Tellyesniczky solution
Zenker solution

In performing an autopsy, the pathologist removes organs one by one and subjects them to an immediate gross examination, opening them with a knife and inspecting their internal features so as to observe any abnormalities of size, shape, color, or consistency and any nodules, injury, hemorrhage, degeneration, scarring, or other significant local changes. Portions of the organ are selected that are most likely to be useful for microscopic study.

The pathologist's initial examination of a surgical or biopsy specimen is usually performed after the specimen has been placed in fixative. Although the fixative alters the color and consistency of the tissue to some extent, gross pathologic features can still generally be recognized. Occasionally specimens are brought directly from the operating room to the pathologist without being placed in preservative or fixative.

The pathologist performs the gross examination of tissue at a cutting board, which protects the top of the workbench from knife cuts and from the chemical action of fixatives. The pathologist handles the specimens with rubber gloves or with forceps, soaking up excess fluid with paper towels or other absorbent materials. Scalpels, razor blades, and scissors are used to open specimens for further examination and to trim them to the proper size for processing. One dimension, at least, of the trimmed specimen must be no more than 3-4 mm to allow penetration of processing chemicals. The trimmed pieces of tissue are placed in small flat round or oblong cassettes of perforated metal or plastic with lids of the same material, in which they will remain during the first stages of processing.

The pathologist dictates findings during or immediately after the gross inspection and cutting of surgical specimens. This dictation typically follows a set pattern:

Identification of the Specimen. The dictation always begins with basic identifying data: the patient's name as shown on the label of the container and on the laboratory requisition accompanying the specimen, and a general indication of what material has been submitted. At every step in the handling of a specimen, care is taken to ensure that it is correctly identified. The container in which it is placed by the pathologist, surgeon, or operating room technician is labeled with the patient's name, the nature of the specimen, and often the date, the name of the person obtaining the specimen, and other information.

Alternatively, a serial number or accession number may be assigned to the specimen container and the pertinent data kept in a register. If only one specimen is taken during an operation, as in an appendectomy, it may be unnecessary to identify it other than by the patient's name. When anatomically indistinguishable specimens are submitted, such as abdominal lymph nodes taken from several areas and possibly containing metastatic malignancy, they must be kept carefully separated and distinguished as to their origins.

In removing a specimen, the surgeon may cut it to a certain shape to indicate its origin or its orientation in the patient's body. Orientation may also be indicated by placement of a suture (surgical stitch) at a certain place in the specimen, such as at the uppermost point of a tumor excised from the skin. In cutting autopsy specimens from paired organs such as the lungs and the kidneys, the pathologist may indicate by the shape of the specimen which side it came from—for example, triangular for left, square for right.

After identifying the specimen, the pathologist may include clinical information (patient's medical history) in the dictation if this is available; often it is entered on the requisition.

Dimensions. The size of each specimen as submitted is usually determined and recorded in three planes in metric units (cm or mm). Solid organs or tumors may be weighed, if practicable, and the weight recorded in grams (g). The volume of any contained fluid (as in a cystic cavity) may be measured or (more often) estimated, and recorded in milliliters (mL) or cubic centimeters (cm^3).

Gross Description. The pathologist then describes the physical features of the specimen, with particular attention to any abnormalities such as swelling, hemorrhage, scarring, or tumor. The description typically includes mention of the color, texture, and consistency of both the exterior and the cut surfaces of the specimen. Any well-defined abnormality (nodule, cyst, ulcer, perforation, scar, pigmentation) is measured as precisely as possible. Not only the exact size and location of any tumor, but also its relation to the margins of the surgical specimen, must be carefully determined to document the adequacy of removal.

Microscopic examination of certain kinds of surgical specimens is routinely omitted unless the pathologist's gross examination shows abnormalities needing further study. Surgically removed tissues that are not usually sectioned for microscopic study include hernia sacs, blood clots, varicose veins, healthy bone (e.g., a section of rib removed for access to thoracic organs), and teeth. If microscopic examination will not be done, the pathologist dictates a diagnostic impression at the conclusion of his report on gross findings.

Because the tissue specimens taken by the pathologist in the autopsy room are generally too large to be handed over directly to a histology technician for preparation of microscope slides, these specimens are subjected to further examination and selective cutting in the pathology laboratory, just as with surgical specimens. Ordinarily, however, the pathologist does not dictate a report after this second inspection and cutting of autopsy specimens, since gross findings are included in the report of the autopsy.

Histopathology Procedures and the Microscopic Examination of Tissue

Histopathology refers to the study of microscopic changes in tissue induced by disease or injury. In practice, the term **histology** is often applied to the whole range of laboratory techniques used in preparing slides of tissue specimens for microscopic study by a pathologist.

The preparation of microscope slides from a gross tissue specimen is a complex and exacting process consisting of many steps, some of which are performed by automatic machinery. The process actually begins when the specimen is placed in fixative. As mentioned earlier, the fixative arrests decomposition and hardens tissue. Before the tissue can be cut into transparent sections, it is necessary to make it still harder by replacing its water content with a rigid material such as paraffin or cellulose. (Bone, however, is too hard for sectioning. A specimen containing bone must be decalcified with either dilute acid, an ion exchange resin, or a chelating agent, or by electrolysis, before it can be processed. The same is true of teeth and soft-tissue specimens such as sclerotic arteries and scar tissue containing calcium.)

When the paraffin method is used, the tissue specimen is first dehydrated by immersion in a graded series of solutions of an organic solvent such as acetone, Cellosolve, ethyl alcohol, or isopropyl alcohol, which replaces the water. The dehydrated tissue is then immersed in a clearing agent such as xylene (xylol), benzene, cedarwood oil, or chloroform, which replaces the dehydrating agent and renders the tissue transparent. Certain agents (dioxane, tetrahydrofuran) can serve as both dehydrating and clearing agents. After clearing, the tissue is transferred to a bath of melted paraffin, which replaces the clearing agent and infiltrates the tissue spaces. When this infiltration is complete, a technician removes the specimen from the paraffin bath with warmed forceps and embeds it in a cube-shaped mold containing fresh melted paraffin.

When the mold has cooled, the result is a block of paraffin inside which the tissue is embedded with all its water replaced, and its empty spaces filled, by paraffin. This paraffin block is then trimmed to appropriate dimensions and cut on a microtome, a precision instrument

Stains and Staining Methods, Mordants, Decolorizers, and Other Materials

acetic acid
acid alcohol
acid-fast bacilli (AFB) stain
acid fuchsin
acid phosphatase
Alcian blue
alizarin
alpha-naphthol esterase
alum-carmine
ammonium silver carbonate
amyloid stain
aniline blue
auramine-rhodamine
    fluorescent stain
azocarmine
azure
basic fuchsin
Best carmine stain
Biebrich scarlet stain
Bielschowsky stain
Bodian stain
Brown-Brenn Gram stain
Brown-Hopp tissue Gram stain
Bullard hematoxylin
Cajal gold sublimate
Cajal trichrome
carbolfuchsin
carmine
Celani method
Congo red
cresyl fast violet
crystal violet
Dane and Herman keratin
    stain
Darrow red
Davenport stain
Delafield hematoxylin
Del Rio Hortega method
Dieterle silver stain

DOPA (dihydroxyphenyl-
    alanine) stain
Ehrlich acid hematoxylin
elastic (elastin) stain
eosin
eosin azure
eosin-phloxine
fast blue
fast green
fast red
ferric ammonium sulfate
ferric chloride
Feulgen method
Fite-Faraco stain
Fontana-Masson stain
Fontana methenamine-silver
    stain
Foot reticulum stain
Fouchet reagent
fuchsin
Gallego method
gentian orange
gentian violet
Giemsa stain
Gill hematoxylin
Gimenez stain
gold chloride
Golgi stain
Gomori aldehyde fuchsin
Gomori methenamine-silver
    (GMS)
Gram stain
Gridley stain
Grocott methenamine-silver
Hale iron stain
Harris hematoxylin
Heidenhain iron hematoxylin
hemalum
hematoxylin

Hiss capsule stain
Holmes silver nitrate
Holzer method
hydrochloric acid
India ink
indigo carmine
iron hematoxylin
iron stain
Janus green B
Jenner method
Jones kidney stain
Kernechtrot
Kinyoun acid-fast stain
Kleihauer-Betke stain
Langeron iodine solution
Levine alkaline Congo red
    method
lithium carbonate
lithium-carmine
Lorrain Smith stain
Lugol solution
Luna modification of Bodian
    stain
Luxol fast blue
malachite green
Mallory-Azan stain
Mallory iron stain
Mancini iodine technique
Marchi method
Masson trichrome stain
May-Grünwald-Giemsa stain
Mayer mucicarmine
methyl violet
methylene blue
Milligan trichrome
mucicarmine
mucin stain
myeloperoxidase
naphthol-ASD chloroacetate
    esterase

Stains and Staining Methods, Mordants, Decolorizers, and Other Materials *(continued)*

naphthol green B
neutral red
Nissl method
nuclear fast red
oil red O
orange G
orcein
osmic acid
osmium tetroxide
oxalic acid
Pap (Papanicolaou) stain
Pappenheim stain
Paragon stain
Perdrau method
periodic acid-Schiff (PAS)
    stain
peroxidase stain
phloxine
phosphomolybdic acid
phosphotungstic acid
phosphotungstic acid-
    hematoxylin (PTAH)
polychrome methylene blue

potassium metabisulfite
potassium permanganate
Protargol
Ramón y Cajal stain
Ranson pyridine silver stain
rapid mucin stain
reticulin stain
Romanowsky's stain
safranin
scarlet red
Scharlach R
Schiff solution
Scott solution
Seller stain
Shorr trichrome
silver nitrate
silver stain
Snook reticulum stain
sodium bicarbonate
sodium bisulfite
sodium hydroxide
sodium thiosulfate
Sudan black

Sudan black B fat stain
Sudan III
tetrachrome
thionin
Tilden stain
toluidine blue
trichrome stain
Truant auramine-rhodamine
    stain
Turnbull blue
Unna stain
uranium nitrate
van Gieson stain
Verhoeff elastic stain
von Kossa calcium stain
Warthin-Starry stain
Wayson stain
Weigert iron hematoxylin
Weigert-Pal method
Weil myelin sheath stain
Wilder reticulum stain
Wright stain
Ziehl-Neelsen acid-fast stain

on the order of an electric meat slicer, which makes transparent slices that are only about 5 micrometers (0.005 mm) thick. For technical reasons, sections are usually made by cutting across the broadest flat surface of the tissue specimen, unless the pathologist has given special instructions for an edge cut or cross section. Usually only one or two sections from each paraffin block are chosen to be made into slides. Sometimes serial sections (for example, every tenth or twentieth slice) are taken so as to provide the pathologist with a three-dimensional concept of a tissue or lesion.

Immediately after cutting, the paraffin sections are floated on a bath of warm water, which helps to smooth out wrinkles and curled edges. Each section is affixed to a separate microscope slide (a thin strip of clear glass about 1 in x 3 in) by means of a film of albumin solution or other suitable adhesive. The slides are identified with labels bearing names or numbers matching those of the containers in which the gross specimens were submitted.

Substances other than paraffin are sometimes used to infiltrate and embed tissue for sectioning. With Carbowax, which is water-soluble, the dehydration and clearing steps can be omitted. However, obtaining satisfactory sections with Carbowax demands a high degree of technical skill. Celloidin is a suspension of a cellulose derivative in a volatile solvent. Because infiltration and embedding with celloidin do not require heat, there is less distortion of tissue than with the paraffin and Carbowax methods. However, celloidin takes much more time; as much as a month may elapse between fixation and sectioning. Commercially available embedding media besides Carbowax include Epon, Paraplast, and Parlodion.

Microscopic examination of the slide at this stage would yield little information, because all of the tissue spaces are filled with the infiltrating medium. This must be removed and replaced with water or some other suitable fluid by a reversal of the procedures used in making the block. Once the infiltrating agent has been removed and the tissue section rehydrated, the slide is immersed in one or more coloring solutions called stains. These impart a more or less intense coloration to the tissues, which greatly facilitates microscopic examination.

Seldom is only a single color applied. Different stains have affinities for different components of tissue, depending on their chemical properties. Hence it is usual to apply at least two contrasting colors. The use of standard combinations of stains enables the pathologist to recognize normal and abnormal microscopic features of tissue consistently and confidently.

In practice, staining usually involves a number of steps besides immersion of the prepared slide in a coloring agent. First a mordant may be applied to render the tissue chemically more receptive to staining. Many fixatives have mordant properties. After the first stain has been applied, the slide is immersed in or washed with a decolorizer, which removes stain from all parts of the tissue to which it has not become chemically bound. The slide is then treated with a counterstain of a contrasting color, which is taken up by tissues decolorized in the preceding step. A polychrome stain is a mixture of two or more coloring agents in one solution. With a polychrome stain, differential staining of tissue components takes place even though the tissue is exposed to all of the coloring agents simultaneously. A metachromatic stain is one that changes color on becoming chemically bound to certain tissues.

By far the most commonly used combination of stains for routine histopathology work is hematoxylin and eosin (H&E). Hematoxylin is a deep blue stain which imparts various shades of blue and purple to cell nuclei and other tissue components of slightly acidic nature. Eosin stains most of the other components pink to red. Many special stains and techniques are available to bring out certain features (nerve tissue, reticular fibers, lipid material, pathogenic microorganisms) that are not shown by routine stains. In submitting a tissue block to the histology technician, the pathologist may write instructions regarding the use of special stains. Some staining operations can be done by automatic machinery, but often part or all of the staining process is performed manually. Slides are placed vertically in tall narrow glass containers called Coplin jars, which are filled with stain or other solutions.

After staining and drying, the tissue section on the slide is ordinarily protected with a cover slip, a very thin sheet of glass about 7/8 in (2.2 cm) square. A film of balsam or other mounting medium is first placed over the tissue section, and the cover slip is gently dropped into place. The balsam eventually hardens around the edges, but under the cover slip it remains fluid indefinitely, preserving the section in a clear, homogeneous, refractile medium. Mounting media in common use are Apathy medium, (Canada) balsam, Clarite, and Permount.

In most laboratories, slides are available for the pathologist's examination 24 to 72 hours after the tissue is removed from the body. Processing is speeded and simplified by the use of automated machinery that dehydrates, clears, and infiltrates tissue during the night. The preceding day's specimens are then embedded, sectioned, and stained on the following morning.

The pathologist examines or "reads" slides with a light microscope, using various magnifications as needed. The standard magnifications are scanning power (X 35–50), low power (X 100), and high power (X 450–500). The greater the magnification, the more the detail that can be distinguished, but the smaller the zone of tissue that can be viewed without moving the slide. After reviewing the slides, the pathologist dictates microscopic findings and then states one or more diagnoses or diagnostic impressions.

Since gross and microscopic reports are dictated on different days, they are seldom transcribed at the same session. Ordinarily the gross report is transcribed on the top half of a standard surgical pathology form, which is then made available to the pathologist at the time the slides are examined microscopically. The dictated microscopic findings and diagnoses are then transcribed on the bottom half of the form, and the form is returned to the pathologist for review and signature.

Having described gross and microscopic findings, the pathologist usually records a diagnosis or diagnostic impression, summarizing and coordinating those findings. The diagnoses listed at the end of an autopsy report may number ten, twenty, or more. The diagnoses may be accompanied by code numbers referring to some standard system of disease nomenclature. In a case of malignancy, the pathologist's diagnosis will often include an estimate of the extent of the malignant process according to a standard grading or staging system.

Biopsy, Cytology, Smear, Aspiration, Frozen Section

The term **biopsy** refers to the removal of tissue from a living patient for pathologic examination. Many factors, including the location of the tissue to be studied, the presumptive diagnosis, and the patient's general condition, influence the choice of a biopsy procedure.

An **excisional** biopsy is the surgical removal of an entire tumor, lesion, or diseased organ from a living patient. The difference between the surgical removal of a tumor or abnormal tissue—which is routinely submitted to a pathologist for examination—and an excisional biopsy is merely one of viewpoint, the latter phrasing emphasizing the diagnostic intent of the procedure. Many surgical pathology specimens are, in effect, excisional biopsies. The term **incisional** biopsy refers to the surgical removal of part of a tumor, lesion, or diseased organ for pathologic study. Incisional biopsy may be preferred to complete removal of an abnormal tissue or organ for technical or cosmetic reasons, and of course total excision of a vital organ or tissue is never feasible.

The majority of biopsies are done in cases of suspected or known malignancy in order to clarify the nature and extent of disease. In the examination of an excisional biopsy specimen, one of the main concerns is to determine whether all abnormal tissue has in fact been excised. Hence the pathologist pays close attention to the periphery of the specimen and, in preparing the tissue for embedding and sectioning, selects and orients the material in such a way that microscopic examination can verify whether or not all abnormal tissue is surrounded by an adequate margin of normal tissue. These findings will guide the surgeon in determining what further treatment is appropriate—chemotherapy, radiation therapy, more surgery, or simply observation.

Sometimes a surgeon needs feedback from the pathologist while an operation is actually in progress. The histologic character of a tumor may determine whether the surgeon can be content with simple excision or whether a more radical procedure must be performed at once. When the resection of a malignancy involves extensive, mutilating surgery, the surgeon may choose to remove tissue in stages, submitting a specimen from each stage for pathologic study before deciding whether to close the incision or remove more tissue. Clearly, the routine methods of preparing specimens for histologic study cannot be used in this setting because of time limitations.

The frozen section technique makes it possible for a pathologist to perform a histologic examination of tissue within minutes after it is removed from the patient. This method substitutes rapid freezing of the water in the tissue for infiltration and embedding with paraffin or another artificial medium. The tissue may be frozen solid on a chilled platform called a cryostat, and then sectioned with a microtome in the usual way. With the freezing microtome, tissue is placed on a perforated stage, frozen with blasts of carbon dioxide gas, and sectioned in place with a blade that is an integral part of the instrument. Frozen sections are mounted on slides and stained rapidly. There is more distortion of tissue than with routine methods of slide preparation, and some histologic details are poorly shown, but sufficient information can be gleaned for the immediate purpose. Tissue examined by frozen section is always submitted for routine processing as well.

In addition to these "open" biopsy procedures, a number of techniques have been devised for removing small pieces of tissue for study without making a surgical incision. These techniques are often performed by physicians who are not surgeons—sometimes even by the pathologist who will examine the specimen. A **punch biopsy** consists of the removal of a plug of skin or mucous membrane with a cylindrical punch 2-5 mm in diameter. In a **shave biopsy**, a thin layer of skin consisting mostly or entirely of epidermis is removed with a blade held approximately parallel to the surface. **Curettage** is a surgical scraping. Sometimes it is done for therapeutic reasons, as in curettage of the uterine lining for excessive menstrual bleeding. Curettage of a lesion on any accessible surface may also be done to procure biopsy material. Tissue may also be snipped or snared from the lining of an internal organ or cavity with an instrument passed through an endoscope. Percutaneous needle biopsy of the liver and kidney are standard procedures. A

biopsy needle consists of two parts, an outer hollow cannula of large bore that is passed through the skin directly into the organ to be studied, and an inner cutting needle that slices and removes a core of tissue.

All of the biopsy procedures discussed above yield specimens of tissue that, however small and fragmentary, can be embedded and sectioned in the routine manner already described. Other standard techniques for sampling living tissue yield specimens that require special processing before they can be examined microscopically.

The term **smear** refers generically to any type of laboratory study in which material is thinly spread over the surface of a microscope slide for examination. A smear may consist of blood, sputum, feces, pus, or any other liquid or semisolid material, and it may either be examined in its natural state or stained to show cellular details, microorganisms, parasites, or foreign material. A smear may be air-dried or it may be sprayed with or immersed in fixative before further processing or staining. Most examinations of smears pertain to clinical rather than to anatomic pathology. However, when a smear consists of cellular material removed from the body by scraping or aspiration, it is stained in much the same way as a slide made by sectioning a block of tissue, and may be examined by an anatomic pathologist.

Cytology is the study of cells. Cytology is often used in the narrow sense of a study of cells that have been detached from a surface for microscopic study, as in a Pap (Papanicolaou) smear (*see box on p. 264*).

The **Pap smear** for detection of abnormal cells from the uterine cervix is the most frequently performed cytologic test. In this technique cells are detached from mucous surfaces (the vaginal walls, the squamocolumnar junction, and the endocervical canal) by means of a specially shaped wooden spatula (Ayre spatula), a suction pipet, an endocervical brush (Cytobrush), a Cervex-Brush (designed to sample the endocervical canal and the squamocolumnar junction simultaneously), or any other suitable instrument, spread on a slide, and immediately fixed by spraying with, or immersion in, a fixative solution. The slide thus prepared by the examiner is delivered to the cytology laboratory, where the cells are stained and examined by a cytologist.

In a newer technique, called the thin-layer (mono-layer) or liquid-based method, cells obtained by the usual means are not smeared on a slide by the examiner but are immersed in a fixative liquid. This liquid, transferred to the laboratory, is filtered to remove debris and then distributed by a mechanical device in an even layer over a small area on a microscope slide before staining and examination.

Reporting of findings on cervical Pap smear follows the Bethesda system (named for Bethesda, Maryland, the site of the National Institutes of Health). The basic format of the report consists of three parts: (1) a statement of the adequacy of the specimen; (2) general categorization (negative for intraepithelial lesion or malignancy; epithelial cell abnormality; or other); (3) descriptive diagnosis, elaborating on the general categorization and including mention of all significant abnormalities (e.g., evidence of inflammation or infection with *Candida* or *Trichomonas*) as well as of the patient's hormonal status (when vaginal cells are present in the smear).

Mild dysplasia of squamous cells, including cellular atypia characteristic of HPV infection, is designated a low-grade squamous intraepithelial lesion (LGSIL or LSIL). Moderate to severe dysplasia is termed a high-grade squamous intraepithelial lesion (HGSIL or HSIL). Squamous intraepithelial lesions that do not meet criteria for either of these categories may be called atypical squamous cells of undetermined significance (ASC-US) or atypical squamous cells suggestive of high-grade lesions (ASC-H).

The finding of ASC-H, LGSIL, or HGSIL is an indication for colposcopy. Women with ASC-US may undergo repeat Pap smear after an interval, colposcopy, or testing for high-risk HPV types (see Chapter 23). The thin-layer method yields a significantly higher percentage of LGSIL and HGSIL and a significantly lower percentage of ASCUS and "unsatisfactory" readings. Computer screening of Pap smears, or rescreening of smears that have been read as negative, can also improve the yield of abnormal findings.

Fine-needle aspiration is a technique used to remove cells by suction from certain structures such as the prostate, subcutaneous lymph nodes and other neck masses, and breast masses. The material obtained is smeared on a slide and stained in the same way as a Pap smear. Another way of obtaining cells for study is by washing a surface, such as the interior of the stomach, with saline or some other suitable fluid and collecting the washings. This method can be used to obtain cellular material from the respiratory tract and many parts of the digestive tract. Sometimes gentle brushing is used to augment the yield of cells.

Various normal and abnormal body fluids—amniotic fluid, joint fluid, and pleural, pericardial, and peritoneal effusions—can be withdrawn from the body by aspiration with needle and syringe and subjected to cytologic study, as well as other examinations such as culture and chemical analysis. When it is desired to subject a clear fluid with a low cell count to cytologic study, the cells may be concentrated by centrifugation or separated by filtration. Aspiration and biopsy of bone marrow are discussed in Chapter 19.

Spinning the fluid in a centrifuge drives the cells to the bottom. The resulting sediment can either be smeared on a slide or processed as if it were a solid piece of tissue, yielding a cell block of paraffin. Alternatively, the fluid may be forced through a filter with very fine openings that trap the cells. The filter paper is then mounted on a slide and stained like a tissue section. In the Nuclepore method, fluid is forced through a filter

Sample Pathology Report

Concordia Hospital Department of Pathology

TISSUE NO: D04-8366
PATIENT: Smith, John
SURGEON: Jones, Mary
PHYSICIAN: Robinson, Jack

DATE: May 15, 2004
AGE: 61
HOSPITAL NO: OP-24387
ROOM NO: N/A

CLINICAL DIAGNOSIS:
Multiple skin lesions.

PREOPERATIVE DIAGNOSIS
Benign skin tags, rule out basal cell carcinoma.

POSTOPERATIVE DIAGNOSIS
Same.

HISTORY AND OPERATIVE FINDINGS
Benign-appearing skin tags, patient requests removal for cosmetic reasons. No history of cutaneous or other malignancy.

TISSUES
1. Lesion, right thumb.
2. Lesion, right thigh.
3. Lesion, left elbow.
4. Lesion, left forearm.

GROSS
The specimen is submitted in four parts.

Part #1, right thumb, is an ellipsoid portion of cutaneous tissue measuring 1.5 x 1.0 x 0.2 cm, centrally showing sessile white papillary lesion measuring 0.3 x 0.3 x 0.1 cm, sectioned and totally submitted "A."

Part #2, right thigh, is an ellipse of skin measuring 1.3 x 0.5 x 1.0 cm, centrally showing an ovoid brown papillary lesion measuring 0.2 x 0.2 x 0.2 cm, sectioned and totally submitted "B."

Part #3, left elbow, consists of a cutaneous ellipse measuring 1 cm on which is mounted an ovoid tan papillary lesion measuring 0.3 x 0.2 x 0.1 cm, totally submitted "C."

(continued)

Sample Pathology Report

PATHOLOGY REPORT, page 2

SMITH, JOHN
PATIENT #OP-24387

Part #4, left forearm, consists of a cutaneous ellipse measuring 0.8 x 0.5 x 0.3 cm, centrally showing a poorly defined gray area of roughened epithelium, totally submitted "D."

MICROSCOPIC

Sections of the first specimen, right thumb, show a centrally thickened epidermis with basal layer of hyperplasia, acanthosis, marked focal hyperkeratosis. Atypical changes are not evident.

Sections of the second specimen, right thigh, show sections of cutaneous tissue with centrally thickened epidermis, showing acanthosis and focal marked hyperkeratosis.

The third specimen, left elbow, shows sections of cutaneous tissue with a centrally slightly thickened epidermis showing acanthosis and rounded keratin inclusions.

The fourth specimen, left forearm, shows sections of cutaneous tissue with a slightly thickened epidermis showing slight acanthosis, basal pigmentation, rounded keratin inclusions. None of the sections show malignant change.

DIAGNOSIS:
SPECIMEN #1: BENIGN SQUAMOUS PAPILLOMA.
SPECIMEN #2: BENIGN SQUAMOUS PAPILLOMA.
SPECIMEN #3: SEBORRHEIC KERATOSIS.
SPECIMEN #4: SEBORRHEIC KERATOSIS.

under pressure; in the Millipore method it is drawn through by suction.

The Autopsy

The autopsy, necropsy, or postmortem examination (sometimes called simply a "post") is the pathologic examination par excellence. During an autopsy, every part of the body can be opened and exhaustively studied, and any organ or tissue can be removed as necessary for processing and microscopic evaluation. Fluids and other materials are readily collected for culturing, chemical testing, and other clinical pathologic studies.

The purposes of the autopsy were set forth briefly in a previous chapter. In nearly every case, the chief reason for doing an autopsy is to determine as precisely as possible the cause of death. It may already be known with a fair degree of certainty on clinical grounds that death was due, for example, to myocardial infarction or to irreversible brain damage sustained in an automobile accident. But an autopsy provides objective anatomic evidence to confirm the clinical diagnosis and to show the exact pathophysiologic mechanism of death. Sometimes two life-threatening conditions are both present at the time of death—for example, severe pneumonitis and meningitis, both due to pneumococcus. The autopsy may supply information as to which condition actually proved lethal. Occasionally the autopsy discloses an unsuspected cause of death—for example, fatal hemorrhage from a peptic ulcer in a patient under treatment for acute myocardial infarction.

An exhaustive search for the cause of death may seem like misplaced effort, since no amount of information generated by an autopsy can bring the patient back to life. But the attempt to secure full, detailed, accurate information about the cause of death is not a mere academic exercise. In every jurisdiction in the United States, a death certificate listing the cause of death must be signed by a physician and filed with the authorities before a dead body may be embalmed and buried or cremated. Although by no means all deaths are investigated by autopsy, certification of the cause of death is more likely to be accurate and complete in those that are. The validity of public health statistics compiled from data entered on death certificates depends on the caution, diligence, and thoroughness with which the certifying physicians investigated the cause of death.

In certain cases (homicide, suicide, fatal accident, death due to poison or drug overdose, and others), the law requires that an autopsy be performed by or under the auspices of a coroner or medical examiner. In addition, an autopsy may be ordered by legal authorities when a person dies during the first 24 hours after hospital admission or after surgery, or when a person with no known health problems dies suddenly. Data supplied by a medicolegal autopsy may become evidence in a criminal prosecution, a wrongful death suit, or both. Statistics on accidental death gleaned from coroners' reports have been used to support legislation concerning, for example, automobile seat belts, motorcycle helmets, drunk driving, and legal drinking age.

In a teaching hospital (one whose mission includes the training of residents, medical students, nurses, and other health professionals), the autopsy serves as a unique learning experience. Physicians at all levels of training can profit by attending autopsies. Organs and tissues removed at autopsy may be preserved and reviewed days later at a pathology conference. Microscope slides made from these tissues may be used as teaching aids for years. For the physician or physicians who were responsible for the treatment of the patient, the autopsy provides invaluable, if not always comforting, feedback on the thoroughness and accuracy of diagnostic evaluation and the appropriateness of treatment. When death occurs in the postoperative period, an autopsy may show that it resulted from surgical complications or errors of technique. Recently implanted grafts, heart valve replacements, pace-

Cervical Cancer and the Pap Smear

Carcinoma of the uterine cervix is the most common gynecologic malignancy in women under 50. The great majority of cervical cancers (90%) are squamous cell carcinomas. These are most likely to arise at the squamocolumnar junction, the line of demarcation between the columnar epithelial cells that line the endocervical canal and the squamous cells that cover the portion of the cervix that faces into the vagina. Invasive cervical carcinoma is the final stage of a series of cellular changes that begin with dysplasia and atypia, progress to intraepithelial neoplasia, then to carcinoma in situ, and finally invade surrounding tissues by penetrating the basement membrane of the cervical epithelium.

This process may take 10-20 years to run its full course. Cervical cancer is rare before age 30 and invasive cancer is rare before age 40. Nearly every case of cervical carcinoma represents the culmination of cellular changes triggered by cervical infection with certain types of human papillomavirus. This is a sexually transmitted disease. Risk factors for the development of cervical carcinoma include early age at first intercourse, having many sexual partners, and low socioeconomic status.

Bleeding, vaginal discharge, and pelvic pain occur relatively late in the evolution of cervical cancer. As many as one-fifth of women with invasive cervical carcinoma have no symptoms. During the 1930s the Greek-born American physician and pioneer cytologist George Papanicolaou (1883-1962) developed techniques to prepare, stain, and interpret smears of cells from the uterine cervix in order to detect dysplastic changes likely to culminate in invasive cancer if left untreated. Thanks largely to the widespread use of the Pap smear to screen asymptomatic women, the number of cervical cancer deaths in the U.S. declined by 74% between 1955 and 1992. Despite the decline, more than 12,000 cases of invasive cancer are still diagnosed in the United States each year, and more than 4000 women die of cervical cancer in this country each year.

A Pap smear is recommended for every woman when she reaches the age of 18 or becomes sexually active, whichever occurs first. Most authorities currently advise that a woman who has had negative annual Pap smears for three consecutive years need not continue to have annual smears, unless she is at high risk for cervical dysplastic changes because of sexual exposure. A history of an abnormal Pap smear or HIV infection may warrant Pap smears at more frequent intervals than annually.

makers, and other materials or devices must be examined for signs of rejection or malfunction. When death follows the use of any experimental treatment, an autopsy is of crucial importance.

Except in those cases where an autopsy is mandated by law and performed by a coroner or medical examiner, written permission must be obtained from the next of kin before an autopsy can begin. The law makes special provision for autopsy permission when the deceased had no known family. Generally it is the responsibility of the attending physician to solicit and obtain autopsy permission. However, the pathologist must assure himself that a permission has been duly signed and witnessed before performing any examination of the body; otherwise he could be subject to legal reprisals for unauthorized mutilation of the dead. The permission form may restrict the pathologist to certain procedures only. For example, permission to open the skull may be withheld. Because microscopic examination of autopsy specimens is an integral part of the procedure, the form must specify that the pathologist may remove and retain such tissues and body parts as he deems necessary.

Autopsies are usually performed in a hospital department set aside for that purpose. The autopsy room or morgue is usually located on a ground floor adjacent to a loading area for the convenience of undertakers, and is equipped with refrigerated lockers for the storage of bodies pending autopsy or removal. Strong illumination and adequate ventilation are essential. The autopsy is performed on a specially designed operating table provided with running water and suction equipment. Attached to the table or immediately available in the room is a cutting board for the gross examination of organs as they are removed from the body. A scale is provided for weighing organs, and graduated containers for determining the volume of fluids. The instruments used are similar to surgical instruments—scalpels, scissors, forceps, clamps, and, for cutting bone, electric saws, chisels, and hammers. In addition, a knife with a very long flat blade is used to cut sections of uniform thickness from large organs such as the spleen and kidney. Specimen containers prefilled with fixative are on hand for immediate preservation of tissues removed.

The subject of an autopsy may be called the body, the cadaver, the deceased or decedent, the patient, the remains, or the subject. The person performing the autopsy is called the prosector, the dissector, the operator, the autopsy surgeon, or simply the pathologist. The prosector is usually assisted by a morgue attendant or diener (German *Diener* 'servant'), who looks after the autopsy facility and its equipment, moves bodies to and from the autopsy table, and helps with the actual autopsy procedure as needed.

The autopsy room is usually equipped with a pedal- or voice-activated dictating machine so that the pathologist can dictate findings while performing the autopsy. An autopsy report or protocol so dictated will naturally follow the sequence of examination procedures as they are actually done. This sequence varies from one prosector to another and may be modified in individual cases for various reasons. In virtually all cases, however, the autopsy follows the same basic plan.

After confirming the identity of the body by means of a wrist tag, a toe tag, or both, and ensuring that a valid consent for the performance of the autopsy has been given in writing, the pathologist weighs the body, if equipment is available for that purpose, and determines its length from crown to heel. The entire body surface is inspected and palpated, and note is made of the color and consistency of the skin, the color and distribution of head and body hair, any deformities, swellings, or injuries (open wounds, discolorations, needle punctures), surgical or traumatic scars, and any other departure from normal and expected appearances. The presence of endotracheal tubes, intravenous lines, and catheters is noted. **Rigor mortis** refers to the stiffening of the muscles that comes on within a few hours after death and passes off after another few hours. **Livor mortis** (postmortem lividity, hypostasis) is a purplish discoloration of the skin due to engorgement of capillaries that occurs shortly after death. Lividity affects whatever parts of the body are lowermost, but does not appear in areas of the skin that have been in firm contact with a supporting surface.

The eyes and the cavities of the mouth, nose, and ears are inspected for evidence of disease, injury, or foreign material. If the eyes have been removed to provide corneal transplants, this fact is noted. The external genitalia are inspected for developmental abnormalities and signs of disease or injury. The body is turned over for inspection of the back and anus.

The thoracic and abdominal cavities are now opened. The prosector makes a Y-shaped incision through the skin and subcutaneous fat of the anterior body surface, the extremities of the Y being at the two shoulders and the pubic region. Some operators make the upper limbs of the Y above the breasts and nearly parallel to the clavicles; others cut below the breasts. Over the thorax the scalpel cuts all the way through skin and fat to the underlying breastbone and ribs. Below the level of the breastbone the operator inserts two fingers into the peritoneal cavity and lifts skin, fat, and peritoneum away from the abdominal organs so that they will not be injured as the incision is carried down to the pubes (veering around the umbilicus).

The skin is retracted from the line of the incision on each side and dissected free of the underlying tissues until wide flaps have been reflected. The thickness of the subcutaneous fat is noted and recorded. The breasts and axillary structures are examined from within and specimens are cut from any abnormal or suspicious areas. The ribs and clavicles are then cut through near their attachments to the breastbone, and the front of the bony thorax is removed in one piece.

The thoracic and abdominal organs are first inspected in their natural positions and then removed for further study. The membranous surfaces of the thoracic and abdominal cavities—pleura, pericardium, peritoneum, diaphragm, omentum—are examined for abnormalities of color or texture, adhesions, or tumors. Any blood or fluid in a body cavity is noted and if possible measured. Each organ is severed from its attachments, weighed, and opened. As the heart is removed, ligatures are placed around the stumps of the great vessels to facilitate embalming of the body by the undertaker. The intestine is removed in its entirety from just below the stomach to just above the rectum. Both solid and hollow organs are opened for inspection of internal detail. Selected features—for example, the thickness of the walls of the cardiac chambers—are measured.

Representative pieces of tissue from each organ are immediately placed in fixative. Entire organs may be preserved in large jars or buckets of fixative if they are needed for a pathology conference or "organ recital" to be held later. Blood may be withdrawn directly from the chambers of the heart for testing. Specimens may be taken for culture or other laboratory procedures, and the contents of the digestive tract may be submitted for chemical analysis. Before incising a solid organ to take material from inside for a culture, the prosector sears the surface with a hot spatula to destroy any microorganisms there, which might contaminate the culture. Any solid material removed from the body and not needed for subsequent study is placed in a large plastic bag, which is sealed at the conclusion of the autopsy and placed inside the body before it is closed.

If an examination of the brain ("head post") is to be performed, the operator makes an incision across the top of the head from ear to ear, turns flaps of scalp forward and backward, and removes the top of the skull like a cap by cutting around it with an electric saw and detaching the cap with a chisel. The brain and its membranes are observed, and any swelling, deformity, tumor, or hemorrhage is noted. The brain is cut free of its attachments and placed intact in fixative. Because brain tissue is extremely soft in its natural state, it is usually allowed to harden in fixative for several days before being cut for gross and microscopic study. If necessary, the spinal cord or specimens of bone can be removed by further manipulation of the saw and chisel. At the conclusion of the autopsy, the attendant sews the incisions shut with heavy thread or cord in a continuous or "baseball" stitch and washes the body.

Occasionally an autopsy is performed on a body that has already been embalmed. In this case, the pathologist's examination will disclose evidence of the embalmer's activities. Embalming consists of two basic procedures: replacement of the blood in the circulatory system with a preservative fluid that incidentally imparts to the skin a cosmetically acceptable hue, and introduction of a similar fluid into the thoracic and abdominal cavities through one or more punctures made with a hollow instrument. Before instilling cavitary fluid, the embalmer removes as much as possible of the contents of the digestive tract by suction through the instrument. After the instrument is withdrawn, the skin puncture site is closed with a plastic plug to prevent leakage.

Exercises

Fill in the Blanks

1. An anatomic pathologist examines two major classes of materials: _____ and _____.

2. Pathologic specimens from living patients are either _____ removed during surgical operations or _____.

3. As soon as possible after being removed from the body, the specimen is placed in container containing a fluid called a _____.

4. Formalin may be referred to as "formaldehyde" because _____.

5. At autopsy, after the organs are removed, they are first subjected to an _____.

6. At least one dimension of the trimmed specimen must be no more than 3-4 mm in order _____.

7. As an alternative to writing identifying information such as patient name, type of specimen, date, and so forth on a specimen container, a _____ may be assigned to the specimen container and the pertinent data kept in a register.

8. The size of each specimen as submitted is usually determined and recorded in _____ in metric units (cm or mm).

9. _____ refers to the study of microscopic changes in tissue induced by disease or injury.

10. Before tissue can be cut into transparent sections, it is necessary to make it hard by replacing its water content with a rigid material such as _____ or _____.

11. The paraffin block is trimmed to appropriate dimensions and cut on a _____, a precision instrument which makes transparent slices that are only about 5 micrometers (0.005 mm) thick.

12. Microscopic examination of a freshly prepared slide would yield little information, because _____,

13. _____ impart a more or less intense coloration to the tissues, which greatly facilitates microscopic examination.

14. Before staining a slide, a _____ may be applied to render the tissue chemically more receptive to staining.

15. A _____ is a mixture of two or more coloring agents in one solution.

Exercises

16. A _____ is a stain of a contrasting color which is taken up by tissues not stained by the first color.

17. A _____ is a stain that changes color on becoming chemically bound to certain tissues.

18. The most commonly used combination of stains for routine histopathology work is _____.

19. Hematoxylin imparts various shades of _____ to cell nuclei and other tissue components of slightly acidic nature.

20. Eosin stains most of the other components _____.

21. Under the cover slip, the _____ remains fluid indefinitely, preserving the section in a clear, homogeneous, refractile medium.

22. The greater the magnification of the microscope, the _____ that can be distinguished, but the _____ that can be viewed without moving the slide.

23. An _____ is the surgical removal of part of a tumor, lesion, or diseased organ for pathologic study.

24. An _____ is the surgical removal of an entire tumor, lesion, or diseased organ from a living patient.

25. In the examination of an excisional biopsy specimen, one of the main concerns is _____.

26. The term _____ refers generically to any type of laboratory study in which material is thinly spread over the surface of a microscope slide for examination.

27. _____ is a technique used to remove cells by suction from certain structures such as the prostate, subcutaneous lymph nodes and other neck masses, and breast masses.

28. The chief reason for doing an autopsy is _____.

29. An autopsy provides _____ to confirm the clinical diagnosis and to show the exact pathophysiologic mechanism of death.

30. The subject of an autopsy may be called the _____, the _____, the _____, the _____, the _____, or the _____.

31. The person performing the autopsy is called the _____, the _____, the _____, the _____, or simply the _____.

Exercises

32. A morgue attendant or _____ ('servant'), looks after the autopsy facility and its equipment, moves bodies to and from the autopsy table, and helps with the actual autopsy procedure as needed.

33. _____ is a purplish discoloration of the skin due to engorgement of capillaries that occurs shortly after death.

34. _____ refers to the stiffening of the muscles that comes on within a few hours after death and passes off after another few hours.

35. _____ affects whatever parts of the body are lowermost, but does not appear in areas of the skin that have been in firm contact with a supporting surface.

36. "Organ recital" is slang for _____.

Multiple Choice: Circle the letter of the best answer from the choices given.

1. Which of the following statements best expresses the purpose of using a fixative.
   A. To arrest the process of decomposition that begins almost at once in devitalized tissue
   B. To kill bacteria and fungi in or on the specimen.
   C. To begin hardening the tissue to facilitate preparation for microscopic study.
   D. All of the above.
   E. None of the above.

2. The most commonly used fixative is which of the following?
   A. Acetone.
   B. Formalin.
   C. Glutaraldehyde.
   D. Zenker solution.
   E. Bouin solution.

3. Which of the following findings could NOT be detected on gross examination?
   A. Abnormalities of size, shape, color, or consistency of an organ.
   B. Nodules.
   C. The cell nucleus.
   D. Injury or hemorrhage.
   E. Degeneration or scarring.

Exercises

4. The patient's name and a general indication of the type of specimen submitted is contained in what portion of a pathology report?
   A. The gross examination.
   B. The histology examination.
   C. The microscopic examination.
   D. The dimensions.
   E. The identification.

5. Of the following specimens, which one is placed into paraffin or cellulose before being cut into transparent sections?
   A. Bone.
   B. Teeth.
   C. Sclerotic artery containing calcium.
   D. Scar tissue containing calcium.
   E. Portions of organs and other soft tissues.

6. The first step in preparing a tissue specimen for sectioning is
   A. To place it in a fixative.
   B. To dehydrate by replacing the water with organic solvents.
   C. To replace the organic solvents with clearing agents to make the specimen transparent.
   D. To place the specimen in a paraffin bath which replaces the clearing agent and fills the tissue spaces.
   E. To embed the specimen in a cube-shaped mold containing fresh melted paraffin.

7. The second step in preparing a tissue specimen for sectioning is
   A. To place the specimen in a paraffin bath which replaces the clearing agent and fills the tissue spaces.
   B. To replace the organic solvents with clearing agents to make the specimen transparent.
   C. To embed the specimen in a cube-shaped mold containing fresh melted paraffin.
   D. To place it in a fixative.
   E. To dehydrate by replacing the water with organic solvents.

8. The third step in preparing a tissue specimen for sectioning is
   A. To embed the specimen in a cube-shaped mold containing fresh melted paraffin.
   B. To replace the organic solvents with clearing agents to make the specimen transparent.
   C. To place the specimen in a paraffin bath which replaces the clearing agent and fills the tissue spaces.
   D. To dehydrate by replacing the water with organic solvents.
   E. To place it in a fixative.

9. The fourth step in preparing a tissue specimen for sectioning is
   A. To dehydrate by replacing the water with organic solvents.
   B. To place it in a fixative.
   C. To place the specimen in a paraffin bath which replaces the clearing agent and fills the tissue spaces.
   D. To replace the organic solvents with clearing agents to make the specimen transparent.
   E. To embed the specimen in a cube-shaped mold containing fresh melted paraffin.

Exercises

10. The final step in preparing a tissue specimen for sectioning is
    A. To place it in a fixative.
    B. To dehydrate by replacing the water with organic solvents.
    C. To place the specimen in a paraffin bath which replaces the clearing agent and fills the tissue spaces.
    D. To embed the specimen in a cube-shaped mold containing fresh melted paraffin.
    E. To replace the organic solvents with clearing agents to make the specimen transparent.

11. Before a tissue specimen affixed to a slide can be stained, what must happen to it?
    A. It must be replaced in a fixative.
    B. It must be rehydrated with some fluid by reversing the procedures used to place it in the block.
    C. It must be cleared with special agents to make it transparent.
    D. It must be dehydrated with organic solvents.
    E. It must be sliced very thin.

12. Because different stains have affinities for different components of tissue, depending on their chemical properties, it is customary to apply stains of
    A. At least 2 contrasting colors.
    B. Only 1 color.
    C. Three or more colors.
    D. At least 2 complementary colors.
    E. One light and one dark stain.

13. The first step in staining tissue on a slide is
    A. To immerse or wash the slide with a decolorizer.
    B. To treat the slide with a metachromatic stain.
    C. To treat the slide with a counterstain of a contrasting color.
    D. To treat the slide with a polychrome stain.
    E. To apply a mordant to render the tissue chemically more receptive to staining.

14. After immersing a slide in a stain, the next step is likely to be
    A. To treat the slide with a counterstain of a contrasting color.
    B. Immersing or washing the slide with a decolorizer.
    C. To treat the slide with a polychrome stain.
    D. To treat the slide with a metachromatic stain.
    E. To apply a mordant to render the tissue chemically more receptive to staining.

Exercises

15. After removing the first stain from all parts of the tissue to which it has not become chemically bound, the next step would be
    A. To treat the slide with a polychrome stain.
    B. Immersing or washing the slide with a decolorizer.
    C. To treat the slide with a counterstain of a contrasting color.
    D. To treat the slide with a metachromatic stain.
    E. To apply a mordant to render the tissue chemically more receptive to staining.

16. Differential staining of tissue components may be achieved by exposing tissue components to all of the coloring agents simultaneously using what kind of stain?
    A. A metachromatic stain.
    B. A polychrome stain.
    C. A counterstain.
    D. A fixative prior to staining.
    E. A mordant prior to staining.

17. The removal of a plug of skin or mucous membrane with a cylindrical instrument 2-5 mm in diameter is
    A. An excision biopsy.
    B. A shave biopsy.
    C. An incisional biopsy.
    D. A punch biopsy.
    E. A smear.

18. Removal of a thin layer of skin consisting mostly or entirely of epidermis with a blade held approximately parallel to the surface is
    A. A shave biopsy.
    B. A smear.
    C. An incisional biopsy.
    D. A punch biopsy.
    E. An excision biopsy.

19. On a Pap smear examination, mild dysplasia of squamous cells, including cellular atypia characteristic of HPV infection, is designated
    A. Atypical squamous cells of undetermined significance (ASC-US)
    B. Atypical squamous cells suggestive of high-grade lesions (ASC-H).
    C. A high-grade squamous intraepithelial lesion (HGSIL or HSIL).
    D. A low-grade squamous intraepithelial lesion (LGSIL or LSIL).
    E. A or D.

Exercises

20. On a Pap smear examination, moderate to severe dysplasia is termed
    A. Atypical squamous cells of undetermined significance (ASC-US)
    B. Atypical squamous cells suggestive of high-grade lesions (ASC-H).
    C. A high-grade squamous intraepithelial lesion (HGSIL or HSIL).
    D. A low-grade squamous intraepithelial lesion (LGSIL or LSIL).
    E. B or C.

21. On a Pap smear examination, squamous intraepithelial lesions that do not meet criteria for either of the first two categories may be called
    A. Atypical squamous cells of undetermined significance (ASC-US)
    B. Atypical squamous cells suggestive of high-grade lesions (ASC-H).
    C. A high-grade squamous intraepithelial lesion (HGSIL or HSIL).
    D. A low-grade squamous intraepithelial lesion (LGSIL or LSIL).
    E. A or B.

22. A technique used to remove cells by suction from certain structures such as the prostate, subcutaneous lymph nodes and other neck masses, and breast masses is
    A. Curettage.
    B. Fine needle aspiration.
    C. Smear.
    D. Thin-layer smear.
    E. Washing the surface.

23. A way of obtaining cells for cytologic study of a structure such as the interior of the stomach or lungs is by
    A. Curettage.
    B. Fine needle aspiration.
    C. Thin-layer smear.
    D. Washing a surface.
    E. Smear.

Short Answers

1. Define or explain:
    a. Bethesda system _____
        _____

    b. biopsy _____
        _____

    c. counterstain _____
        _____

Exercises

    f.   mordant _____

         _____

    g. Pap smear _____

         _____

    h. polychrome stain _____

         _____

2. What is the most widely used fixative?

    _____

3. What does the pathologist do with a surgical specimen after completing the gross examination?

    _____

    _____

4. What are some ways by which a surgeon might indicate the origin or anatomic orientation of a specimen taken for pathologic study?

    _____

    _____

    _____

    _____

5. Name some kinds of surgical specimens that are not routinely sectioned for microscopic study.

    _____

    _____

    _____

    _____

6. Why must embedding of tissue in paraffin be preceded by dehydration and clearing?

    _____

    _____

    _____

    _____

Exercises

7. What is meant by making serial sections of a specimen?

   _____

   _____

   _____

   _____

8. What two methods can be used to obtain cells for study from fluids with low cell counts?

   a. _____

   b. _____

9. What is the principal advantage of the frozen section technique?

   _____

   _____

   _____

   _____

10. List several reasons for performing an autopsy.

    _____

    _____

    _____

    _____

11. What two points must always be verified by the pathologist before an autopsy is begun, except in a forensic setting?

    a. _____

    b. _____

12. What is postmortem lividity?

    _____

    _____

Exercises

13. Which major organ is sometimes removed but not opened at the time of autopsy? Why?

_____

_____

_____

_____

14. List two reasons why a frozen section might be requested during surgery?

   a. _____

   b. _____

15. What are the three components of the Bethesda system of reporting Pap smear findings?

   a. _____

   b. _____

   c. _____

Activities for Application and Further Study

1. Why do you think paraffin is the more common embedding media for tissue specimens in spite of the stated advantages of celloidin and Carbowax? (You may need to do a little research outside the text to answer this.)

2. A pathology report is prepared in two steps, the first being the dictation and transcription of the gross findings with that report being returned to the pathologist before the microscopic findings are dictated. Why do you think this procedure has been developed?

3. If, as your textbook says, "the attempt to secure full, detailed, accurate information about the cause of death is not a mere academic exercise," then what purposes does the autopsy serve?

4. Call your local coroner or the pathologist at your local hospital and see if you can obtain a film of an autopsy for the class to see. As you watch the film, compare the procedure to that described in the text. Are there any differences?

Pathologic Change and Pathologic Diagnosis

18

Introduction

This chapter surveys the various types of change that can be observed on gross and microscopic examination of tissue specimens, and discusses their causes and diagnostic implications.

In performing a gross examination of a tissue specimen, the anatomic pathologist looks for departures from expected color, size, shape, surface texture, internal consistency, and homogeneity, as well as for any tumors, cysts, hemorrhage, exudate, tissue death, scarring, or abnormal deposition of materials such as fat or calcium. In examining microscopic sections of tissue the pathologist observes the type, size, shape, number, and distribution of cells present, the configuration and staining properties of their nuclei, cytoplasmic granules, vacuoles, or deposits, the type and distribution of intercellular material such as connective-tissue fibers, extravasated blood, fibrinous or other exudates, and any variations from expected tissue architecture.

Arriving at a pathologic diagnosis is not simply a question of recognizing certain patterns that are characteristic of certain diseases. This visual recognition is only the starting point for an analysis of all available data leading to a diagnostic formulation that includes, when possible, the cause of the disorder in this particular patient, its chronology and degree or extent, and its relation to other abnormal conditions, past and present. In examining tissue from a living patient, the pathologist regards the specimen not as a static product of past events but rather as a momentary glimpse of a dynamic process that is still going on.

The diagnosis may be purely local, referring only to the specimen submitted—for example, a basal cell carcinoma of the cheek, completely excised and contained in its entirety in the surgical specimen submitted. On the other hand, assessment of a small piece of tissue may enable the pathologist to diagnose a widespread or systemic condition. For example, certain findings in a lymph node may indicate a malignant process affecting the entire lymphatic system, and certain changes in the kidney may point to a diagnosis of diabetes mellitus.

Disorders of Development

Developmental disorders are those that are built into the body during fetal development. Here it is important to distinguish clearly between two terms that overlap and are therefore often confused. A hereditary disorder affects an individual's genetic makeup and hence it exists from the moment of conception. Examples are Down syndrome and muscular dystrophy. A congenital disorder is present at birth. Although all hereditary disorders are also congenital (though they may not be evident at birth), many congenital disorders are not hereditary, but are caused by adverse environmental factors during fetal development. Examples are fetal alcohol syndrome due to maternal alcoholism and congenital blindness due to maternal rubella.

A developmental disorder may affect only one organ or tissue—indeed, it may be microscopic—or, on the other hand, it may produce striking deformities and lethal or life-threatening dysfunctions affecting the whole body. Abnormal formation of a tissue or organ is called **dysplasia**. (The term is also applied to acquired malformations or changes in cells.) **Hypoplasia** refers to underdevelopment of a structure, **aplasia** to extreme underdevelopment, and **agenesis** is complete failure of formation (congenital absence).

Many genetic disorders exist only at the cellular or biochemical level. These have been called inborn errors of metabolism. For example, hemophilia is a hereditary inability to form coagulation Factor VIII, a plasma protein needed for normal blood clotting. Sickle cell anemia is a genetically transmitted disorder in which an abnormal hemoglobin (hemoglobin S) is synthesized instead of the normal kind, with the result that erythrocytes are malformed and unduly fragile. Even though an inborn error of metabolism may be molecular in nature and difficult or impossible to detect except by laboratory testing, it can have widespread and devastating effects on health. Both of the examples given above are life-threatening diseases. Numerous inherited metabolic errors have been identified. The subject of inherited disease is discussed more fully in Chapter 23.

During the third week following conception, the embryo differentiates into three primitive layers of cells. Each of these **germ layers** will give rise to a specific group of tissues and organs as development proceeds. The **ectoderm**, or outer layer, forms the epidermis, the nervous system including the specialized sensory structures of the eye and ear, and the enamel of the teeth. The **mesoderm**, or middle layer, forms connective tissue (including cartilage and bone), muscle (all types), the circulatory and genitourinary systems, and the spleen. The **endoderm**, or inner layer, forms the epithelial linings of the respiratory, digestive, and excretory systems, the liver, and the pancreas. Some congenital disorders affect derivatives of only one of these germ layers. Thus an ectodermal dysplasia may result in abnormalities of the skin, the eyes, and the central nervous system.

Further embryonic development involves a complex series of divisions, foldings, and fusions as the basic plan of the body is laid down and the organs begin to form. Any disturbance during this critical period can result in faulty development or in complete fusion. Examples of such disorders are an abnormal communication between two heart chambers, incomplete closure of the spinal column (spina bifida), and cleft palate. Flaws of development may result in zones of essentially normal tissue forming in the wrong places, or in abnormal proportions or combinations of normal tissue. Tissue that appears at an abnormal site is said to be ectopic or heterotopic. For example, implants of thyroid tissue may appear in the ovary. An abnormal combination of tissues in their normal location is called a **hamartoma**.

Disturbances of fetal development can result from maternal malnutrition or infection or from intrauterine exposure to drugs, chemical poisons, or ionizing radiation. Harmful influences acting early in pregnancy, particularly during the first trimester, typically cause spontaneous abortion or severe fetal malformation (failure of organs or limbs to develop; cardiac and neural anomalies). Once the major organ systems are formed, adverse influences on the fetus can cause defects in tissue differentiation, low birth weight, premature birth, or stillbirth.

A **teratogen** is any substance or condition that can induce congenital malformations. Recognized teratogens include drugs (radiopharmaceuticals, anticancer agents, hormones), chemicals (lead, ethyl alcohol), and maternal infections that spread to the fetus. Tetracycline antibiotics administered during pregnancy can cause discoloration and hypoplasia of dental enamel. Intrauterine exposure of a female fetus to the estrogen diethylstilbestrol has resulted in deformities of the genital tract and increased risk of clear cell adenocarcinoma of the cervix or vagina. Fetal alcohol syndrome, which occurs in at least one-half of infants born to women who abuse alcohol chronically during pregnancy, includes mental and growth retardation, spinal defects, cardiac valvular and septal defects, and pixielike facial features (broad flat nose, hypoplastic upper lip, and short palpebral fissures).

The risk of teratogenesis is particularly high with four maternal infections: toxoplasmosis, rubella, cytomegalovirus disease, and herpes simplex, represented by the acronym TORCH. All of these can cause malformations of the brain and the eye. In addition, rubella, which unlike the other TORCH infections does the most damage when contracted during the first trimester, causes malformations of the ear and the heart.

Disorders of Growth and Nutrition

Growth refers generally to an increase in the number of cells rather than to differentiation of cells or increase in cell size. Even when not due to hereditary factors, disorders of growth can begin early in fetal development if the maternal environment is deficient in essential nutrients. Low birth weight is a common feature of many prenatal nutritional syndromes. Deficient maternal intake of folic acid is associated with a risk of neural tube defects (anencephaly, spina bifida).

But most nutritional disorders begin after birth. Good health requires a regular intake of water, proteins, carbohydrates, fats, vitamins, and minerals. Dietary deficiencies of any of these during infancy and childhood may result in stunting of growth or in abnormalities of development. For example, inadequate vitamin D intake can lead to rickets, in which bones are improperly formed. Deficient intake of iron at any age can lead to anemia, a deficiency of red blood cells in the circulation. Even when dietary intake is adequate, the absorption of certain nutrients can be blocked by congenital or acquired abnormalities of the digestive system. Such blockages are the basis for several malabsorption syndromes. In sprue, for example, the absorption of fat in the small intestine is deficient, so that dietary fat passes out of the body in the stools (steatorrhea).

A general deficiency of all nutrients results in cachexia (inanition, starvation), manifested by depletion of fat stores, wasting of muscles, and widespread deterioration of cellular functions. In our culture, overnutrition or exogenous obesity is a more frequently encountered threat to health than inanition. In obesity the amount of adipose tissue in the body, particularly in the subcutaneous fat layer, is increased. Obesity is associated with a higher incidence of many diseases, including hypertension, diabetes, coronary artery disease, degenerative joint disease, and some malignancies. The mortality rate in morbid obesity (twice the ideal weight or greater) is ten times that of the nonobese population.

Hormonal factors play a vital role in nutrition and growth. Abnormal increase or decrease of hormone levels due to disease of endocrine glands can induce local or generalized disturbances of growth and development. Growth hormone from the pituitary gland regulates increase in long bone length and other developmental changes during childhood and adolescence. Deficiency of growth hormone during childhood results in dwarfism. Deficiency of thyroid hormone in childhood causes a nutritional and metabolic retardation known as cretinism. Adrenal disease causing a decline in cortisol levels (Addison disease) is associated with muscle wasting. Endocrine abnormalities are more fully discussed in Chapter 20.

Hypertrophy and hyperplasia refer to excessive growth or development of a tissue or organ. **Hyperplasia** is an increase in the number of cells or other structural elements, **hypertrophy** an increase in the size of cells or fibers. In practice this distinction is often ignored. Overdevelopment may be hormonally induced. An excessive amount of growth hormone in childhood leads to gigantism, or abnormally increased stature. If growth hormone levels rise only after closure of the growth centers in the long bones, the result is a deforming enlargement of the hands, feet, and face called acromegaly. Overdevelopment can also be genetically induced, as in excessive growth of the long bones in arachnodactyly. Increased local circulation, as in arteriovenous fistula, can cause enlargement of an extremity. Compensatory, adaptive, or reactive hyperplasia occurs when part of an organ (e.g., liver or thyroid) is lost and the remaining part enlarges to compensate for the loss. An organ may hypertrophy to meet increased demands placed on it, as when the muscular wall of the left ventricle thickens to compensate for a leaky mitral valve.

Dystrophy refers to abnormal (not necessarily deficient) development as a result of inappropriate nutrition. (The term is also applied to congenital or acquired disorders not directly resulting from nutritional causes.) The abnormal transformation of one fully differentiated tissue type into another—for example, the transformation of columnar epithelium into squamous epithelium—is known as **metaplasia**.

Classical Pathology

The Greek physician Hippocrates (460–377 BC) is honored as the father of medicine because he argued that disease is a purely natural phenomenon, subject to rational explanation and amenable to rational treatment. The doctrines of Hippocrates, as modified and augmented by Galen (AD 129–199), dominated Western medical thought until the beginning of the modern scientific era. According to Hippocratic medicine, health depends on a proper balance of four bodily "humors" (blood, phlegm, yellow bile, and black bile), and disease results when there is an excess of one or more of these with respect to the others. This abortive attempt to formulate reasons for the changes that take place when a person gets sick became the basis for a system of therapeutics that relied heavily on phlebotomy (bloodletting) and the administration of violent emetics and cathartics to rid the body of excessive or "corrupt" humors.

Inflammation

Inflammation is a general term for the reaction of living tissue to injury or irritation. It is the most commonly encountered pathologic process and frequently occurs along with, or as a consequence of, other patterns of response. The gross features of inflammation—redness, heat, swelling, and pain—have been recognized for many centuries. The biochemical and histologic correlates of these phenomena are still under study today. Although, in certain diseases, inflammation occurs in many organs and tissues throughout the body, the pathology of inflammation is best understood as a local event or series of events.

A wide variety of injuries and irritations can elicit an inflammatory response from living tissue—a response that is always strikingly similar, with only minor variations depending on the nature of the stimulus. Causes of inflammation can be divided into two broad categories: pathogenic (disease-causing) microorganisms, and physical or chemical injury. The latter category includes cutting, crushing, burning, freezing, electrical shock, radiation, various types of foreign body, and irritation or poisoning by chemical agents. In addition, certain processes originating inside the body—tissue death due to circulatory impairment, the formation and spread of a malignant tumor, the production of abnormal antibodies that attack normal tissue—can set off an inflammatory response.

For convenience, inflammation is usually thought of as involving two distinct processes: an acute response to injury or irritation, in which the body seeks to contain or limit the damage; and a repair phase in which destroyed tissue is regenerated or replaced by scar tissue. Actually these processes overlap, one grading imperceptibly into the other.

The acute phase of inflammation consists of a response on the part of capillaries and certain cells to chemical substances released by damaged tissue. The capillaries in a zone of inflamed tissue dilate. Although many of the channels in a capillary bed are normally shut down, they all tend to open as part of an inflammatory reaction. In fact, if inflammation persists for more than a few hours, endothelial buds begin to form from capillaries and give rise to new capillaries. At the same time, capillary walls thicken, so that the net effect is congestion or engorgement of tissues with blood rather than an increased flow of blood through the tissues. This increased amount of blood in the tissues, or hyperemia, accounts for the familiar observation of redness and heat in an inflamed part, and is the basis for the word *inflammation*—literally, 'a fire inside'. As a result of vascular engorgement, plasma leaks from capillaries and venules into the tissue spaces producing swelling or edema.

Of more obvious benefit is the cellular component of the inflammatory response. Substances released by damaged tissue attract certain types of cells into the area of injury, a process called chemotaxis. Phagocytic cells assemble with remarkable speed, engulfing, breaking down, and removing dead tissue, foreign material, or invading microorganisms. The principal phagocytes are the histiocytes (macrophages) of connective tissue and the neutrophils and monocytes of the circulating blood. Histiocytes migrate into the battle zone from surrounding tissue. Leukocytes, particularly neutrophils, arrive via the circulation and emerge through capillary walls by a process called diapedesis. In the presence of large fragments of foreign material, many histiocytes may join together to form a syncytium or multinucleate giant cell to deal with the invader more efficiently.

Variable numbers of mast cells, plasma cells, eosinophils, and other cells of blood and tissue may also participate in the cellular response, depending on the inciting cause. Lymphocytes, whose function is to produce antibodies, appear in increasing numbers as the inflammatory response continues, and in chronic inflammation they are usually the principal cell found. Plasma cells (which evolve from lymphocytes) and eosinophils are also more likely to appear in chronic inflammation.

The pathologist refers to a collection of unusual numbers of cells in tissue as an **infiltrate**. An infiltrate of neutrophils and histiocytes will generally be interpreted as a sign of acute inflam-

mation; a lymphocytic infiltrate ("small round cell infiltrate" or "mononuclear cell infiltrate") suggests a more chronic process. The term **exudate** is used in a somewhat general way for any abnormal collection of fluid formed by release of plasma from the circulation into the tissues. A serous exudate is low in protein; a fibrinous exudate is rich in protein, including fibrin. Generally an exudate tends to localize injurious material and limit its spread. An exudate may form on and cling to an epithelial surface; it may accumulate in a body cavity; or it may simply filter into and distend the intercellular spaces of tissue, producing local swelling (edema). When an exudate contains a large amount of dead tissue along with large numbers of neutrophils, it is called **pus**, and its formation is known as **suppuration**. In severe inflammation, damaged capillaries may allow red blood cells to leak into tissue spaces. This local hemorrhage is not part of the inflammatory reaction but rather becomes part of the problem: the extravasated erythrocytes must now be engulfed and broken down by macrophages along with other degenerated tissue elements.

The repair phase of inflammation may begin before the acute phase has reached its peak. Repair of damaged tissue takes place in two distinct ways. Some tissues are able to replace lost or destroyed cells through **regeneration**—an increase in the number of cells by mitosis and division of existing cells (reactive hyperplasia). The liver and epithelial tissues in general have a high potential for regeneration. Peripheral nerves and skeletal muscle have some; cardiac muscle, cartilage, and fat have little; and nerves in the central nervous system have none. When cells cannot be replaced by regeneration, the body does the next best thing and produces a patch of scar tissue.

Wound repair begins with proliferation of capillaries along the wound edges. Loops of newly formed capillaries form minute but grossly visible red granules on the surface of this healing tissue, hence the term **granulation tissue**. Meanwhile, a fibrin-rich exudate forms in any open spaces.

Fibroblasts migrate into this medium from surrounding tissue and produce collagenous fibers, bridging the wound or tissue defect with a zone of scar. This process is known as **fibrosis**. The composition of scar tissue is essentially the same whether it is formed in burned skin, cardiac muscle devitalized by blockage of a coronary artery, or a lung segment ravaged by tuberculosis. The formation of scar tissue in an exudate, a blood clot (thrombus), or a mass of necrotic (dead) tissue is known as **organization**. Sometimes fibrosis results in the "walling off" of a mass of foreign material that cannot be broken down (e.g., a bullet) or of a cavity in tissue left by injury or sloughing.

Once the scar is formed, the capillaries within it are gradually obliterated. With the passage of time, scar tissue tends to shrink and become more dense. Mature scar tissue has no circulation, no feeling, no ability to contract, no sweat glands or hair follicles; it is just fibrous tissue. Generally this is better than nothing, but when fibrosis is excessive it can become a liability. Scar tissue can produce deformity, obstruct normal passages, and compress nerves, causing pain or paralysis. Scar tissue that forms in an area of exudate between two serous surfaces can result in adhesions—such as between the lung and the chest wall, or between adjacent loops of intestine. Fibrosis is a lasting marker of past inflammation. The degree of fibrosis is generally in proportion to the severity and extent of the original injury and the duration of the inflammatory response. A smoldering inflammatory reaction that is kept going by chronic infection or retained foreign material may result in the formation of granulomas—microscopic or grossly evident nodules of excessive fibrous reaction.

Allergy

Allergy or anaphylaxis is a condition of induced hypersensitivity to certain foreign substances (allergens), such as inhaled pollens or swallowed foods or medicines. After an initial exposure to these substances, certain persons form complex proteins called antibodies. On subsequent exposure, a reaction occurs between the allergen and the antibody, culminating in a release of histamine from mast cells. The local effect of histamine release is capillary dilatation and edema. In the skin this can take the form of hives (urticaria) or other types of eruption. In the respiratory tract, allergy can cause congestion of mucous membranes, excessive production of mucous and serous secretions, and bronchiolar spasm and edema (asthma). Serum sickness is a syndrome of fever, urticaria, and joint inflammation due to allergy to foreign protein, such as in serum or antivenin of animal origin. Severe anaphylaxis can cause widespread vascular collapse, shock, and death (anaphylactic shock). Many allergic reactions are transitory, leaving no visible change in tissue specimens. Severe or chronic allergy can cause inflammatory changes, in which eosinophils are conspicuous.

In a number of diseases (rheumatoid arthritis, lupus erythematosus, periarteritis nodosa), the basic abnormality is formation of an antibody that reacts with the body's own tissues to induce local inflammation and destruction. These autoimmune disorders are also called collagen diseases because they attack principally connective tissue.

Infection

Infection means the proliferation of microscopic organisms within the living body, with more or less harmful consequences. Infectious diseases are also called contagious, communicable, or transmissible diseases because, with important exceptions, they can be transmitted in one way or another from one person to another. It is customary and convenient to discuss infection along with inflammation because in most infectious diseases there is a marked inflammatory response, which accounts for the most striking and characteristic signs and symptoms.

The clinical picture and pathologic findings in an infectious disease depend chiefly on the

Modern Pathology

Developments in anatomy, chemistry, and particularly microscopy during the eighteenth century led to a revolution in pathologic thinking. The old Hippocratic-Galenic theories were rejected in favor of a rigorously scientific pathology based on correlation of symptoms and physical findings with gross and microscopic changes detected on postmortem examination. The pioneer of this new anatomic pathology was an Italian physician and anatomist, Giovanni Battista Morgagni (1682–1771), whose epoch-making work, *The Seats and Causes of Disease*, was published in 1761. The German pathologist Rudolf Virchow (1821–1902) carried the science further by explaining disease in terms of changes in the behavior and interrelations of cells. His *Cellular Pathology* was published in 1858.

It was also during the nineteenth century that the French chemist Louis Pasteur (1822–1895) and the German physician Robert Koch (1843–1910) demonstrated conclusively that some diseases are caused by microorganisms that multiply in the body, produce toxic wastes capable of interfering with normal functions, and induce similar disease on being transmitted to healthy persons.

biological properties of the infecting organisms, but also on the route by which they enter the body, their number and virulence, and such host factors as general health and the possession of protective antibodies. Some microorganisms that a normal body can harbor without ill effects are capable of invading tissues and causing disease when host defenses are impaired by nutritional deficiency, disturbances of the immune system, or preexisting infection with another organism. Infectious agents that lie in wait for a breakdown in host defenses are called opportunistic.

Many infections are purely local, as in the case of a dental abscess or a fungal infection of the feet. Others are systemic, spreading through the body by the blood or lymphatic channels and producing widespread, perhaps fatal, disease. Regional spread can also occur, as in the familiar example of a head cold that evolves into a chest cold. Not every infection is due to a single species of organism in pure strain; mixed infections are common in certain parts of the body and in debilitated patients.

In response to some infections, the immune system produces antibodies, complex substances that react chemically with invading organisms or their toxic products in a lock-and-key fashion, inactivating them and bringing the infection to an end. In some cases, protective antibodies continue to be formed throughout life (as, for example, after chickenpox and infectious mononucleosis). In other diseases (the common cold, staphylococcal abscess), any antibodies formed either are not protective or do not continue to be formed after recovery.

The following remarks refer to the pathology of various types of infection. Aspects of infectious disease and the immune response pertaining to clinical pathology are more fully discussed in Chapters 21 and 22 respectively.

Bacterial Infection

Bacteria are one-celled organisms capable of multiplying rapidly by cell division. By no means all bacteria are harmful, and some are even beneficial, including those that live in the normal human colon. Pathogenic bacteria vary greatly in structure, growth characteristics, and ability to harm a human host, and they cause a correspondingly broad range of diseases, including boils, streptococcal pharyngitis, some kinds of pneumonia and meningitis, most urinary tract infections, tetanus, cholera, typhoid fever, tuberculosis, syphilis, and gonorrhea.

Bacteria are classified on the basis of shape, staining properties, cultural characteristics, and other variables. Cocci are round, bacilli rod-shaped. Staphylococci are cocci which form in grape-cluster shapes. Streptococci are cocci that occur as pairs or chains. Spirochetes are spiral-shaped bacteria.

Pathogenic bacteria do much of their harm by producing waste products called toxins. Toxins vary widely in their capacity to damage tissue and to break down normal defenses against the growth and spread of bacteria. Some toxins work locally, such as the streptococcal toxins that break down bridges between cells and allow the bacteria to infiltrate tissue more readily. Others have remote or systemic effects, such as toxins produced by tetanus organisms, which can induce generalized convulsions and paralysis. The presence of toxins (not necessarily of bacterial origin) in the circulation is known as toxemia.

Pathogenic bacteria multiply generally in intercellular fluid, occasionally in cavities and tissue spaces such as the urinary bladder, the pericardium, or a joint space. A suppurative infection which remains localized—"walled off" by tissue reaction—is called an abscess. This type of infection is commonly caused by staphylococci and some other organisms. Infection that spreads readily through tissue spaces, causing diffuse swelling, such as that induced by some streptococci, is called cellulitis. Septicemia is the invasion of the blood stream by significant numbers of virulent organisms from a focal infection. This may result not only in severe systemic symptoms—fever, chills, and circulatory collapse—but also in the formation of secondary abscesses remote from the original focus.

Only a few types of bacteria are capable of invading cells. Rickettsiae are very small bacilli that reproduce inside host cells and cause a variety of diseases, including typhus and Rocky Mountain spotted fever, most of them characterized by fever and rash. Chlamydias, which cause ocular and genital infections, are also intracellular bacteria. None of these intracellular organisms can be detected in routine histologic preparations. Indeed, the diagnosis of infectious disease generally requires cultures, serologic testing, and special staining procedures that pertain to clinical rather than to anatomic pathology.

Fungi

Fungi are less important than bacteria as causes of human disease. Most of the pathogenic fungi cause only superficial infections of skin and mucous membranes, hair, and nails (such as athlete's foot and ringworm of the skin), but a few are capable of systemic spread to produce severe, even life-threatening disease of the lungs, central nervous system, or other tissues. Two forms of fungi are recognized. A yeast is a unicellular organism that reproduces by budding. A mold consists of multicellular, filamentous masses (mycelia) of branching tubules called hyphae, which reproduce by various means. A few fungi can exist in either form, but most occur in only one form.

Several types of fungi may be present on normal skin and in other areas of the body, and only invade tissue when there is some impairment of local or general defenses. In fact, all fungi possess only slight invasive abilities. Typically a fungus elicits only a mild inflammatory reaction, but often a very chronic one. Fungi cannot be identified in tissue sections without special staining procedures.

Viruses

Unlike bacteria and fungi, viruses are not living organisms. A virus is a very small segment of genetic material (DNA or RNA) encased in a protective protein shell. Upon entering a living cell, the virus assumes control of that cell's function and reproduction. The normal operations of the cell are suspended and it becomes a factory for the synthesis of more virus. Finally the cell disintegrates, releasing hundreds of thousands of new virus particles, which can then invade other cells. Viral infection typically elicits an acute, self-limited inflammatory response, without suppuration or fibrotic reaction. Viruses show a predilection for skin and mucous membranes, and even those that cause systemic disease often produce eruptions of papules or vesicles (as in measles and chickenpox).

Viruses cause many important diseases, including the common cold, influenza, measles, mumps, chickenpox, warts, herpes simplex, hepatitis, poliomyelitis, AIDS, and rabies. Virus particles are much too small to be seen by light microscopy, but cells infected with virus show characteristic changes that may enable the pathologist not only to recognize that infection is present but even to identify the specific virus involved. Among these changes may be mentioned cytoplasmic and intranuclear inclusion bodies and the formation of multinucleate giant cells.

Parasites

Parasites are a heterogenous group of organisms that spend part or all of their life cycles on or in the human body, causing varying degrees of disease by depriving the host of nutrients, invading or disrupting tissues, and eliciting allergic and inflammatory reactions. Some parasites, such as the protozoans that cause malaria and amebic dysentery, are microscopic; others, such as liver flukes and intestinal worms, are not. Parasites are more of a health problem in the tropics than in the temperate zone, but a few (pinworms, *Trichomonas*) are found in all latitudes, and any of them can appear in returned travelers. Many parasites, or their cysts or eggs, can readily be identified in tissue sections.

Disorders of Circulation

Hyperemia, Edema

The critical importance of a normal circulation for the health and functioning of all bodily tissues is emphasized by the variety and severity of disorders that can result when this circulation is altered or impaired.

As noted above, inflammation is accompanied by hyperemia (increased blood in tissues, due to engorgement of capillaries) and edema (tissue swelling due to leakage of plasma from the circulation into intercellular spaces). Hyperemia or edema or both can occur in various other conditions as well.

Hyperemia (congestion) may be either active or passive. **Active hyperemia** occurs when the flow of blood into an area is increased by widespread dilatation of arterioles. Besides being part of an inflammatory reaction, this arteriolar dilatation can result from increased environmental temperature, emotional stimuli (blushing), or local or systemic disease or poisoning that impairs vascular tone. In active hyperemia, tissues are redder than normal because of their increased content of oxygenated blood.

Passive hyperemia is caused by a slowing or stoppage of the venous outflow of blood from an organ or tissue. Such a slowing of venous return of blood to the heart can be caused by anything that obstructs or compresses a major vein, including a blood clot, a tumor, scar tissue, or a pregnant uterus. Local impairment of venous drainage induces a condition called stasis, in which blood stagnates in a capillary bed. A more generalized slowing of venous return occurs in congestive heart failure. When the pumping action of the heart is reduced by valvular disease, coronary artery disease, or any other cause, it fails to empty itself completely with each contraction. As a consequence, back-pressure builds up in the veins, and the tissues become congested. When the left ventricle fails, congestion occurs in the lungs; with right ventricular failure, the entire systemic circulation becomes congested. In long-standing heart failure, many organs develop changes known collectively as chronic passive congestion.

Unlike active hyperemia, passive congestion results in a decrease of oxygen supply to tissues and a buildup of waste products. Passively congested tissues and organs become cyanotic (blue) because of their increased content of nonoxygenated blood. Capillaries must dilate to accommodate the increased volume of blood. Edema results from both the rise in capillary pressure and increased permeability of capillaries and venules. Red blood cells as well as plasma may leak into intercellular spaces. In time, edema fluid may be replaced by fibrosis. All of these changes tend to impair the function of an organ such as the liver or the lung more or less severely, and once fibrosis occurs the impairment may be irreversible.

Edema (also known as hydrops or dropsy) may be local or generalized, depending on its cause. Lymphedema is an increase in tissue fluid due to local obstruction of lymphatic channels by a tumor, scarring, or chronic inflammation in lymph nodes. Angioneurotic edema is a local allergic response resulting from a sudden change in vascular tone and permeability. A variety of other conditions can produce increases in capillary permeability of a more widespread distribution. These include severe systemic infections, asphyxia, and intoxication with various chemicals. Osmotic edema results from retention of sodium in cardiac, renal, hepatic, or endocrine disease or from a decrease in the concentration of albumin in plasma. The osmotic effect of a normal level of albumin is to hold the water content of the blood in the circulation despite the pressure within the system. A decline in the production of albumin (as from starvation or liver disease) or loss of albumin from a diseased kidney (nephrotic syndrome) results in leakage of plasma water into tissue spaces.

Ascites is the presence of edema fluid in the abdominal (peritoneal) cavity; pericardial and pleural effusions are called, respectively, hydropericardium and hydrothorax. Edema that is most prominent in the lower extremities is called dependent. Anasarca is a generalized edema of the whole body.

Ischemia, Thrombosis, Embolism

Ischemia is a reduction in the supply of blood to a tissue or organ. It can result from obstruction of a single major artery by a clot or external compression, or from generalized narrowing of arterioles by vascular disease. An organ or tissue that is suddenly and completely deprived of its blood supply cannot long survive the lack of oxygen and essential nutrients and the accumulation of harmful waste products. However, tissues vary greatly in their ability to tolerate ischemia, and the more slowly it develops, the less devastating its effects. Many tissues are able to compensate for ischemia of gradual onset by developing a collateral circulation, consisting of newly formed arterioles and capillary beds. Ischemic tissue is abnormally pale and may become edematous because of increased capillary permeability. Prolonged ischemia may result in atrophy (reduction in size), fibrosis, and permanent loss of function. Severe acute interruption of blood supply to any tissue may culminate in infarction (necrosis, death of tissue).

Blood coagulates when the soluble plasma protein called fibrinogen is converted to fibrin, an insoluble gel that forms strands in which blood cells become enmeshed. The formation of fibrin depends on the presence of calcium and certain other plasma or tissue components. Several alternative series of biochemical reactions, some of them involving platelets, can lead to clotting of blood. A clot that forms within the circulatory system is called a thrombus, and the process of its formation is called thrombosis. This can result from local disease or injury of a vessel wall, circulatory stasis, or an increase in the coagulability of the blood.

A thrombus may completely obstruct the vessel in which it forms. If this is an artery, thrombosis will result in ischemia or infarction of the tissue supplied by the artery; if a vein, in passive congestion of the tissue or organ drained by the vein. Meanwhile, the thrombus undergoes a gradual process of organization. Capillary buds and inflammatory cells enter it from the vessel wall and eventually break it down, leaving behind a mass of fibrous tissue. Canalization (recanalization)—the opening of a new passage through the obstructed vessel—may occur in time. Thrombosis is particularly common in the veins of the pelvis and lower extremity. A thrombus can also develop on the interior wall of a cardiac chamber (mural thrombus) under certain conditions.

Because blood in some parts of the circulatory system normally clots after death, it is important for the pathologist to distinguish between thrombi and postmortem clots. A thrombus is adherent to the vessel wall, tough, and friable; a postmortem clot is soft, homogeneous, and easily separated from the wall of the vessel in which it forms. Depending on their color, postmortem clots may be called either currant jelly clots or chicken fat clots.

Anything other than fluid blood moving through the circulatory system is called an embolus, and the process of its formation or release into the circulation is called embolism or embolization. A thrombus detached from its site of formation is by far the most common kind of embolus, and thromboembolic disease is an important cause of disability and death. A thrombus from a systemic vein passes through the right atrium and right ventricle to lodge in a branch of the pulmonary artery (pulmonary embolism). This can result in fatal circulatory collapse—a common cause of death in elderly and debilitated persons and those suddenly immobilized by injury or surgery. A patient who survives the embolic episode may develop a pulmonary infarction—a zone of tissue death in the affected lung. A mural thrombus from the left atrium or left ventricle can pass through the aorta to block a major artery, producing ischemia or infarction of an organ or an extremity. The release of many thrombotic fragments into the circulation is called a "shower" of emboli. Septic emboli are fragments of an infected thrombus which, upon being released into the circulation, can not only obstruct small vessels but carry infection to sites remote from the original focus.

Materials other than thrombi can enter the circulation and cause embolic phenomena. Air embolism occurs when a substantial volume of air is introduced into a vein as a result of injury, misadventure during certain surgical procedures, or in a deliberate attempt to cause death. Air that reaches the right ventricle interrupts blood flow through the heart. Fat embolism results when fat from injured adipose tissue or marrow from a fractured bone enters the circulation. Extensive fat embolism may lead to a syndrome of respiratory failure, neurologic dysfunction, and petechial rash occurring 1–3 days after long-bone fracture. Amniotic fluid embolism due to entrance of amniotic fluid into the maternal circulation before or during labor usually causes respiratory distress and circulatory collapse (possibly anaphylactic) and may be accompanied by disseminated intravascular coagulation. The mortality rate is high. At autopsy the pulmonary vessels are stuffed with epithelial cells, hair, and amorphous debris of fetal origin. Drugs and other materials injected for recreational purposes can also act as emboli.

Hemorrhage, Shock

The escape of whole blood from the circulation is called hemorrhage. Generally this results from direct injury to one or more vessels, but it can also occur when the wall of a vessel is weakened by disease such as arteriosclerosis or inflammation. Ecchymosis is the release of blood into the skin after injury. Purpura refers to widespread zones of skin hemorrhage due to generalized vascular disease, deficiency of platelets, or circulating toxins. A hematoma is a collection of extravasated blood in tissue.

Shock is an acute, life-threatening state of hypotension (subnormal blood pressure) with inadequate blood flow through vital organs. In shock there is a disparity between the volume of the circulatory system and the volume of blood it contains. A reduction in blood volume is known as **hypovolemia**. The sudden loss of a large amount of blood from the circulation triggers various compensatory mechanisms, including an increase in the force and rate of the heartbeat, a shift of fluid from intercellular spaces into the circulation, and a shutting down of less important capillary beds such as those in the skin and the digestive system. These compensatory mechanisms account for some of the more conspicuous features of hemorrhagic (hypovolemic) shock, such as pallor and coldness of the skin and increased pulse rate. After the rapid loss of about 40% of total blood volume, adequate perfusion of vital organs cannot be maintained by compensatory mechanisms, and death occurs. Hypovolemic shock can also occur when a large volume of plasma is lost from the circulation, as in dehydration and severe burns. Shock can occur in a person with normal blood volume if the arteries undergo widespread dilatation. This happens in severe septicemia (septic shock) and in various chemical intoxications.

Atrophy

Atrophy is a decrease in the bulk of a tissue or structure that was formerly of normal size and development. Generally it results from the reduction or withdrawal of some essential substance. Hence atrophy may be caused by impairment of blood supply, deficiency in the intake or absorption of nutrients, or failure of hormone stimulation. Atrophy implies both a grossly evident decrease in the size of a structure and a reduction in the number of cells composing it. Microscopic examination usually shows a change not only in the absolute number of cells but in their proportion and arrangement.

Many cells, especially those of cardiac muscle, acquire yellow or brown pigment granules (lipofuscin) on undergoing atrophy. This coloration is evident on gross inspection of tissue. Secretory epithelium, such as that of the liver and kidney, is particularly susceptible to reduction in cell number and disturbance of cellular organization. Connective tissue is less subject to atrophy and in fact the fibrous and fatty stromal elements of an atrophic organ may increase, offsetting in some degree the gross reduction in its bulk. Skeletal muscle atrophy involves a reduction in cell size. Some kinds of atrophy may be considered normal. The thymus gland usually undergoes atrophy during infancy, the tonsils after puberty. Atrophy of the ovaries and breasts normally follows menopause.

Cachexia (wasting) or general atrophy has already been described as a consequence of starvation. Cachexia can also result from any severe systemic disease (chronic infection, widespread malignancy) that impairs general metabolism. Fat and muscle are the tissues that are most conspicuously reduced in cachexia. Senile atrophy refers to a group of irreversible chemical changes that take place with aging. Certain tissue elements—elastic fibers, bone, and nerve cells—are particularly subject to senile atrophy, though the type and degree of change vary greatly from person to person. Some features of senile atrophy are probably due to impairment of circulation by vascular disease, itself often a form of senile change.

Many forms of atrophy are purely local. Chronic ischemia from any cause can lead to atrophy of the affected organ or tissues. Pressure atrophy results when a tissue is subject to constant or intermittent pressure, as from a swelling, tumor, or deformity in an adjacent structure. The basis of pressure atrophy is generally a disturbance of the blood and the lymphatic circulation. Obstruction of a duct, such as the ureter or the hepatic duct, can result in such a buildup of pressure within the organ normally drained by that duct that atrophy ensues.

Disuse atrophy results when a part is subjected to prolonged inactivity or immobilization. Muscle and bone are especially vulnerable to this kind of atrophy. Neurotrophic atrophy affects skeletal muscle whose nerve supply has been interrupted by injury or disease. Endocrine atrophy is a reduction in parenchymal elements, with decline in function, of a tissue or organ whose normal hormonal stimulation has been lost. For example, the thyroid and adrenal glands undergo atrophy when the pituitary gland (the source of thyroid stimulating hormone and adrenocorticotropic hormone) is destroyed by disease or surgically removed.

Degeneration

Degeneration is a broad term referring to a heterogeneous group of disorders characterized by changes in tissue chemistry. In most of these disorders, microscopic examination reveals swelling of cells and accumulation or deposition in their cytoplasm of substances not normally seen there. Abnormal deposits of material may also occur in intercellular spaces. Special staining may be required to show or to identify abnormal materials in and among cells. Degenerations are classified according to which of these materials are present.

Degenerative changes involving alteration of tissue proteins are among the most common. Abnormal deposits of protein are identified in microscopic sections by their eosinophilic staining properties, that is, their attraction for eosin and other acidic stains. **Albuminous, hyaline, and waxy degeneration** occur in various tissues, usually as a result of chronic or systemic disorders of tissue chemistry.

Amyloid is a hyaline protein material that can be distinguished from similar substances by staining with Congo red or by application of iodine. Immunoperoxidase staining using antibodies to various amyloid proteins provides more specific identification. In primary amyloidosis, which is of unknown cause, deposits of amyloid appear chiefly in cardiac and skeletal muscle. Secondary amyloidosis, occurring as a sequel or complication of chronic infection (especially tuberculosis) involves primarily the spleen, kidneys, liver, and adrenals. Amyloid deposits are particularly likely to occur in blood vessel walls. Severe amyloidosis can impair organ function.

Mucinous degeneration refers to any tissue disorder accompanied by abnormal accumulation or deposition of mucin, the protein component of mucus. Excessive mucin can be found in tumors formed from mucus-producing glands, or in glands whose ducts have been obstructed. **Mucoid** is a similar substance produced by connective tissue and found in increased amounts in myxedema (resulting from deficiency of thyroid hormone) and in myxoma (a type of connective tissue tumor). Fibrinoid, a breakdown product of diseased collagen, may be seen in various degenerative processes affecting connective tissue, particularly autoimmune disorders.

Degenerative changes involving abnormal deposition of adipose or lipid material (fat) are also common. Routine techniques of tissue preparation remove fat, leaving empty spaces in the sections. Treatment of tissue with osmic acid before dehydration, clearing, and infiltration fixes the fat and colors it black. Sudan III and other stains are useful for showing adipose material, especially in frozen sections. **Fatty infiltration** is an increase in the fat content of connective-tissue (stromal) components of various organs, which occurs in obesity and other disturbances of lipid metabolism. In contrast, **fatty degeneration** refers to the appearance of fat inside parenchymal cells, such as those of the heart, liver, and kidneys, which have sustained metabolic damage as a result of anemia, toxemia, chronic infection, certain chemical intoxications, and other severe systemic disorders. Fatty changes in the liver commonly occur in chronic alcoholism and in both obesity and undernutrition.

Cholesterol is a lipid (fatlike) material normally present in blood and tissues. Deposits of cholesterol can occur in certain tissues, particularly blood vessels, when circulating levels are elevated as a result of diabetes, hypothyroidism, kidney disease, or hereditary disturbance of cholesterol metabolism. Atherosclerosis, a deposition of cholesterol in the lining of arteries accompanied by fibrosis, is a major cause of stroke and heart attack. Cholesterol is a normal component of bile and may form deposits in the wall of the gallbladder, especially when the gallbladder is chronically inflamed. In addition, cholesterol is an important constituent of gallstones.

Several other normal substances may appear in abnormal amounts or locations in tissue as a reflection or accompaniment of biochemical dysfunction. Deposition of calcium in tissues other than bones and teeth is abnormal, except that the pineal gland normally shows some calcification after age 20. Calcium appears in microscopic sections as irregular masses of basophilic (blue) material. Dystrophic calcification is a deposition of calcium in chronically inflamed, fibrotic, or degenerating tissue, as in tendinitis, osteoarthritis, pulmonary tuberculosis, and in aging blood vessels with or without cholesterol deposits. Metastatic calcification is deposition of calcium in normal tissues as a result of an excessive level of calcium in the blood. The lungs, kidneys, and blood vessels are most susceptible; calculi (stones) may also form within the urinary tract. **Ossification** implies not only pathologic calcification but formation of bone tissue with haversian systems.

Glycogen is a starchlike carbohydrate that serves as a storage form of glucose, the principal sugar used by the body in energy metabolism. Glycogen is synthesized by the liver and stored in liver and skeletal muscle cells, to whose cytoplasm it normally imparts a finely granular appearance. Abnormal deposition of glycogen in cells occurs in diabetes mellitus and in hereditary abnormalities of glycogen storage. Special stains may be used to show glycogen.

Salts of **uric acid**, a normal breakdown product of certain foods, accumulate in the blood and tissues in gout and other metabolic disorders. Formation of urate crystals in joints causes the pain and swelling of acute gouty arthritis. Nodular urate deposits in subcutaneous tissue are called tophi. Urates may also contribute to the formation of urinary calculi.

Hemosiderin is an iron-containing breakdown product of hemoglobin. Normally, small amounts of hemosiderin are present in macrophages of the liver and spleen and in other cells. Excessive hemosiderin deposits (hemosiderosis) may be found in macrophages and other cells in any condition in which many red cells are broken down (hemolysis), in chronic passive congestion, and after local hemorrhage into tissues. In hemochromatosis, large amounts of iron and hemosiderin are deposited in the skin and cardiac muscle and in parenchymal cells of the liver and pancreas, as a result of a disturbance of iron metabolism.

Bilirubin, the principal pigment of bile, is formed by the further degradation of hemoglobin in the liver. Disease of the liver or obstruction of its ducts can cause a rise in the level of bilirubin in the blood. When this rise is sufficient to impart a yellow or green color to tissues, the condition is known as jaundice. **Porphyrins** (coproporphyrin and uroporphyrin), additional breakdown products of hemoglobin, may accumulate in tissue and impart a pink to purple color to urine, teeth, bones, and even the skin in persons with various metabolic and hematologic disorders (porphyrias).

Melanin, the normal pigment of the skin and of the iris, may be increased in certain abnormal conditions. Sun exposure, pregnancy, and adrenocortical deficiency (Addison disease) cause bronzing of the skin due to increase of melanin. Melanin is responsible for the tan, brown, or black color of pigmented lesions such as freckles, moles, and malignant melanoma. Melanin pigmentation may occur at sites of chronic inflammation or trauma in the skin and in the cartilage and urine (ochronosis) of persons with alkaptonuria, an uncommon inborn error of metabolism. Deposits of foreign material, such as injected inks (tattoos) and absorbed heavy metals (lead, silver), can also cause pigmentation in skin and other tissues.

Necrosis

Necrosis refers to a group of physical and chemical changes in a cell, tissue, or organ that reflect total and permanent cessation of all biological processes and functions—in a word, death. Severe trauma, chemical poisoning, severe or chronic inflammation or degeneration, and any interruption in the supply of oxygen and nutrients can lead to necrosis. On gross examination, necrotic tissue appears white, gray, or yellow, and opaque. On microscopic examination, necrotic cells have more intensely eosinophilic cytoplasm than living ones and their nuclei may show shrinkage and distortion (pyknosis), fragmentation (karyorrhexis), or dissolution (karyolysis). As time passes, cell membranes rupture and architectural details of tissue are lost.

Various types of necrosis are described on the basis of associated physical changes. In **coagulation necrosis**, the usual pattern, plasma proteins gel and solidify, whereas in **liquefaction necrosis** (characteristic of the central nervous system) the dead tissue becomes fluid. **Caseous necrosis**, seen in tuberculosis, involves the conversion of tissue into microscopic masses of homogeneous, cheesy material. A zone of necrotic tissue typically acts as an irritant and elicits an inflammatory reaction in adjacent tissue. It may also show zones of hemorrhage. **Fat necrosis**, a local necrosis of adipose tissue, may result from trauma or ischemia. It is also seen in pancreatic disease, in which local

release of fat-digesting enzymes may convert fatty tissue to whitish, opaque, nodular material, which is subject to calcification.

Gangrene is an extensive local necrosis, usually in an extremity, due to circulatory impairment. Dry gangrene is a purely ischemic disorder; wet gangrene implies secondary infection of a necrotic limb.

Infarction is localized necrosis of a zone of tissue due to obstruction of an artery or, occasionally, a vein. In some tissues, such as the kidney, infarction produces a pale, bloodless zone of necrosis (anemic infarct). In others, such as the lung and cardiac muscle, necrosis is preceded or accompanied by considerable hemorrhage from damaged vessels (hemorrhagic infarct). Typically an infarct assumes a wedge shape with the narrow end pointing toward the obstructed vessel.

Putrefaction or decay refers to the decomposition of the body as a whole after death. It is due in part to the action of bacteria normally resident in the intestine. Another element in the decomposition of the dead body is autolysis, or breakdown of cells and tissues by the action of their own chemical components. This is particularly conspicuous in the stomach; gastric juice begins to digest the stomach lining within minutes after death. Gases generated in a putrefying body (cadaverine, putrescine, and others) have an oppressive, nauseating odor. They may cause marked swelling of soft tissues and may distend or even rupture the bowel and other body cavities and spaces. Blood and tissue fluids in which gases of putrefaction are dissolved have a foamy or frothy appearance.

Physical Trauma

Physical injury and chemical poisoning are important causes of tissue damage, disease, and death. Physical trauma, broadly conceived, includes any damage to tissues caused by exposure to excessive kinetic, thermal, electrical, or radiant energy. Friction, stretching, compression, cutting, tearing, or crushing of tissue by physical force causes damage in proportion to the amount of force applied and the type and volume of tissue exposed to it. Disruption of capillaries or larger vessels with focal or diffuse hemorrhage is a feature of most physical trauma. Rigid tissues such as bone, cartilage, and teeth are subject to cracking or shattering (fracture). In soft tissues, distortion of normal architecture occurs at gross and microscopic levels, with tearing or bursting of cell membranes, separation of connective tissue fibers, loss of cellular organization, collapse or disruption of ducts, passages, and other tissue spaces with escape of secretions or contained fluids and gases, and general fragmentation of tissue. In cutting and puncturing wounds due to sharp objects, injury may be largely limited to separation of tissues without extensive damage beyond the margins of the wound.

An inflammatory response begins promptly in any injured tissue whose blood supply has not been critically impaired. Destroyed or devitalized tissue undergoes necrosis and is removed by macrophages or by sloughing, while surrounding tissues supply endothelial buds and fibroblasts for regeneration and repair. Infection is a common consequence of trauma, especially when bacteria from the skin, the bowel, or the respiratory tract are introduced into areas of hemorrhage, exudate, degeneration, or necrosis. Fibrotic scarring as a late result of extensive injury may cause severe deformity and dysfunction.

Damage due to excessive heat is usually confined to the skin. Depending on the amount of heat and the duration of exposure, a burn can induce a spectrum of injury ranging from hyperemia and edema to coagulation and carbonization (charring) of protoplasm. Vesication (blistering) occurs when there is an effusion of fluid under the epidermis. Chilling of tissue causes a general retardation of biochemical reactions and a reduction of blood flow through capillary beds, and may lead to edema, vesication, and denaturation of protein.

Electrical shock results from a flow of electrical current through tissues. This may generate enough heat to produce local burns. An electrical current can also interfere with the physiology of nerve and muscle cells, causing failure of respiration, fatal disturbance of cardiac rhythm, or both.

Radiant energy of various wavelengths can damage tissue. Ionizing radiation (x-rays, gamma rays) can not only alter the chemistry of cytoplasm and intercellular fluid but also block cell mitosis and induce aberrant cell division and tumor formation. Cells in mitosis are much more vulnerable to the effects of ionizing radiation than other cells. Sunlight and ultraviolet radiation from other sources can produce acute burns not unlike thermal burns. Prolonged exposure to lower doses of solar irradiation causes tanning (increase in pigment cells), accelerates degeneration and atrophy of both dermis and epidermis, and may promote malignant change.

Chemical Poisons

The variety of ways in which chemical poisons can do harm is almost as broad as the variety of poisons. Chemical poisons in gas, liquid, or solid form can exert their effects on contact with skin and mucous membranes or by being swallowed, inhaled, or injected. Strong mineral acids (sulfuric acid, nitric acid) have an immediate and undiscriminating corrosive action on all tissues. Heavy metals (lead, mercury, arsenic) interfere with the metabolism of any cells to whose cytoplasm they penetrate. Organic solvents (benzene, carbon tetrachloride) have a predilection for nerve tissue because of its high content of fatty material. Carbon monoxide competes with oxygen for binding sites on hemoglobin molecules in red blood cells. Some substances block mitosis in certain types of cells. Benzene, for example, can interfere with formation of red blood cells.

Drugs and certain plant poisons may exert a highly specific action on one type of tissue—for example, the conduction system of the heart—or may interfere with one specific type of biochemical reaction—for example, the synthesis of essential clotting factors. Establishing a diagnosis of chemical poisoning usually depends on identification of the poison by chemical analysis of blood, tissue, secretions, or waste products.

Neoplasia

Neoplasia can be defined as an erratic, uncontrolled growth of cells that serves no useful or beneficial purpose. The product of neoplasia may be called a growth, tumor, or neoplasm. Various explanations have been offered for the occurrence of neoplasia, but none of these fits all cases. Among causes that seem to explain certain types of neoplasms may be mentioned an aberrant repair process after chronic inflammation; alteration of cell genetics by chemical poisons, ionizing radiation, or viral infection; hormonal stimulation; depression of cellular immunity; and hereditary factors.

Neoplastic cells arise from normal cells by abnormal mitosis and generally bear some resemblance to their cells of origin. However, their genetic coding is permanently deranged, and this is often reflected in irregularity of structure (atypia). Moreover, neoplastic tissue generally fails in some measure to duplicate the internal organization and architecture of normal tissue. For example, glandular structures may be ill-formed or nonfunctioning, and the expected proportions and relations between parenchyma and stroma may not be preserved. Neoplasia is sometimes difficult to distinguish histologically from chronic inflammation.

A neoplasm that is capable of causing death by extending into or spreading to normal tissue and destroying it is called cancerous or malignant; one that does not do so is called benign. It is noteworthy that a histologically benign tumor can cause death by compressing some vital structure or eroding a major blood vessel, and on the other hand, a slowly growing malignancy may not prove lethal if a more rapidly progressive fatal condition supervenes. Some tumors are inherently malignant from their earliest origins, while others begin as benign tumors and undergo malignant degeneration. Most benign tumors, however, remain benign.

Much of the day-by-day practice of pathology is concerned with the identification of malignancies and the determination of their extent and expected future behavior. Several features are more characteristic of malignant neoplasms than of benign ones. First, a malignant tumor is more likely to display anaplasia—the presence of primitive cells, or more undifferentiated cells than are normally present in the affected tissue. Second, a malignant tumor typically enlarges by infiltration and invasion of surrounding tissues, whereas a benign tumor expands while remaining sharply localized and readily distinguishable from surrounding normal tissue. Often a benign tumor has a definite capsule.

Third, a malignant tumor tends to grow faster than a benign one. Fourth, a malignant tumor is capable of metastasis—establishing secondary foci of malignant cells at sites remote from the primary tumor. Metastasis can be lymphatic, through lymph channels; hematogenous, through the blood circulation; or by direct implantation, as in the peritoneal cavity and central nervous system, where seeding of a fluid medium with malignant cells can result in development of metastatic tumors over the surface bathed by that fluid (drop metastases). Each type of tumor has its preferred sites for metastasis. In general, tumors of epithelial origin (carcinomas) tend to metastasize by lymphatic channels, tumors of connective tissue origin (sarcomas) by the blood stream. Metastasis to a vital organ such as the brain, the lung, or the liver is a common mechanism of death in malignant disease. The presence of widespread metastases (carcinomatosis) is often associated with cachexia, toxic manifestations, and increased susceptibility to infection.

Malignant cells display a number of distinctive morphologic features. They tend to vary more in size (anisocytosis) and shape (pleomorphism) than normal cells, and to form irregular clusters instead of showing the polarity of normal cell aggregations. The nuclei of malignant cells tend to be larger than the nuclei of nonmalignant cells in proportion to their cytoplasm (high nuclear/cytoplasmic ratio) and to vary more in size, shape, and structure. These nuclei also tend to stain more darkly (hyperchromasia) and to show prominent nuclear membranes and one or more large, acidophilic nucleoli. Mitotic figures are more frequent in malignant tissue, and are often multipolar or otherwise anomalous. The cytoplasm of malignant cells often contains vacuoles. Giant-cell formation is characteristic of some malignancies.

A neoplasm is called hormone-dependent when its development results in part from stimulation by a normal or abnormal level of hormone in the circulation. For example, cancer of the prostate depends on testicular androgen, and does not develop in men who have been castrated. Conversely, both benign and malignant tumors arising from glandular tissue can produce excessive levels of hormone that cause remote or systemic effects (functioning tumors). Hormone-like substances produced by tumors arising from nonglandular cells may also induce remote effects (paraneoplastic syndromes).

Because the proliferation of neoplastic tissue is not subject to normal controls, it often outstrips the available blood supply. Many tumors, especially malignant ones, contain areas of degeneration, necrosis, and hemorrhage. Cysts formed within a tumor may be lined with secretory epithelium and contain serous, mucinous, or other secretion, or they may simply be clefts or spaces formed by degeneration of tissue and filled with necrotic debris. Calcium deposits may develop in degenerating tumor tissue. In a scirrhous tumor, exuberant production of connective tissue fibers (desmoplasia) yields a dense, woody or stony consistency. Some malignancies, particularly rapidly growing ones, elicit intense inflammatory reaction in surrounding tissues. A malignant tumor developing on a surface, such as skin or mucous membrane, may evolve in one of three patterns: as a thickened plaque, infiltrating laterally; as a polypoid or fungating mass growing away from the surface; or as an ulcer formed by undermining and destruction of surface epithelium.

The **grade** of a malignant neoplasm is a quantitative estimate of its malignant potential, generally based on the percentage of anaplastic (undifferentiated) cells it contains. Grading correlates generally with the expected future behavior of a tumor, a high-grade malignancy being more prone to invade and metastasize than a low-grade one. The following widely used grading system is called the Broders index:

Grade 1: one-fourth undifferentiated cells
Grade 2: one-half undifferentiated cells
Grade 3: three-fourths undifferentiated cells
Grade 4: all cells undifferentiated

Staging of a malignancy is a formulation of its current extent, an attempt to describe its behavior up to the present. A tumor that remains confined to its tissue of origin is said to exist **in situ** (carcinoma in situ). A system of staging used for many tumors is the TNM (tumor-node-metastasis) classification. In each class, a number represents the degree of spread, 0 meaning "none" or "undetectable." Thus, T2, N1, M0 would indicate a locally invasive tumor with involvement of regional lymph nodes but no distant metastases. Elaborate TNM codes have been worked out for several types of tumor.

Both grading and staging of tumors are important in prognosis, in choice of therapy, and in statistical recording (tumor registry).

Nomenclature of the Commoner Neoplasms

Origin	Benign Neoplasms	Malignant Neoplasms
Epithelium		
surface epithelium	papilloma	epidermoid carcinoma
secretory epithelium	adenoma	adenocarcinoma
endothelium, lymph vessel	lymphangioma	lymphangioendothelioma
endothelium, blood vessel	hemangioma	hemangioendothelioma
Connective Tissue		
adult fibrous tissue	fibroma	fibrosarcoma
fat	lipoma	liposarcoma
cartilage	chondroma	chondrosarcoma
bone	osteoma	osteogenic sarcoma
embryonic fibrous tissue	myxoma	myxosarcoma
notochord	chordoma	chordoma
nerve sheath	neurofibroma	neurogenic sarcoma
Muscle		
skeletal muscle	rhabdomyoma	rhabdomyosarcoma
smooth muscle	leiomyoma	leiomyosarcoma
Nerve		
neuron	neuroma	neuroma
Hemolymphatic Tissue		
bone marrow		myeloma
lymphoid tissue		lymphoma

Exercises

Fill in the Blanks

1. A _____ disorder affects an individual's genetic makeup and hence it exists from the moment of conception.

2. A _____ disorder is present at birth.

3. All _____ are congenital, but not all congenital disorders are hereditary.

4. Hereditary and congenital disorders (may, may not be) evident at birth. (Choose one.)

5. Abnormal formation of a tissue or organ and acquired malformations or changes in cells are called _____.

6. Disorders that exist only at the cellular or biochemical level have been called _____.

7. Zones of essentially normal tissue forming in the wrong places are said to be _____ or _____.

8. An abnormal combination of tissues in their normal location is called a _____.

9. A _____ is any substance or condition that can induce congenital malformations.

10. Growth refers generally to an _____ in the number of cells rather than to _____ of cells or increase in cell size.

11. Even when dietary intake is adequate, the absorption of certain nutrients can be blocked by congenital or acquired abnormalities of the digestive system and can result in several _____.

12. _____ refers to abnormal (not necessarily deficient) development as a result of inappropriate nutrition.

13. The abnormal transformation of one fully differentiated tissue type into another—for example, the transformation of columnar epithelium into squamous epithelium—is known as _____.

14. In inflamed tissues, substances released by damaged tissue attract certain types of cells into the area of injury, a process called _____.

15. The function of _____ is to produce antibodies.

16. Lymphocytes, plasma cells (which evolve from lymphocytes), and eosinophils are more likely to be increased in _____ inflammation.

17. A collection of unusual numbers of cells in tissue is referred to as an _____.

Exercises

18. The term _____ is used in a somewhat general way for any abnormal collection of fluid formed by release of plasma from the circulation into the tissues.

19. The formation of pus is known as _____.

20. Infection is the _____ within the living body, with more or less harmful consequences.

21. Infectious diseases are also called contagious, communicable, or transmissible diseases because, with important exceptions, _____.

22. _____ organisms are microorganisms that a normal body can harbor without ill effects but that are capable of invading tissues and causing disease when host defenses are impaired by nutritional deficiency, disturbances of the immune system, or preexisting infection with another organism.

23. A virus is a _____ encased in a protective protein shell.

24. Two consequences of inflammation from altered or impaired circulation are _____ and _____.

25. _____ occurs when the flow of blood into an area is increased by widespread dilatation of arterioles and results in tissues being redder than normal because of their increased content of oxygenated blood.

26. Stasis, or local impairment of venous drainage in which blood stagnates in a capillary bed, and congestive heart failure, a more generalized slowing of venous return caused by right ventricular failure, are examples of a condition known as _____.

27. _____, a deposition of cholesterol in the lining of arteries accompanied by fibrosis, is a major cause of stroke and heart attack.

28. Establishing a diagnosis of chemical poisoning usually depends on _____.

29. _____ can be defined as an erratic, uncontrolled growth of cells that serves no useful or beneficial purpose, resulting in a growth, tumor, or neoplasm.

30. A neoplasm that is capable of causing death by extending into or spreading to normal tissue and destroying it is called _____ or _____; one that does not do so is called _____.

Exercises

Multiple Choice: Circle the letter of the best answer from the choices given.

1. Which of the following is an example of a congenital disorder as opposed to hereditary?
   A. Down syndrome.
   B. Fetal alcohol syndrome.
   C. Muscular dystrophy.
   D. Inborn error of metabolism.
   E. Spina bifida.

2. All of the following are hereditary disorders except
   A. Cleft palate.
   B. Down syndrome.
   C. Congenital blindness due to maternal rubella.
   D. Muscular dystrophy.
   E. Spina bifida.

3. The risk of teratogenesis is particularly high after maternal infection with a TORCH organism, which includes all of the following conditions except
   A. Toxoplasmosis.
   B. Herpes simplex.
   C. Cytomegalovirus disease.
   D. Roseola.
   E. Rubella.

4. An excessive amount of growth hormone in childhood leads to an abnormally increased stature, known as
   A. Gigantism.
   B. Acromegaly.
   C. Arachnodactyly.
   D. Hyperplasia.
   E. Hypertrophy.

5. If growth hormone levels rise only after closure of the growth centers in the long bones, the result is a deforming enlargement of the hands, feet, and face called
   A. Gigantism.
   B. Dwarfism.
   C. Addison disease.
   D. Acromegaly.
   E. Cretinism.

Exercises

6. Thickening of the muscular wall of the left ventricle to compensate for a leaky mitral valve is an example of
   A. Addison disease.
   B. Metaplasia.
   C. Compensatory hyperplasia.
   D. Acromegaly.
   E. Dystrophy.

7. The inability of the cells to repair damage to an organ or tissue through regeneration results in
   A. Granulomas.
   B. Anaphylaxis.
   C. Fibrosis.
   D. Granulation.
   E. Scar tissue.

8. Which of the following terms is defined as microscopic or grossly evident nodules of excessive fibrous reaction?
   A. Granulomas.
   B. Scar tissue.
   C. Anaphylaxis.
   D. Fibrosis.
   E. Granulation.

9. Which of the following terms refers to the proliferation of capillaries along the wound edges evidenced by minute but grossly visible red granules on the surface?
   A. Fibrosis.
   B. Granulation.
   C. Anaphylaxis.
   D. Granulomas.
   E. Scar tissue.

10. Fibroblasts migrate into the fibrin-rich tissue in a wound from surrounding tissue and produce collagenous fibers, bridging the wound or tissue defect with a zone of scar in a process known as
    A. Granulomas.
    B. Granulation.
    C. Anaphylaxis.
    D. Fibrosis.
    E. Scar tissue.

Exercises

11. _____ is a condition of induced hypersensitivity to certain foreign substances (allergens), such as inhaled pollens or swallowed foods or medicines.
    A. Granulomas.
    B. Granulation.
    C. Anaphylaxis.
    D. Fibrosis.
    E. Scar tissue.

12. _____ are complex substances that react chemically with invading organisms or their toxic products in a lock-and-key fashion, inactivating them and bringing the infection to an end.
    A. Antibodies.
    B. Antigens.
    C. Granulomas.
    D. Allergens.
    E. Hives.

13. Infection that spreads readily through tissue spaces, causing diffuse swelling, such as that induced by some streptococci, is called _____.
    A. Bacteremia.
    B. Toxemia.
    C. An abscess.
    D. Septicemia.
    E. Cellulitis.

14. _____ is the invasion of the blood stream by significant numbers of virulent organisms from a focal infection.
    A. Bacteremia.
    B. Toxemia.
    C. An abscess.
    D. Septicemia.
    E. Cellulitis.

15. Which of the following are organisms that spend part or all of their life cycles on or in the human body, depriving the host of nutrients, invading or disrupting tissues, and eliciting allergic and inflammatory reactions?
    A. Bacteria.
    B. Parasites.
    C. Viruses.
    D. Antibodies.
    E. Fungi.

Exercises

16. The common cold, influenza, measles, mumps, chickenpox, warts, herpes simplex, hepatitis, poliomyelitis, AIDS, and rabies are examples of diseases induced by which of the following?
    A. Antibodies.
    B. Bacteria.
    C. Fungi.
    D. Parasites.
    E. Viruses.

17. Yeasts and molds which infect primarily the skin and mucous membranes are subdivisions of which of the following pathogens?
    A. Antibodies.
    B. Bacteria.
    C. Fungi.
    D. Parasites.
    E. Viruses.

18. Which of the following is an increase in tissue fluid due to local obstruction of lymphatic channels by a tumor, scarring, or chronic inflammation in lymph nodes?
    A. Lymphedema.
    B. Angioneurotic edema.
    C. Edema.
    D. Congestion.
    E. Passive hyperemia.

19. Which of the following is a local allergic response resulting from a sudden change in vascular tone and permeability?
    A. Lymphedema.
    B. Angioneurotic edema.
    C. Edema.
    D. Congestion.
    E. Passive hyperemia.

20. The presence of edema fluid in the pericardial space is called _____.
    A. Ascites.
    B. Angioneurotic edema.
    C. Congestive heart failure.
    D. Hydropericardium.
    E. Anasarca.

21. Pleural effusion, or the presence of edema fluid in the pleural space, is called
    A. Ascites.
    B. Anasarca.
    C. Hydrothorax.
    D. Angioneurotic edema.
    E. Dependent edema.

22. Which of the following terms denotes generalized edema of the whole body?
    A. Ascites.
    B. Anasarca.
    C. Hydrothorax.
    D. Angioneurotic edema.
    E. Dependent edema.

23. Which of the following terms refers to a collection of extravasated blood in tissue?
    A. Hematoma.
    B. Hemorrhage.
    C. Shock.
    D. Purpura.
    E. Ecchymosis.

24. Which of the terms below refers to widespread zones of skin hemorrhage due to generalized vascular disease, deficiency of platelets, or circulating toxins?
    A. Ecchymoses.
    B. Purpura.
    C. Hematoma.
    D. Extravasation.
    E. Hypovolemia.

25. The escape of whole blood from the circulation is called
    A. Hemorrhage.
    B. Ecchymosis.
    C. Purpura.
    D. Shock.
    E. Hematoma.

Exercises

26. The sudden loss of a large amount of blood from the circulation triggering an increase in the force and rate of the heartbeat, a shift of fluid from intercellular spaces into the circulation, and a shutting down of less important capillary beds results in a condition called _____.
    A. Compensatory shock.
    B. Congestive failure.
    C. Hypovolemic shock.
    D. Septic shock.
    E. Hypotensive shock.

27. Which of the following terms refers to a decrease in the bulk of a tissue or structure that was formerly of normal size and development?
    A. Hypertrophy.
    B. Entropy.
    C. Cachexia.
    D. Degeneration.
    E. Atrophy.

28. Which of the following terms refers to a group of irreversible chemical changes that take place with aging?
    A. Disuse atrophy.
    B. Neurotrophic atrophy.
    C. Endocrine atrophy.
    D. Pressure atrophy.
    E. Senile atrophy.

29. Which of the following results when a tissue is subject to constant or intermittent pressure, as from a swelling, tumor, or deformity in an adjacent structure?
    A. Disuse atrophy.
    B. Neurotrophic atrophy.
    C. Endocrine atrophy.
    D. Pressure atrophy.
    E. Senile atrophy.

30. Which of the following is a type of degeneration characterized by an increase in the fat content of connective-tissue (stromal) components of various organs, which occurs in obesity and other disturbances of lipid metabolism?
    A. Waxy degeneration.
    B. Fatty infiltration.
    C. Mucinous degeneration.
    D. Primary amyloidosis.
    E. Fatty degeneration.

Exercises

31. Which of the following refers to the appearance of fat inside parenchymal cells, such as those of the heart, liver, and kidneys, which have sustained metabolic damage as a result of anemia, toxemia, chronic infection, certain chemical intoxications, and other severe systemic disorders?
    A. Fatty degeneration.
    B. Fatty infiltration.
    C. Mucinous degeneration.
    D. Primary amyloidosis.
    E. Waxy degeneration.

32. Which type of necrosis is seen in pancreatic disease, in which local release of adipose-digesting enzymes may convert adipose tissue to whitish, opaque, nodular material, which is subject to calcification?
    A. Fat necrosis.
    B. Waxy necrosis.
    C. Coagulation necrosis.
    D. Caseous necrosis.
    E. Liquefaction necrosis.

33. Which of the following types of necrosis refers to the form in which plasma proteins gel and solidify?
    A. Waxy necrosis.
    B. Coagulation necrosis.
    C. Fat necrosis.
    D. Liquefaction necrosis.
    E. Caseous necrosis.

34. Which type of necrosis, seen in tuberculosis, involves the conversion of tissue into microscopic masses of homogeneous, cheesy material?
    A. Liquefaction necrosis.
    B. Fat necrosis.
    C. Coagulation necrosis.
    D. Waxy necrosis.
    E. Caseous necrosis.

35. In which of the following types of necrosis does the dead tissue becomes fluid?
    A. Caseous necrosis.
    B. Coagulation necrosis.
    C. Liquefaction necrosis.
    D. Fat necrosis.
    E. Waxy necrosis.

Exercises

Short Answers

1. Define pathology. Name and define its three principal branches.

    _____

    _____

    _____

    _____

2. Define or explain:

    a. anaplasia _____

    _____

    b. ascites _____

    _____

    c. desmoplasia _____

    _____

    d. embolism _____

    _____

    e. thrombosis _____

    _____

    f. hyperchromasia _____

    _____

    g. infarction _____

    _____

    h. ischemia _____

    _____

    i. necrosis _____

    _____

    j. pleomorphism _____

    _____

    k. putrefaction _____

    _____

    l. shock _____

    _____

Exercises

3. What information does a pathologist's report contain besides a record of abnormalities found in the specimen?

    _____

    _____

    _____

    _____

4. What kinds of change in the gross and microscopic features of a tissue specimen are taken into account by the pathologist in arriving at a diagnosis?

    _____

    _____

    _____

    _____

5. Distinguish the following:

    a. hypoplasia _____

    _____

    b. aplasia _____

    _____

    c. agenesis _____

    _____

6. What are the three germ layers?

    a. _____

    b. _____

    c. _____

7. How does hypertrophy differ from hyperplasia?

    _____

    _____

    _____

    _____

Exercises

8. List various causes of inflammation.

_____

_____

_____

_____

9. What is responsible for the redness and heat in inflamed tissue?

_____

_____

_____

_____

10. What is phagocytosis?

_____

_____

_____

_____

11. Distinguish beneficial from harmful types of antibody formation.

_____

_____

_____

_____

12. Name some autoimmune or collagen diseases.

_____

_____

_____

_____

Exercises

13. In what important ways do viruses differ from bacteria and fungi?

_____

_____

_____

_____

14. What are some ways in which a parasite may affect the health of the host?

_____

_____

_____

_____

15. Mention some types of atrophy that are normal or expected.

_____

_____

_____

_____

16. What is the name of the pigment normally found in the skin and the iris?

_____

_____

_____

_____

17. List four major differences between benign and malignant neoplasms.

a. _____

b. _____

c. _____

d. _____

Exercises

18. Distinguish between grading and staging of malignant neoplasms.

_____

_____

_____

_____

19. In what ways do the following substances normally found in the body cause problems?

    a. cholesterol_____

    _____

    b. calcium _____

    _____

    c. glucose _____

    _____

    d. uric acid _____

    _____

    e. bilirubin _____

    _____

    f. melanin _____

    _____

20. List three types of trauma that can cause changes in tissues detectable by gross and microscopic examination.

    a. _____

    b. _____

    c. _____

Exercises

Activities for Application and Further Study

1. "According to Hippocratic medicine, health depends on a proper balance of four bodily 'humors' (blood, phlegm, yellow bile, and black bile), and disease results when there is an excess of one or more of these with respect to the others." Perhaps with the help of your instructor, your terminology book, or a librarian, list medical conditions based on these "humors." For example, the term "exsanguinate" comes from *sanguis* (blood).

2. Using a dictionary, list 5-10 each of common bacteria, parasites, fungi, and viruses that are pathogenic in man. Beside each, list the condition(s) each organism causes and in a third column some of the prominent symptoms of each condition. Do you see patterns of similarity or dissimilarity among the organisms in the same calss. Are there similarities between classes of organisms?

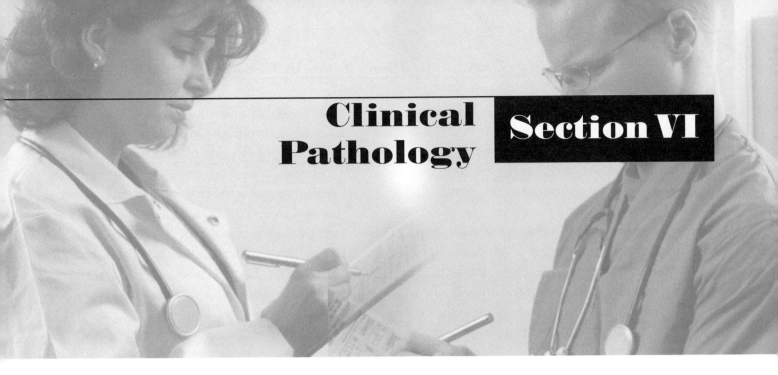

Clinical Pathology

Clinical pathology is the branch of pathology that is concerned with examinations and tests performed on body fluids such as blood and cerebrospinal fluid, wastes such as urine and feces, and abnormal products such as pus and calculi. Most of these examinations yield quantitative data, that is, they count discrete components or measure concentrations, rates, or other features of a specimen that are capable of being expressed numerically. By convention, the terms **laboratory (lab) test**, **laboratory (lab) work**, and so on are limited to procedures pertaining to clinical pathology, even though most of the procedures proper to anatomic pathology are also carried out in laboratories.

Clinical pathology is divided into a number of branches. The names of some of these branches have double meanings, referring both to independent scientific disciplines or medical specialties or subspecialties and also to divisions of medical technology. **Hematology** is the study of blood. The term refers both to a subspecialty of internal medicine concerned with abnormalities in the formation and function of blood cells (such as anemia and leukemia) and to a branch of laboratory technology concerned with the performance of quantitative and qualitative assessments of blood cells.

Biochemistry deals with the chemical properties and interactions of all the substances composing the living body. **Clinical chemistry** is the application of biochemistry to diagnostic medicine. In practice, clinical chemistry refers almost exclusively to quantitative chemical analysis of blood specimens. **Urinology** is a branch of medical technology that involves basic microscopic and chemical examination of urine specimens.

Microbiology is concerned with the study of microscopic living things. Medical microbiology concentrates on bacteria, fungi, and other microorganisms capable of causing human disease. Bacteriology, parasitology, mycology (the study of fungi), and virology are divisions of medical microbiology. **Immunology** studies the defensive mechanisms whereby the body recognizes foreign materials and invading microorganisms as non-self and mobilizes cellular and chemical agents against them. **Serology** (a branch of immunology) studies antigen-antibody reactions, particularly with respect to the diagnosis of infectious diseases. **Molecular biology**, a branch of biochemistry that investigates DNA and RNA, provides diagnostic information about both infectious and inherited diseases.

The practice of clinical pathology thus comprises an extensive range of physical, chemical, and biological procedures. These include microscopic examination of blood and other fluids for an assessment of the number and type of cells present, both normal and abnormal, and for the identification of pathogenic microorganisms, crystals, and foreign material; qualitative and quantitative chemical analysis of body fluids, particularly blood, for electrolytes, carbohydrates, proteins, lipids, vitamins, enzymes, hormones, waste products, dissolved gases, drugs, and poisons; culture of material for bacterial, fungal, or viral growth; and biological testing for antibodies indicative of previous or current infection or of certain autoimmune disorders or other conditions.

In the following chapters, the most important of these tests will be briefly described or explained and their significance in diagnosis will be outlined. Space does not permit the inclusion of all laboratory tests in current use or the exhaustive discussion of any test.

A brief survey of the types of procedures performed in clinical pathology is in order here. One

One of Virchow's most memorable contributions to modern pathologic thinking was his statement, "Disease is life under altered conditions." Although even today we find it hard not to think of a disease as a "thing" that someone "has," disease is merely an abstraction—a state, quality, or condition somehow different from that indefinable state, quality, or condition we call "health."

The major premise of pathology is that specific kinds of disease are consistently associated with specific changes in bodily structure and function. A further premise is that the specimen of blood, urine, or tissue submitted to pathologic study is representative of what remains in the patient's body.

basic type of examination is **inspection of a specimen by light microscopy**. The specimen may be examined either in its natural state or after concentration, centrifugation, or treatment with stains or reagents to bring out features that would not otherwise be visible. Microscopic examination can yield various types of information about the material under study. The shape, grouping, and staining characteristics of cells in a fluid such as blood or urine are examples of purely qualitative observations. The size and relative or absolute numbers of various cells present are quantitative measurements. (Usually such measurements are made electronically rather than optically.) The microscope is also used to identify pathogenic microorganisms in smears made directly from body fluids or from cultures; to detect and study parasites or their eggs, crystals, and foreign material; and to observe reactions such as agglutination (clumping) or lysis (bursting) of cells in various serologic tests.

Quantitative chemical analysis plays a very large role in modern clinical pathology, and new tests are constantly being developed. Most of these tests are performed on blood or its plasma or serum fractions, but urine, cerebrospinal fluid, saliva, sweat, hair, and other body products and secretions can also be subjected to chemical analysis. Chemical tests are done to measure the levels of normal bodily constituents such as blood sugar or serum calcium, and also to detect and measure substances not normally present in the body, such as waste products of diseased tissue and chemical poisons.

Medical microbiology employs two basic methodologic tools. One of these is microscopic examination of fresh or processed **smears** of pus or other materials, as discussed above, and the other is the growth of pathogenic microorganisms under controlled conditions in **cultures**. By providing a large number of microorganisms in pure strain, culturing enhances the microbiologist's ability to identify them. In addition, the growth pattern of the organism in the culture medium, which may contain selective nutrients, chemical indicators, or other additives, provides further identifying information. Culturing methods can also be used to test the effectiveness of various antibiotics against a pathogen. Some culturing techniques, such as a colony count of urine, yield quantitative results.

Besides performing direct examinations, measurements, and analyses of specimens, the clinical laboratory technician uses a variety of indirect methods to gather data about a patient's condition. One important type of laboratory determination is **function testing**, in which the capacity of an organ or tissue to perform its normal function is assessed. For example, a measured quantity of a substance may be introduced into the patient's body as a challenge to an organ such as the liver or kidney to incorporate or excrete the substance. The amount of this substance, or of some chemical product or derivative of it, is then measured in the blood, urine, or other fluid, and the functional integrity of the organ under study determined by appropriate calculations.

Several related tests are often performed on one specimen. A group of tests frequently performed together is sometimes called a **panel** or profile (electrolyte panel, liver profile). There are a number of reasons for the practice of performing several tests as a group. The tests composing an electrolyte panel (sodium, potassium, chloride, and bicarbonate) are performed together on the same specimen of blood because the levels of these substances are closely interrelated, are used to calculate other values, and can change from minute to minute. A liver panel includes several tests of liver function, such as direct and total bilirubin, total protein and albumin, AST, ALT, alkaline phosphatase, LDH, ammonia, and cholesterol. Each of these tests looks at liver function from a different angle. The net result of considering them together is a better balanced and more sharply focused view of the functional status of the liver than could be obtained by doing only one or two of the tests.

Another kind of test panel allows the diagnostician to assess several possibilities simultaneously. For example, an arthritis panel, performed on a patient with acute joint symptoms, might include tests to detect rheumatic fever, rheumatoid arthritis, lupus erythematosus, gout, and metabolic bone disease. Although the patient may have none of these, and certainly does not have all of them, it is more convenient to do the tests simultaneously on a single specimen of blood than to do them one at a time, drawing blood separately for each test and awaiting the result before proceeding to the next test.

Modern laboratory medicine makes use of highly diverse and complex technology, often involving sophisticated and expensive instruments and reagents. Many tests, including frequently performed chemical analyses and counts of blood cells, are done by automatic machinery, which not only performs the requisite tests but prints the results in a standard format.

Frequently a blood specimen is subjected to an automated battery of quantitative analyses for twenty or more substances. A chemistry panel or profile of this type provides a broad range of data from a single specimen, and because it is automated it can be carried out at much lower cost than just two or three of the component tests performed individually by a technician. A chemistry panel is often performed when only one or two of the included tests are relevant to the patient's condition. In this setting, the remaining tests may be considered screening procedures.

Because most clinical laboratory tests yield quantitative results, standardization of units of measure is essential for consistency of reporting and interpretation of tests. As mentioned in Chapter 1, the International System (in French, *Système International d'Unités*, or SI) is a decimal system of weights and measures, based on the metric system, that was adopted in 1960. Prefixes and units used in SI are shown in Appendix I. To the meter, kilogram, and second of the metric system, SI added the ampere (a unit of electrical current), the candela (a unit of luminous intensity), the kelvin (a unit of temperature), and the mole (a unit of amount of matter).

A **mole** is defined as the amount of a substance containing a number of elementary particles (atoms, molecules, or ions) equal to the Avogadro number (6.0225×10^{23}). The mass (weight) of one mole of any substance is the molecular weight of that substance expressed in grams. Because chemical substances react with one another in proportion to their molar masses rather than to their weights in grams, molar equivalents are a more rational and useful measure in quantitative chemistry. Clinical laboratories in the United States are gradually making the transition from grams (milligrams, micrograms, etc.) to moles (millimoles, micromoles, etc.) in reporting test results. A mixture of substances, or a substance whose molecular structure is unknown, cannot be measured in moles. Hence for a few materials, weights continue to be given in grams. Molar equivalents of test results and other values are given in this book in square brackets. For example, the normal serum level of myoglobin is 14-51 mcg/L [0.8-2.9 nmol/L].

The official SI abbreviation for the prefix **micro-** (one millionth) is the Greek letter mu (μ). Thus, the SI abbreviation for **microgram** (0.000 001 g, or one millionth of a gram) is μg. The unavailability of Greek letters on some computers and word processors has sometimes led to the ill-advised expedient of substituting the Roman letter *u* for Greek μ. Of deeper concern, in handwritten material the Greek letter can easily be misread as the Roman letter *m*, in which case the abbreviation μg would be misread as *mg* (milligram, 0.001 g, one thousandth of a gram). A computer can make the same mistake in handling digital material composed with non-congruent software.

In order to prevent such errors, it has been recommended that the name of a unit containing the prefix **micro-** (e.g., **microgram, microliter**) be written in full, in both longhand and in computer work. Alternatively, the abbreviation **mc** can be substituted for the Greek letter mu. That practice has been adopted throughout this book,. Thus, **mcg = microgram, mcL = microliter, mcmol = micromol, mcU =microunit**.

Although the liter, a unit of volume equal to one cubic decimeter, is not part of SI, it has been retained for statements of concentration. Concentrations are expressed only per liter and no longer per deciliter, milliliter, or other fractional unit. For many laboratory determinations, this convention results in very large numbers. For example, the red blood cell count was traditionally reported as cells per cubic millimeter (mm^3) of blood. A normal count is in the range of 4-6 million cells/mm^3. Expanding such a count to the number of cells per liter means multiplying the count per cubic millimeter by 1 million (the number of cubic millimeters in a liter). This yields a normal range for the red blood cell count per liter of 4 to 6 trillion cells. In practice, such large figures are never written out, but are expressed as numbers less than ten multiplied by the appropriate power of ten: $4\text{-}6 \times 10^{12}$. (Ten raised to the twelfth power is one trillion.)

Because the lowercase *l* is easily mistaken for the numeral *1*, it is recommended that, in both handwritten material and computer work, the capital *L* be used as the abbreviation of the unit name **liter**, and that the capital letter also appear in abbreviations of units derived from the liter (**dL, mL, mcL**). Those practices are followed in this book.

Counts and concentrations reported by a clinical laboratory are usually arrived at partly by calculation. Clearly a laboratory technician reporting the red blood cell count in cells per liter did not start with a whole liter of the patient's blood. In actual practice, a small measured volume of blood is diluted, and the cells in a convenient volume of this fluid are then counted, usually by an electronic device. The final figure reported is obtained by calculation.

Results of chemical analysis are usually expressed as concentrations, that is, as a certain weight or volume of the substance in question per unit volume of specimen. Thus, for example, a blood sugar test might be reported as showing 6.9 nmol (nanomoles) per liter. (One nanomole, which is one billionth of a mole, can also be expressed as 10^{-9} mol.) In traditional units, this would be expressed as 124 mg/dL of glucose, meaning that each deciliter (one-tenth of a liter, or 100 mL) of the blood sample was found to contain 124 mg of glucose. Here again, a much smaller volume of blood than a liter, or even than a tenth of a liter, is actually tested, and the concentration as reported is arrived at by calculation.

For some types of chemical test, results are reported neither as the mass (weight) nor as the amount of matter per unit of volume. In determining the concentration of an enzyme in a blood specimen, it may be faster and more economical to measure the chemical activity of the enzyme than to find its actual concentration by quantitative analysis. If the enzyme under investigation is an alkaline phosphatase (an enzyme that breaks down phosphate in an alkaline medium), then a known volume of the patient's serum is allowed to act on a known quantity of phosphate under controlled conditions. The breakdown of phosphate that occurs during a fixed time interval is then determined, and the amount of enzyme activity is expressed in some arbitrary units.

Units of enzyme activity are often distinguished by the name or names of the persons who developed the test. Thus, a serum alkaline phosphatase test result might be reported as 7.5 King-Armstrong units/dL, 3.0 Bodansky units/dL, or 1.8 Bessey-Lowry units/dL, depending on the test procedure used. Because of inherent differences in the tests, results are not directly convertible from one type of units to another. Currently there is a tendency to adopt one test procedure as a standard and to refer to the units used in that test as international units (IU). Reference ranges given in this book for enzyme assays and other tests reported in units may vary widely from reference ranges using different units.

Another type of quantitative test is the serologic titer determined by serial dilutions. Like some enzymes, antibodies are identified in a serum specimen not by chemical analysis but by observation of their activity—for example, their ability to clump (agglutinate) blood cells or particles of latex coated with a specific antigen. In order to form an estimate of the concentration of an antibody in a serum specimen, the technician prepares a series of graded dilutions of the serum. The initial dilution might be 1:7, and each subsequent dilution half of the preceding: 1:14, 1:28, 1:56, 1:112, and so on. The various dilutions are then set out in a row of test tubes and the test material added to each of the tubes. The results of the test are reported as the highest dilution of serum in which antibody activity can still be detected. A report of 1:56 means that antibody activity occurred in all tubes up to and including the one containing the 1:56 dilution of serum, but not at 1:112 or higher dilutions.

The results of two or more tests may be used to calculate rates, ratios, or other derived values. For example, from the three standard measurements of the red blood cell included in the complete blood count—the red blood cell count, the hemoglobin, and the hematocrit—three other values, called red cell indices, are routinely determined: mean corpuscular volume (hematocrit ÷ red blood cell count), mean corpuscular hemoglobin (hemoglobin ÷ red blood cell count), and mean corpuscular hemoglobin concentration (hemoglobin ÷ hematocrit).

The principal proteins of the serum are albumin and globulin. Although these two fractions could be separately measured by chemical analysis, it is technically simpler to determine first the total protein and then the albumin concentration. The globulin concentration is then calculated as the difference between the albumin fraction and total protein.

As discussed in Chapter 1, a crucial factor in the interpretation of any diagnostic test is the concept of **normal**. For most tests, a range of results called a normal range or reference range has been established as being compatible with normal function or absence of disease or impairment. This range is ordinarily based on a statistical analysis of large numbers of results obtained by testing apparently healthy persons. Test results above or below this range are considered abnormal. For some tests, one set of normals is appropriate for women and another for men. Various sets of normal values may be applied depending on the patient's age.

Most laboratories publish sets of normal ranges based on their own experience and equipment. Normal ranges quoted in the following chapters are average figures based on specific test methods. Normal ranges for some laboratories may vary widely from these figures, particularly when different methods are used. In testing for a substance not normally present in the body, such as lead or arsenic, any amount at all is considered abnormal. The results of a qualitative test—for example, a urine pregnancy test—may be reported as simply positive or negative.

The choice of method for performing a given test may be governed by such considerations as cost, speed of performance, availability of special equipment or reagents or of appropriately trained technicians, as well as the comparative sensitivity and specificity of the various methods available. It may be appropriate to accept a method yielding only 90% sensitivity if a more sensitive test costs fifty times as much. Similarly, a test that can be performed by a person having no special training in medical technology may be preferred to a test of higher specificity because of the greater convenience of doing the simpler test at a doctor's office or in the patient's home. Many types of laboratory test equipment are available in kit form for use by untrained personnel outside of a laboratory setting, or even by patients themselves. Such kits may contain premeasured reagents and are often designed to yield unequivocal positive or negative results by means of a color change instead of quantitative results requiring interpretation.

The operation of most clinical laboratories is streamlined and highly efficient, and the performance of most tests quite routine. The **turnaround time** for a given laboratory to perform a given test is the time that elapses between submission of the specimen and release of the report of test results. A few tests are performed only on hospitalized persons, but most tests can also be performed on outpatients, from whom blood or other specimens are obtained at a physician's office or at the laboratory. Most hospital laboratories perform testing on outpatients as well as inpatients. In addition, many free-standing or independent clinical pathology laboratories serve an exclusively outpatient population, generally on referral from physicians' offices.

Securing a specimen for laboratory study may require special techniques and special preparation of the patient. For certain tests, the subject must have fasted for several hours before blood is drawn. For others, certain medicines or foods must be withheld for hours or days before testing.

Blood is ordinarily obtained for testing by venipuncture (phlebotomy), that is, by inserting a needle into a vein in the forearm, after antiseptic preparation of the skin, and withdrawing a sufficient volume of blood by means of a syringe or sealed vacuum tube. Other sites of venipuncture may be appropriate in some patients. A specimen for determination of blood gases (oxygen and carbon dioxide) is obtained by arterial puncture. When only a small quantity of blood is needed, an adequate specimen may be obtained by pricking a finger or, in infants, a heel (pinprick). At autopsy, blood can be obtained directly from the heart for diagnostic or forensic studies.

For serologic studies and most blood chemistries, the blood is allowed to clot naturally in the specimen tube. For hematologic testing and some chemical tests, clotting is prevented by the addition of a small amount of anticoagulant. Various anticoagulants are used depending on the tests to be done. Anticoagulants in common use are EDTA (ethylenediaminetetraacetic acid), sodium fluoride, sodium oxalate, sodium citrate, and heparin. All blood specimens and most others, including those for microbiologic study, are collected and stored in sterile containers to prevent deterioration caused by the growth of contaminating microorganisms. In addition, blood and most other specimens are refrigerated as an added precaution against chemical or biological change if some time will elapse between obtaining the specimen and performing the test. For a few tests, however (e.g., cold agglutinins, blood culture), refrigeration is avoided because it can alter test results.

A specimen of pus, drainage, or secretions for microbiologic study is ordinarily obtained with a sterile swab of cotton or similar material, which is then transmitted in a sterile tube to the laboratory. The tube may contain a nutrient solution (transport medium) to favor the survival of organisms until they reach the laboratory. Alternatively, the person obtaining the specimen may immediately inoculate a culture plate with the swab. The plate is then transmitted to the lab-

oratory for incubation. Specimens of pleural, peritoneal, and joint fluid are obtained by surgical aspiration of the anatomic region of origin with a sterile syringe and needle.

Regardless of where a specimen is obtained, it must be accompanied by a **requisition** when it is submitted to a laboratory for study. The requisition is a printed form on which the person obtaining the specimen records the patient's name and other identifying data, the nature of the specimen and the manner of its collection, the test or tests required, the date, the physician requesting the test, the person or place to which the report is to be sent, and perhaps information about billing and insurance. Often the requisition is prepared in triplicate or quadruplicate on variously colored sheets, each sheet having a specific purpose or destination.

Proper **identification** of the source of a specimen is of paramount importance in all laboratory work. The specimen container must be labeled with full identifying information, and at every step from the arrival of the specimen at the laboratory to the release of the completed report, procedures are strictly followed to ensure accuracy of identification.

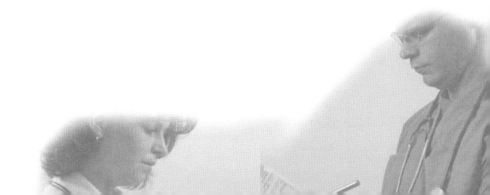

Hematology, Coagulation, and Blood Typing

19

Hematology

The field of hematology embraces the study of the formed elements of the blood (red blood cells, white blood cells, platelets) as well as blood typing and blood coagulation. Red blood cells, white blood cells, and platelets are formed in stationary organs or tissues and released into the circulation as needed.

Red blood cells or erythrocytes are unique among body cells in having no nuclei throughout the entire course of their functional existence (*see Fig. 19.1*). They are formed in bone marrow by repeated divisions of large cells called erythroblasts. Through successive generations, developing erythrocytes become smaller, finally losing their nuclei just before being released into the circulation. The circulating erythrocyte is a round disc with both sides slightly hollowed, so that when seen on edge it has a dumbbell profile. The cytoplasm stains lightly with acidic stains. Erythrocytes are elastic and readily compressible. When found in groups they tend to form rouleaux (singular, rouleau) like stacks of coins.

The function of the erythrocyte is to carry oxygen from the capillaries of the lungs to the capillaries of the rest of the body, and carbon dioxide from the tissues to the lungs for excretion. Each erythrocyte consists of a colloidal complex of lipid and protein material of which hemoglobin is the most important constituent. This iron-containing substance, which is responsible for the red color of blood, forms a loose chemical union with oxygen in the lungs and releases it in the tissues. An erythrocyte survives for about 120 days after entering the circulation. Then it disintegrates and is removed from the blood, principally by phagocytes in the spleen, which conserve and recycle its iron content. Breakdown products of hemoglobin that are not recycled are responsible for the color of bile, urine, and feces.

White blood cells (leukocytes) are larger than erythrocytes and much less numerous in circulating blood, the ratio being about 600:1.

Unlike erythrocytes, which perform their only function in circulating blood, leukocytes appear in the blood only when in transit from their point of production to their destination in tissues. All leukocytes have nuclei. They are divided into two major classes on the basis of the sites where they develop.

Although all leukocytes arise from precursor cells in the bone marrow, only myeloid leukocytes develop to maturity there. Leukocytes that undergo most of their development in lymphoid tissue are called lymphoid. Leukocytes of myeloid origin are further divided into granulocytes, which show conspicuous granules in their cytoplasm, and monocytes, which do not. Granulocytes are also called polymorphonuclear leukocytes (PMNs) because their nuclei are typically divided by shallow clefts into two to five lobes. Granulocytes are subdivided according to the staining properties of their granules into neutrophils, eosinophils, and basophils.

Neutrophils, the most numerous of all white blood cells, have granules that show approximately equal affinity for acidic and basic stains. The function of neutrophils is to engulf and digest devitalized tissue, invading microorganisms, and other foreign material. Within minutes after injury, neutrophils begin to migrate from the blood into the affected tissue. The nuclei of immature neutrophils are elongated but not lobed. Such cells are called unsegmented neutrophils, stab cells, band cells, or simply bands.

Eosinophils, normally making up no more than 5% of circulating white blood cells, have coarse granules that attract eosin and other acid dyes. Their function is unknown but their numbers increase in parasitic infestation and allergic disorders, and decrease after administration of adrenocortical steroid drugs. **Basophils** constitute 1% or less of circulating leukocytes. Their coarse granules stain with basic dyes. They produce histamine, serotonin, and other biochemically active substances. These three types of granulocytes (polymorphonuclear leukocytes) are

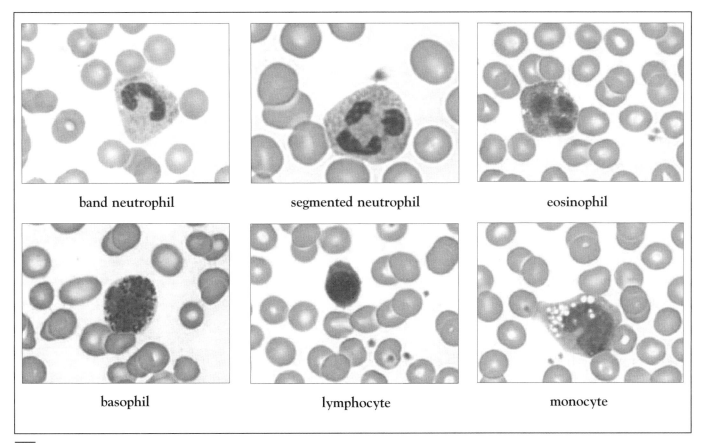

band neutrophil   segmented neutrophil   eosinophil

basophil   lymphocyte   monocyte

Fig. 19.1. Formed elements of blood. Courtesy and copyright, Clinical Chemistry and Hematology Laboratory, Wadsworth Center, NY State Dept. of Health (http://www.wadsworth.org/chemheme).

formed in bone marrow by differentiation of precursor cells called myelocytes.

Monocytes are large cells that make up 5-8% of total circulating leukocytes. Their nuclei are large, kidney- or horseshoe-shaped, and eccentrically placed. Monocytes function as phagocytes in tissues, and are perhaps identical with histiocytes.

Lymphocytes are found in lymphoid tissue (spleen, lymph nodes) and in circulating blood. Normally they make up about 25% of circulating white blood cells. Lymphocytes are slightly larger than erythrocytes and have relatively large, dark-staining nuclei. Their function is to produce antibodies, to modulate immune processes, and to perform other protective functions. Lymphocytes develop from precursor cells in bone marrow, but migrate to other tissues before maturing. Lymphocytes are divided into two major popula-

tions, distinguished by letters referring to their sites of development in birds: B lymphocytes from the bursa of Fabricius (an intestinal pouch), T lymphocytes from the thymus. Although they function in different ways, their activities are closely interrelated.

B cells (B lymphocytes) migrate in an immature state from the marrow to lymphoid tissue. Here they undergo differentiation and maturation before moving to other lymphoid tissues via the bloodstream, where they constitute 5-15% of circulating lymphocytes. A mature B cell can synthesize antibodies in small amounts, but these remain attached to the cell surface. Under appropriate circumstances, however, B cells evolve into plasma cells, which produce antibodies in large amounts and release them into the circulation.

T cells (T lymphocytes) migrate from the marrow to the thymus for maturation before proceeding to other lymphoid organs and tissues. They make up 55-65% of circulating lymphocytes. On the basis of their surface proteins, T cells are subdivided into several types, each with its specific function.

Helper (or inducer) **T cells** stimulate or augment the production of antibody by B cells and plasma cells. **Suppressor T cells** modify or curb this production. **Cytotoxic (killer) T cells** destroy cells they recognize as antigenic.

A few large, granular lymphocytes that are neither B nor T cells are known as null cells. Their functions are unknown, but some of them seem to operate as natural killer cells, attacking foreign cells directly without any true immune response.

Besides these distinctions based on function, lymphocytes can be classified on the basis of their surface proteins, which can be detected by testing with antibodies produced in mice or other non-human species. Surface proteins are subdivided by cluster of differentiation (CD). All lymphocytes carry the CD11a surface protein molecule, but only T cells have CD2 and CD3 proteins, only helper T cells have CD4 protein, and only suppressor and cytotoxic T cells have CD8 protein. Hence alternative designations for helper T cells are CD4+ cells (that is, cells that are positive when tested for CD4 proteins) and, more simply, T4 cells.

Plasma cells, as already mentioned, are specialized lymphocytes that produce antibodies and release them into the circulation. Plasma cells are somewhat larger than lymphocytes and have more abundant and darker-staining cytoplasm. Their nuclei are round, with a cartwheel pattern due to the distribution of chromatin. They are found chiefly in bone marrow but small numbers circulate in the blood.

Platelets are very small round or oval bodies found in circulating blood. They are formed in bone marrow as extrusions from the cytoplasm of giant cells with lobed nuclei called megakaryo-cytes. Platelets are not cells and do not have nuclei. They function in blood clotting.

Procedures performed routinely in the hematology laboratory include counts of blood cells and platelets, examination of stained smears of blood, and certain basic chemical tests. Typing and crossmatching of blood for transfusion are ordinarily performed in a separate laboratory associated with a blood bank where blood intended for transfusion is stored.

Most hematologic procedures can be performed on blood obtained by either fingerstick or venipuncture. Some tests, however, require more blood than can be obtained by fingerstick. Unless testing is performed as soon as the blood is removed from the body, the specimen must be treated with anticoagulant.

The basic tool of hematologic diagnosis is a group of tests called the **complete blood count** (CBC). The complete blood count comprises enumerations of red blood cells, white blood cells, and platelets; a differential count of white blood cells; and determination of the hematocrit and the hemoglobin. A stained smear of blood may be examined to confirm the differential count or to observe red or white blood cells for abnormalities of appearance. The term **hemogram** is inconsistently applied to the complete blood count or to some of the tests composing it.

As a preliminary to counting red or white blood cells, the technician combines a known volume of the whole blood specimen with a known volume of diluent. Different diluents and different dilutions are used for red blood cells and for white blood cells. The diluted specimen is passed through an electronic counter that rapidly registers each cell in the specimen. Different settings enable the counter to distinguish between white and red blood cells on the basis of their size, and further to distinguish among the various types of white blood cell (differential count). Cell counts are reported either per cubic millimeter (traditional) or per liter (SI).

Red Blood Cells

The three basic examinations of the **erythrocyte** (red blood cell), nearly always performed together, are the red blood cell count, the hemoglobin, and the hematocrit. Normal ranges for all three of these tests are 5-10% lower in women than in men. The normal **red blood cell count** is 4 800 000 to 5 600 000/mm^3 [4.8-5.6 x 10^{12}/L]. Elevation of the count (polycythemia or erythrocytosis) occurs as part of acclimation to life at high altitude, in compensation for certain forms of pulmonary and cardiovascular disease that impair oxygenation of tissues (pulmonary hypertension, pulmonary emphysema, cardiac valvular lesions), as a feature of some hematologic malignancies, in clear cell carcinoma of the kidney, and as an idiopathic overproduction of red blood cells (polycythemia vera). Reduction of the red blood cell count (anemia or erythrocytopenia) reflects either diminished production of red blood cells (deficiencies of iron, protein, or vitamins; disease or destruction of bone marrow), increased hemolysis (hemolytic anemias, chemical poisoning, transfusion reaction, toxemia, burns, malaria), or acute or chronic hemorrhage.

The **hemoglobin** content of blood (all of it normally within red blood cells) is determined by a quantitative chemical test. The normal hemoglobin level is 12 to 16 g/dL [7.5-10 mmol/L]. Broadly speaking, changes in this level are due to changes in the red blood cell count, and occur for the same reasons.

The **hematocrit** is that fraction of whole blood that consists of cells. A tube of blood is spun at high speed in a centrifuge. This causes the cells to settle rapidly by centrifugal force. The column of cells is then measured as a fraction of the total column of blood in the tube. The normal hematocrit reading is 40 to 48% [0.40-0.48]. The hematocrit is sometimes referred to as the volume of packed cells. When the procedure is carried out on a specimen of fingerstick blood in a capillary tube, it is called a microhematocrit. Because the hematocrit measures roughly the same thing as the preceding two tests, changes in hematocrit occur for the same reasons as in those tests.

It is, however, possible to obtain more specific information about abnormalities in red blood cells by determining the **red blood cell indices**. These values involve no additional testing of blood but are derived by calculation from the three tests just described. Normal ranges for red cell indices are the same for men and women.

The **mean corpuscular volume** (MCV) is found by dividing the hematocrit by the red blood cell count. The normal range is 82 to 92 mcm^3 (cubic micrometers) [82-92 fL (femtoliters)]. An increase in the mean corpuscular volume (macrocytosis) means that red blood cells are larger than normal. Because this generally results from defective synthesis of red cells due to lack of vitamin B$_{12}$, folic acid, or both, macrocytosis is frequently accompanied by reduction in the red blood cell count (macrocytic anemia). Macrocytosis occurs in pernicious anemia and in some anemias associated with pregnancy, alcoholism, hepatic cirrhosis, and malabsorption syndromes. Reduction in mean corpuscular volume (microcytosis) occurs in anemias due to deficiency of iron or to chronic blood loss or hemolysis.

The degree of variation in red blood cell size can be measured by the electronic counter at the same time as the red blood cell count. The **red cell distribution width** (RDW) is normally less than 15%, which means that the smallest cell counted varies less than 15% in size from the largest cell counted. Greater variation in red cell size (anisocytosis) occurs in many disorders associated with abnormal erythropoiesis, including congenital hemolytic anemias and anemias occurring in deficiency states or chronic disease.

The **mean corpuscular hemoglobin** (MCH) is found by dividing the total hemoglobin by the red blood cell count. The normal range is 27 to 31 pg (picograms) per cell. This value, representing the average weight of hemoglobin per red blood cell, is of limited significance. A more useful figure is the **mean corpuscular hemoglobin concentration** (MCHC), computed by dividing the hemoglobin by the hematocrit. The mean corpuscular hemoglobin concentration is normally between 32 and 36 g/dL [320-360 g/L]. An increase in this concentration (hyperchromia) occurs in hereditary spherocytosis. Reduction of MCHC (hypochromia) is characteristic of anemias due to deficiency or malabsorption of iron, certain hereditary anemias, and chronic blood loss.

Abnormalities of red cell shape include spherocytosis (spherical shape), ovalocytosis (oval shape), and sickling (sickle shape). Each of these indicates abnormality in the chemical structure of the red blood cell. Target cells are erythrocytes with a bull's-eye appearance due to flattening of the cell with a prominent spot of hemoglobin in the center. Burr cells have a crinkled profile because of abnormal chemical structure.

Abnormalities may be noted in the cytoplasm of red blood cells. Nucleated red blood cells are marrow forms released prematurely into the circulation. Recently formed erythrocytes may contain remnants of nuclear chromatin called Howell-Jolly bodies. They are found in increased numbers in some hemolytic anemias and after splenectomy. Siderocytes are red blood cells containing discrete iron (siderotic) granules. They are found normally in newborns. In older children and adults siderocytes may indicate hemolytic anemia, pernicious anemia, or lead poisoning.

A large number of hereditary disorders in the synthesis of hemoglobin and the formation of red blood cells have been identified. Some of these disorders can be diagnosed on the basis of red cell indices and red cell morphology, but for most of them diagnostic confirmation depends on **hemoglobin electrophoresis**. This test is performed by placing a chemically treated specimen of blood in an electric field and noting the rates at which various components migrate from one pole to the other.

Numerous variants of normal hemoglobin, differing in the amino acid sequences of the globin fraction, occur in the red blood cells of persons with hereditary disorders of hematopoiesis. Often several abnormal hemoglobins are found in the same person. Some hereditary disorders of hemoglobin formation (hemoglobinopathies) are without symptoms, but many are associated with diminished production of red blood cells, and most with excessive hemolysis. Hence they are characterized by mild to severe anemia and are often classed as hereditary (or congenital) hemolytic anemias.

Normal adult hemoglobin is designated hemoglobin A. The most commonly encountered abnormal hemoglobin is hemoglobin S, which is characteristic of sickle cell anemia. Hemoglobins C, D, and E are associated with varying degrees of impairment. In some persons, fetal hemoglobin (hemoglobin F) continues to be formed in significant proportions throughout life.

Although persons with some congenital hemolytic anemias may remain asymptomatic, all are at increased risk of certain pathologic changes. Jaundice may appear at times of increased hemolysis. Since most of this hemolysis occurs in the spleen, chronic enlargement of that organ is common. Splenomegaly and hepatomegaly may also indicate extramedullary hematopoiesis (formation of red blood cells in tissues other than the bone marrow). Heightened hemolytic activity raises the bilirubin content of bile and predisposes to cholelithiasis (formation of bilirubin gallstones) and cholecystitis (inflammation of the gallbladder). Persons with severe hemolytic disease are subject to widespread thrombosis in small vessels and to ischemic ulcers of the legs. A hemolytic crisis (sudden breakdown of many red blood cells) may be precipitated by reduction in atmospheric oxygen, impairment of pulmonary gas exchange, infection, or other severe physical stress.

The most frequently encountered congenital hemolytic anemia is sickle cell anemia, which affects 1 in 400 African-Americans. Persons with sickle cell trait (the heterozygous form) produce some red blood cells containing hemoglobin S, and persons with sickle cell disease (the homozygous form) produce more. Red cells containing hemoglobin S tend to assume a sickle shape, particularly under conditions of reduced oxygen tension, and to rupture. Although sickle cell trait is often asymptomatic, sickle cell disease commonly causes developmental abnormalities (cardiomegaly; long, thin extremities), splenomegaly, and recurrent bouts of abdominal and extremity pain. Persons with sickle cell disease are also subject to aseptic necrosis of long bones and to infections with *Salmonella* organisms.

Thalassemia (Mediterranean anemia, Cooley anemia) is more common in persons of Mediterranean or Far Eastern ancestry. It is associated with abnormal structure of the red blood cell (target cells) and with varying amounts of hemoglobin C, E, and F. Like sickle cell anemia, it occurs in a milder heterozygous form (thalassemia minor) and a more severe homozygous form (thalassemia major). Symptoms and complications are, however, generally milder than in sickle cell anemia. In hereditary elliptocytosis (ovalocytosis, Dresbach syndrome), some red blood cells have an oval or cigar shape, and variable amounts of hemoglobin C are present. Because some of the red blood cells in hereditary spherocytosis are rounded instead of flattened, they are more readily hemolyzed by changes in osmotic environment.

Hereditary deficiency of **glucose-6-phosphate dehydrogenase** (G-6-PD) in red blood cells, also called favism, is a type of hemolytic anemia in which red cells are subject to hemolysis after exposure to certain drugs (primaquine, sulfonamides, nitrofurans), chemicals (methylene blue, toluidine blue), and foods (fava beans). This disorder, perhaps the commonest inborn error of metabolism, affecting as many as 10% of

African-American males, is frequently asymptomatic.

Hemolysis, the breakdown of red blood cells with release of hemoglobin into the plasma, occurs in many of these congenital hemoglobinopathies, in transfusion reactions, and in certain toxic states. Small amounts of free hemoglobin normally occur in the blood and are removed by normal physiologic mechanisms without doing harm. Extensive hemolysis with high concentration of free hemoglobin can cause hemolytic jaundice by overtaxing the ability of the liver to break it down and excrete it, and can damage the kidney.

Haptoglobin is an $alpha_2$-globulin, normally present in circulating blood, that binds any free hemoglobin released by hemolysis. Hemoglobin bound by haptoglobin is removed from the circulation by the liver and its iron content recovered and recycled. Determining the concentration of haptoglobin is thus an indirect measure of hemolysis. The normal haptoglobin concentration is 20-165 mg/dL [0.20-1.65 g/L]. Levels are low after hemolysis and also in severe liver disease.

In addition to electrophoresis to detect aberrations in amino acid structure, hemoglobin can be subjected to chemical testing to identify the presence of abnormal products or compounds resulting from various intoxications. **Methemoglobin** is a form of hemoglobin in which ferrous iron has been oxidized to the ferric state. This form of hemoglobin does not function in oxygen transport. A small amount of methemoglobin (less than 3% of total hemoglobin) is normally present. The level is increased in rare hereditary metabolic errors and after absorption of certain oxidizing agents (nitrobenzene, phenylhydrazine, primaquine, nitrates).

The potential gravity of carbon monoxide poisoning is due largely to the fact that hemoglobin shows a greater affinity for carbon monoxide than for oxygen. Measuring the concentration in the blood of **carboxyhemoglobin** (the compound formed by hemoglobin and carbon monoxide)

provides evidence of carbon monoxide intoxication and permits assessment of its severity. A level above 5% of total hemoglobin indicates carbon monoxide poisoning. Similarly, hydrogen sulfide poisoning can be detected by determination of **sulfhemoglobin** (sulfmethemoglobin), and cyanide poisoning by determination of **cyanmethemoglobin**.

Other tests performed on red blood cells in the hematology laboratory include the sickle cell preparation, the osmotic fragility test, the erythrocyte survival time, the reticulocyte count, and the erythrocyte sedimentation rate. In a **sickle cell preparation**, blood is incubated at reduced oxygen tension and the red cells are observed through a microscope for sickling. The **osmotic fragility test** involves incubating specimens of blood in tubes of sterile saline solution of varying osmotic concentration (osmolality), and observing in which tubes hemolysis occurs. Osmotic fragility is increased—that is, hemolysis occurs at osmolalities more nearly normal—in spherocytosis and most other congenital and acquired hemolytic anemias, including those accompanying certain malignancies. Osmotic fragility is reduced—that is, hemolysis occurs at lower osmolalities than with normal red blood cells—in sickle cell anemia, thalassemia, and iron deficiency anemia and some other microcytic anemias.

A normal erythrocyte survives for about 120 days before being broken down in the spleen. Survival time is shortened in hemolytic disorders or any cause. The measurement of **erythrocyte survival time** is performed with a radioisotope of chromium. A specimen of the patient's blood is labeled with chromium Cr 51 sodium chromate and reinjected into the patient. Specimens of blood obtained at intervals during the next several weeks are tested to determine what percent of the cells in the specimen remain in the circulation. Nuclear imaging may also be performed to detect any sites of high concentration of radioisotope.

As mentioned earlier, very young erythrocytes (erythrocytes recently released from the bone marrow into the circulation) may show remnants of nuclear material in their cytoplasm in a stained blood smear. Vital staining (addition of a stain such as methylene blue to whole blood that has been treated with anticoagulant) provides a more distinctive visualization of this material. A smear made of blood after vital staining shows basophilic material forming an irregular network in the cytoplasm of younger red blood cells, which are called reticulocytes. The normal **reticulocyte count** is 0.5 to 1.5% of all red blood cells. Increase in this count (reticulocytosis) suggests heightened erythropoiesis in response to blood loss or hemolysis.

The **erythrocyte sedimentation rate** (ESR, sed rate) is the rate at which red blood cells in a specimen of whole blood, treated with anticoagulant and allowed to stand in a glass column of standard dimensions, settle by gravity to the bottom of the tube. The sedimentation rate (corrected for abnormalities in the hematocrit) is reported as mm/h (millimeters per hour) of settled red blood cells. The normal range depends on the procedure used but is always higher for women than for men. The erythrocyte sedimentation rate is not primarily a reflection of red cell structure or function. It is increased in many acute and chronic inflammatory conditions (viral hepatitis, tuberculosis, acute rheumatic fever, rheumatoid arthritis), acute myocardial infarction, various toxic states, and various malignancies including particularly those accompanied by production of abnormal globulins. Although highly nonspecific, the sedimentation rate is useful in monitoring the course of certain disorders such as rheumatic fever and some malignancies.

White Blood Cells

The normal **white blood cell count** is 5000 to 10 000/mm^3 [5-10 x 10^9/L]. Elevation of the white blood cell count (leukocytosis) occurs in acute or chronic inflammation of any cause and in leukemia and some lymphomas. Depression of the white blood cell count (leukopenia) results from suppression of their production by toxic substances, chemotherapy, radiation, or disease of hematopoietic tissue.

The white blood cell count is of limited usefulness in diagnosis. Interpretation of variations in this count depends on the relative numbers of the various white blood cells present. This information is obtained by performing a **differential white blood cell count** (often called simply a **differential**), a tally of the various types of white cells as identified by a technician examining a stained smear of blood or by an electronic counter programmed to distinguish among cell types by detecting their nuclear and cytoplasmic features.

For optical counting, a smear is made by spreading two or three large drops of fresh whole blood very thinly across a microscope slide. The smear is air-dried and flooded with a methanol-based polychrome stain such as Wright (methylene blue and eosin) or Giemsa (azure II and azure II eosin), which quickly and simultaneously colors nuclear material blue and cytoplasm pink. Usually one hundred white blood cells are counted and the number of each cell type found is expressed as a percent. Differential counting can also be performed electronically, but this method, which distinguishes cells by size, cannot precisely identify abnormalities of cell structure or maturity.

The table on p. 332 shows normal ranges for the six types of cell encountered in a smear of normal blood. The figures in the middle column are percents obtained by differential counting. Those in the right column are absolute counts of the various cell types, computed by multiplying the percent of each type by the total white blood cell count.

Variations in the relative numbers of mature (segmented) and immature (band) forms of neutrophils may result from the use of different criteria for segmentation of the nucleus. Some observers consider any constriction in a neutrophil nucleus as evidence of segmentation, while others count all neutrophils as band cells unless their nuclei are separated into at least two lobes with only filamentous connections.

Increase in the absolute number of neutrophils (neutrophilia) occurs in acute bacterial infections, toxemia, uremia, acidosis, burns, and myeloproliferative diseases (leukemia, lymphoma). The more acute and intense the neutrophilic response, the greater the number of immature cells (bands) that are likely to be present. An increase in the percent of band cells is called a **shift to the left** or a left shift because at one time cell counts were recorded on a form in which the column for band cells was to the left of the column for mature neutrophils. Relative neutrophilia (increased percent of neutrophils in the differential count without absolute increase) occurs when the absolute number of lymphocytes is reduced.

Reduction in the absolute neutrophil count (neutropenia) occurs in toxic states, chemical poisoning (arsenic, antimetabolites, sulfonamides), typhoid fever, some viral infections (measles, influenza), overwhelming bacterial infection, and miliary tuberculosis, and after irradiation. A relative neutropenia without reduction in absolute number of circulating neutrophils appears when there is a marked increase in the absolute number of lymphocytes.

An increase in the number of eosinophils (eosinophilia) occurs in various allergic states (asthma, urticaria), parasitism (trichinosis, echinococcosis), polyarteritis nodosa, sarcoidosis, diseases of hematopoietic tissue (Hodgkin disease, chronic myelogenous leukemia), and after splenectomy. A decrease in the number of eosinophils (eosinopenia) occurs after chemotherapy, irradiation, or treatment with adrenocortical steroid.

An increase in the number of basophils (basophilia) is seen in chronic myelogenous leukemia, polycythemia, Hodgkin disease, and after splenectomy. A decrease in the number of basophils (basopenia) occurs in hyperthyroidism and after chemotherapy, irradiation, or administration of adrenocortical steroid.

An increase in the absolute number of lymphocytes (lymphocytosis) is typical of many viral infections (mumps, infectious hepatitis, infectious mononucleosis), tuberculosis, brucellosis, thyrotoxicosis, and lymphatic leukemia. Relative lymphocytosis accompanies marked neutropenia. Absolute reduction in lymphocytes (lymphopenia) is seen in autoimmune disorders, particularly systemic lupus erythematosus, and in some congenital and acquired immune deficiencies including AIDS. Relative lymphopenia occurs with absolute neutrophilia.

The principal mechanism by which the human immunodeficiency virus (HIV), the cause of AIDS, impairs immunity and renders the patient vulnerable to opportunistic infections is by gradual destruction of CD4 lymphocyte. Serial determination of the CD4 count is a means of monitoring immune compromise in AIDS and assessing the effects of treatment. The normal CD4 count is 500-1500 cells/mm^3 [0.5-1.5 x 10^9 cells/L], representing approximately 40% of all circulating lymphocytes. Decline of the CD4 count below 200 cells/mm^3 [0.2 x 10^9 cells/L] or of the relative proportion of CD4 lymphocytes below 20% indicates severe immune compromise and the need for prophylaxis against opportunistic infections.

An increase in the number of monocytes (monocytosis) occurs in some infections due to bacteria (tuberculosis, infective endocarditis), rickettsiae (typhus, Rocky Mountain spotted fever), or protozoa (malaria, trypanosomiasis), and in some collagen diseases, sarcoidosis, Hodgkin disease, polycythemia vera, and monocytic leukemia. Reduction in the number of monocytes (monocytopenia) is not often recognized but may accompany conditions involving destruction or suppression of bone marrow.

A marked rise in the white blood cell count (over 50 000/mm^3 [50 x 10^9/L]) usually indicates leukemia. Occasionally, however, such a rise reflects a very severe infection or toxemia with intense cellular response. Extreme leukocytosis in the absence of leukemia is called a leukemoid reaction. Myelocytic, lymphocytic, and monocytic forms are recognized.

In addition to the six normal types of cell discussed above, several others are occasionally identified in the stained blood smear. Immature

Cell Type	Differential Count	Absolute Count
Neutrophils, segmented	40–70%	2000–6500/mm^3 [2000-6500 x 10^6/L]
Neutrophils, bands	4–8%	200–800/mm^3 [200-800 x 10^6/L]
Eosinophils	2–4%	100–400/mm^3 [100-400 x 10^6/L
Basophils	0–1%	40–60/mm^3 [40-60 x 10^6/L]
Monocytes	4–6%	200–600/mm^3 [200-600 x 10^6/L]
Lymphocytes	25–40%	1250–4000/mm^3 [1250-4000 x 10^6/L]

cells of the myelogenous line not normally found outside the marrow, and immature lymphatic cells not normally found outside lymphoid tissue, may appear in the blood in leukemias or lymphomas or as part of a leukemoid reaction. Atypical lymphocytes (also called Downey cells or virocytes) are large lymphocytes with pale or foamy cytoplasm and prominent oval or horseshoe-shaped nuclei resembling those of monocytes. These occur in lymphatic leukemia, brucellosis, viral hepatitis, and various other viral infections. When they exceed 10% of all white blood cells they are virtually diagnostic of infectious mononucleosis. Plasma cells appear in peripheral blood in multiple myeloma, plasma cell leukemia, and some viral infections. Coarse basophilic stippling in the cytoplasm of neutrophils, known as toxic granulation, usually indicates severe infection or toxemia.

Platelets and Coagulation Factors

Blood coagulates (clots) when the soluble plasma protein fibrinogen is converted to insoluble fibrin. Normally this occurs after another plasma protein, prothrombin, is converted to thrombin. Activation of prothrombin can come about through a number of alternative biochemical pathways, variously involving platelets, tissue factors, and plasma proteins other than prothrombin and fibrinogen. All known coagulation mechanisms require the presence of calcium. In addition, Factor V (labile factor), Factor VII (stable factor, proconvertin), Factor VIII (antihemophilic globulin, AHG), Factor IX (Christmas factor), Factor X (Stuart-Prower factor), and Factor XI (plasma thromboplastin antecedent) are all necessary for normal coagulation.

Disorders of coagulation (coagulopathies) can be either congenital or acquired. Deficiency or lack of any of the plasma clotting factors, including fibrinogen and prothrombin, can occur as an isolated genetic defect. Classical hemophilia (hemophilia A), due to congenital deficiency of Factor VIII, is transmitted as a sex-linked recessive trait, carried by females but expressed only in males. Hemophilia B (Factor IX disease, Christmas disease) shows a similar pattern of inheritance. Acquired deficiency of prothrombin (hypoprothrombinemia) is more frequent than congenital deficiency. It can result from deficiency of vitamin K (an essential chemical building block for prothrombin), hepatic disease (particularly biliary obstruction, which blocks absorption of vitamin K by preventing passage of bile salts into the bowel), or treatment with coumarin anticoagulants. Acquired or congenital deficiency of plasma clotting factors causes a hemorrhagic tendency of variable severity characterized by prolonged bleeding from wounds, hematoma formation, hemarthrosis (bleeding into joints), and hematuria (blood in the urine).

In contrast, congenital or acquired deficiency of platelets (thrombocytopenia) is associated with petechiae (pinpoint hemorrhages in the skin) or purpura (larger skin hemorrhages). Frank or severe hemorrhage occurs less frequently. Idiopathic thrombocytopenic purpura (ITP) is an autoimmune disorder of children, usually benign and self-limited. In thrombotic thrombocytopenic purpura (TTP), deficiency of platelets may be accompanied by hemolytic anemia, renal impairment, and bizarre neurologic manifestations. The acute form may progress rapidly to a fatal termination. In Glanzmann disease (thrombasthenia), the platelet count is normal but platelet function is impaired.

Hemorrhagic manifestations, usually purpuric, also occur in certain diseases of blood vessels. In hereditary hemorrhagic telangiectasia (Osler-Weber-Rendu disease), recurrent bleeding occurs from telangiectases in the skin and mucous membranes. Von Willebrand disease is a hereditary hemorrhagic disorder, often mild, characterized by deficiency of Factor VIII, abnormal platelet function, and vascular abnormalities. Examples of acquired vascular disorders accompanied by purpuric bleeding include Henoch-Schoenlein purpura, Cushing syndrome, and scurvy.

Disseminated intravascular coagulation (DIC), which results from imbalance between the mechanisms of coagulation and of fibrinolysis, can be induced by infection (meningococcal meningitis, Rocky Mountain spotted fever, septicemia), trauma, shock, complications of pregnancy and parturition, and myelocytic leukemia. Clinical manifestations range from widespread bleeding to widespread intravascular thrombosis, and both of these may occur together.

Precise diagnosis of a hemorrhagic disorder depends on the results of several basic tests, which are often performed together as a coagulation panel: platelet count, bleeding time, clotting time, prothrombin time, partial thromboplastin time, and clot retraction. In addition, plasma assay for specific coagulation factors is possible.

The **platelet count** is performed by methods analogous to those for the red and white blood cell counts (optical or electronic). The normal platelet count is 150 000 to 300, 000/mm³ [15-30 x 10⁹/L]. The platelet count may be increased in collagen diseases and some malignancies, particularly those of the bone marrow. The platelet count is decreased in idiopathic thrombocytopenic purpura, thrombotic thrombocytopenic purpura, and disease or toxic states associated with damage to the bone marrow.

One of the ways in which platelets aid in controlling bleeding is by forming a mechanical plug at the site of vascular injury. Since platelet aggregation or clumping is essential to this process, laboratory testing of **platelet aggregation** can indicate abnormal platelet function. In this test a specimen of plasma is treated with an agent that normally stimulates platelet aggregation. As aggregation occurs and platelets settle, the specimen becomes clearer. Serial measurements of the amount of light transmitted by the specimen are used to graph the rate of platelet aggregation. Abnormal test results occur in von Willebrand disease, idio-

pathic thrombocytopenic purpura, and other disorders of platelets.

Bleeding time, clotting time, and capillary fragility tests are performed directly on the patient. **Bleeding time** tests are crude, semiquantitative measurements of hemostasis after a penetrating injury of the skin. In the Duke method a small puncture wound is made with a sterile lancet in a convenient place such as an earlobe or fingertip. In the Ivy method, a blood pressure cuff is placed on the arm and inflated to 40 mmHg, and a spring-loaded lancet is used to make a standard-sized incision in the forearm. For both tests, filter paper or other absorptive material is touched to the wound every 30 seconds to determine whether bleeding continues. The bleeding time is the interval between puncture and cessation of bleeding. A normal bleeding time is 4 minutes or less. The time is prolonged in deficiencies or abnormalities of platelets and in von Willebrand disease.

The **clotting time** is the time required for a specimen of whole blood, obtained by venipuncture, to coagulate. The normal clotting time by the standard Lee-White method is 6 to 17 minutes. The clotting time is prolonged in deficiency of fibrinogen or of some other plasma clotting factors and after administration of heparin. This test is used to monitor heparin therapy.

The **Rumpel-Leede test** (tourniquet test) assesses capillary fragility and platelet function. A blood pressure cuff is applied to the arm and inflated to a pressure that is midway between the subject's systolic and diastolic pressures. After a test period of 5 minutes, the number of petechiae (pinpoint subcutaneous hemorrhages) on the forearm below the cuff is counted. Normally fewer than 10 petechiae should be noted. An abnormally high number may occur in thrombocytopenia, von Willebrand disease, disseminated intravascular coagulation (DIC), and vitamin K deficiency.

Congenital deficiencies of **coagulation factors** are diagnosed by specific assay of those factors. Assays are available for Factor I (fibrinogen),

Factor II (prothrombin), Factor V (labile factor), Factor VII (stable factor), Factor VIII (antihemophilic globulin [AHG]), Factor IX (plasma thromboplastin component [PTC], Christmas factor), Factor X (Stuart-Prower factor), Factor XI (plasma thromboplastin antecedent [PTA]), Factor XII (Hageman factor), and Factor XIII (fibrin stabilizing factor [FSF]).

Often it is simpler and less expensive to measure the activity of a coagulation factor in the laboratory than to determine its concentration in the blood. The **prothrombin time** (pro time or PT) test is performed by adding a combination of calcium and thromboplastin to a specimen of plasma previously treated with an anticoagulant to bind the calcium that is naturally present. (Thromboplastin is a generic term for substances that convert prothrombin to thrombin.) The prothrombin time is the time required for a clot to form. The results of the prothrombin time test are expressed as both a time (for example, 14 seconds) and a ratio (more correctly, a quotient) obtained by dividing the patient's prothrombin time by a control value for normal serum.

Because the potency of thromboplastins varies from one source or batch to another, the precision of the prothrombin time test is enhanced by multiplying the test ratio by a sensitivity index determined for each lot. The resulting International Normalized Ratio (INR) has worldwide applicability regardless of the source of the thromboplastin, and makes possible international dialog and accord on diagnostic and therapeutic standards referring to coagulation and its disorders.

Prolongation of the prothrombin time, and hence increase of the ratio above 1.0, occurs in deficiency of prothrombin (which may be due to hepatic disease or deficiency of vitamin K), Factor V, Factor VII, Factor IX, or fibrinogen, and after administration of coumarin anticoagulants. This test is used to monitor therapy with coumarin anticoagulants.

When a blood specimen coagulates under laboratory conditions, all the prothrombin present should be converted to thrombin. Determining the prothrombin time of the serum that remains after clotting is thus a way of assessing the coagulation process. This test is called the **prothrombin consumption time**. A high concentration of prothrombin (shortened prothrombin consumption time) is found in deficiencies of platelets or of Factors VIII, IX, XI or XII.

The **thrombin time** test determines the speed with which a clot forms in a specimen of the patient's blood to which thrombin has been added. Prolongation of this time indicates a deficiency or abnormality of fibrinogen or the presence of some substance such as heparin that inhibits conversion of fibrinogen to fibrin.

The activated **partial thromboplastin time (PTT)**, a modification of the prothrombin time test in which a phospholipid preparation is substituted for thromboplastin, is a more sensitive indicator of deficiency of plasma coagulation factors. The normal PTT is 22 to 37 seconds. Prolongation may be due to deficiency of fibrinogen or of Factor IX, X, XI, or XII.

One hour or less after a clot forms in a specimen of whole blood, it begins to retract, that is, to shrink and separate from the portion of the plasma that is still fluid, which is known as serum. Normally this retraction is complete in about six hours, but it may take as long as 24 hours. Clot retraction is a function of platelet activity. Prolongation or failure of **clot retraction**, as measured under standard conditions in the laboratory, indicates either deficiency of platelets or impaired platelet function (thrombasthenia).

Plasminogen is a normally occurring substance that is converted to plasmin after a fibrin clot has formed in the body. The function of plasmin is to break down (degrade) fibrin chemically so as to prevent excessive clotting. A disturbance of this mechanism can lead to excessive plasmin activity and a rise of **fibrin degradation products** in the circulating blood, with both abnormal bleeding and abnormal clotting (disseminated intravascular coagulation, DIC). Testing for fibrin degradation products, also called fibrin split products (FSP), is therefore a means of diagnosing DIC. The normal level is less than 3 mcg/mL [3 mg/L]. Other conditions besides DIC that can elevate this level include myocardial infarction, deep vein thrombosis and pulmonary embolism, toxemia of pregnancy, and renal disease.

D-dimer is a specific fibrin degradation product whose level in the blood is elevated in about 95% of patients with pulmonary embolism A normal level is therefore helpful in ruling out that diagnosis. False positive results occur in other disorders, including myocardial infarction, infection, and malignant disease.

Antithrombin (antithrombin III) is another naturally occurring substance that modulates blood coagulation by inhibiting the action of thrombin and several other coagulation factors. Congenital or acquired deficiency of this substance can result in localized or disseminated intravascular coagulation.

Cryofibrinogenemia is an acquired disorder occurring in association with malignant disease, collagen diseases such as scleroderma, renal dialysis, and thromboembolic disease. The blood of persons with this disorder contains an abnormal substance, **cryofibrinogen**, which precipitates when an appropriately prepared blood specimen is chilled.

Bone Marrow Studies

Examination of bone marrow can give information about the formation, normal or abnormal, of red blood cells, white blood cells, and platelets; the relative proportions of the various precursor cell lines; the cellularity of the marrow, as opposed to replacement of hemopoietic (blood-forming) elements by fibrosis or fat; marrow iron stores; and the presence of malignant cells, as in leukemias, multiple myeloma, and cancers metastatic to the marrow.

Liquid marrow may be obtained for examination by aspiration with a large-bore needle, or a solid core of tissue may be removed with a biopsy needle. In either case the surface is disinfected as for a surgical procedure and local anesthetic is injected. The usual site for marrow aspiration is the sternum. For biopsy the iliac crest is preferred and, in infants and small children, the anterior tibia. Ribs and vertebrae may also be used. Specimens may be obtained from more than one site.

A marrow aspirate is smeared and stained like a blood smear, while a biopsy is processed as solid tissue. Besides evaluating the appearance of all cellular elements present, the pathologist or cytologist calculates the myeloid/erythroid ratio, that is, the ratio of leukocyte to erythrocyte precursors in the marrow. The normal ratio is 2.0-4.0; values at the higher end of this range are usual in children. The ratio is increased in chronic myelogenous leukemia and in disorders resulting in loss of erythroid elements. The ratio is decreased in agranulocytosis and in disorders resulting in overgrowth of erythroid elements. Special stains may be applied to assess marrow iron stores or to detect abnormal accumulation or storage of certain substances (amyloid, glycogen). Marrow specimens can also be cultured or subjected to histochemical, serologic, or molecular biology procedures.

Blood Typing

Although all normal blood has approximately the same chemical composition, the antigenic properties of blood vary from person to person. That is, the plasma of some persons contains antibody that will agglutinate (clump) and hemolyze the erythrocytes of some other persons. The classification of blood according to the antigenic properties of the red blood cells is known as blood typing or grouping. The blood type of an individual is genetically determined and remains unchanged throughout life. Blood typing is of paramount importance in blood transfusion and in the diagnosis and treatment of certain conditions associated with pregnancy.

Blood Type	Agglutinogens in Red Cells	Agglutinins in Serum
A	A	anti-B
B	B	anti-A
AB	A and B	none
O	none	anti-A and anti-B

The most important antigen-antibody relationships of the red blood cell are those involved in the ABO system. The essential facts regarding this system are set forth in the table above.

If blood from a type A donor is given to a type B recipient, the anti-A agglutinin in the recipient's serum will agglutinate the donor's red blood cells. To a lesser extent, donor anti-B agglutinin will agglutinate the recipient's red blood cells. A hemolytic reaction due to transfusion of incompatible blood is manifested by fever, chills, shock, and renal failure. The mortality rate is high.

A second kind of erythrocyte antigen is that of the **Rh system**. About 85% of the population are Rh positive, that is, their red blood cells contain the Rh antigen, which the other 15% lack. Persons who are Rh positive have no antibody to the Rh antigen, and do not form it. Although persons who are Rh negative also lack such antibody at birth, they are capable of forming it after challenge with Rh positive blood. A person who is Rh negative may receive a first transfusion of Rh positive blood with impunity. After forming antibody to the Rh antigen in this blood, however, such a person may not receive further transfusions of Rh positive blood without risk of hemolytic reaction.

Because the Rh positive blood type is transmitted genetically as a dominant trait, an Rh negative woman can conceive and bear an Rh positive child if the father is Rh positive. Although mixing of fetal and maternal whole blood does not normally occur, it may result from minor trauma or during labor and delivery. The mother may then form anti-Rh antibody and continue to do so throughout life. During subsequent pregnancies this antibody, diffusing across the placenta, will hemolyze fetal Rh positive red blood cells, causing the condition known as hemolytic disease of the newborn or erythroblastosis fetalis. An Rh positive child born to a previously sensitized Rh negative mother develops jaundice at birth or shortly thereafter because of extensive hemolysis, and nucleated (immature) red blood cells appear in the fetal circulation. Hemolytic disease of the newborn can also result from incompatibility in the ABO system, but this is seldom serious.

Serologic testing can be used to identify acquired hemolytic anemias, including those arising from Rh incompatibility. In the **direct Coombs test**, the patient's red blood cells are tested with antiserum to determine whether they have become coated with an antiglobulin. This test is positive in a newborn with erythroblastosis fetalis and in persons with acquired hemolytic disease due to production of abnormal globulins, as in leukemia, lymphoma, and collagen diseases.

In the **indirect Coombs test**, the patient's serum is tested for antiglobulin by incubation with erythrocytes. The indirect Coombs test is positive in the mother of an infant with erythroblastosis fetalis and in any person with anti-Rh antiglobulins or other acquired hemolyzing antibodies, as in hematopoietic malignancies and collagen diseases. Both direct and indirect Coombs tests are negative in hereditary hemoglobinopathies.

Other blood groups that may be of clinical importance are Duffy (Fy), Kell (K), Kidd (Jk), Lewis (Le), and Lutheran (Lu). Testing for these and other minor groups finds its principal application in attempts to disprove paternity. If blood specimens are available from the child, its mother, and the putative father, nonpaternity can be proved in a majority of cases by exhaustive blood grouping. DNA testing, however, is more conclusive.

All blood intended for transfusion is typed in the ABO and Rh systems by application of specific agglutinins (anti-A, anti-B, anti-Rh) and observation for clumping of cells. The blood of a prospective transfusion recipient is also typed. Before transfusion, each unit of blood is crossmatched with the blood of the prospective recipient. That is, donor cells are mixed with recipient serum (major crossmatch) and recipient cells are mixed with donor serum (minor crossmatch). Any agglutination or hemolysis in either major or minor crossmatch is evidence of incompatibility and a contraindication to transfusion of that unit of blood to that recipient. In the standard crossmatch procedure, separate major and minor cell-serum mixtures are made in saline, in albumin solution, and in a solution containing antiglobulin to enhance sensitivity.

Exercises

Fill in the Blanks

1. _____ deals with the chemical properties and interactions of all the substances composing the living body. (Section VI.)

2. _____ studies the defensive mechanisms whereby the body recognizes foreign materials and invading microorganisms as non-self and mobilizes cellular and chemical agents against them. (Section VI)

3. _____, a branch of biochemistry that investigates DNA and RNA, provides diagnostic information about both infectious and inherited diseases. (Section VI)

4. Medical microbiology employs two basic methodologic tools—microscopic examination of fresh or processed _____ of pus or other materials and the growth of pathogenic microorganisms under controlled conditions in _____ enhancing the microbiologist's ability to identify them. (Section VI)

5. Culturing methods can also be used to test the effectiveness of various _____ against a pathogen. (Section VI)

6. A group of tests frequently performed together is sometimes called a _____ or _____.

7. In determining the concentration of an enzyme, such as _____, in a blood specimen, it may be faster and more economical to measure the chemical activity of the enzyme than to find its actual concentration by quantitative analysis. (Section VI)

8. Like some enzymes, _____ are identified in a serum specimen not by chemical analysis but by observation of their activity—for example, their ability to clump (agglutinate) blood cells or particles of latex coated with a specific antigen. (Section VI)

9. The globulin concentration of serum is calculated as the difference between the _____ fraction and _____. (Section VI)

10. Blood is ordinarily obtained for testing by _____, also called _____, that is, by inserting a needle into a vein in the forearm, after antiseptic preparation of the skin, and withdrawing a sufficient volume of blood by means of a syringe or sealed vacuum tube. (Section VI)

11. A specimen for determination of blood gases (oxygen and carbon dioxide) is obtained by _____ puncture. (Section VI)

12. When only a small quantity of blood is needed, an adequate specimen may be obtained by _____.

13. Another word for red blood cell is _____.

Exercises

14. When found in groups erythrocytes tend to form _____ like stacks of coins.

15. Another name for white blood cells is _____.

16. Granulocytes are also called _____ because their nuclei are typically divided by shallow clefts into two to five lobes.

17. The type of white blood cell which does not show conspicuous granules in its cytoplasm is the _____.

18. Immature neutrophils with elongated but not lobed nuclei are called _____, _____, _____, or simply _____.

19. Under appropriate circumstances, certain lymphocytes known as _____ evolve into plasma cells, which produce antibodies in large amounts and release them into the circulation.

20. _____, which make up 55-65% of circulating lymphocytes, migrate from the marrow to the thymus for maturation before proceeding to other lymphoid organs and tissues.

21. _____ destroy cells they recognize as antigenic.

22. A few large, granular lymphocytes of unknown function, some of which seem to operate as natural killer cells but that are neither B nor T cells, are known as _____.

23. Only helper T cells have _____, and only suppressor and cytotoxic T cells have _____.

24. Alternative designations for helper T cells are _____ and, more simply, _____.

25. The term _____ is inconsistently applied to the complete blood count or to some of the tests composing it.

26. Reduction of the red blood cell count is known as _____ or _____.

27. The term _____ refers to the formation of red blood cells in tissues other than the bone marrow.

28. The white blood cell count is of limited usefulness in diagnosis, but the _____ contains more useful information.

29. An increase in the percent of band cells is called a _____ because at one time cell counts were recorded on a form in which the column for band cells was to the left of the column for mature neutrophils.

Exercises

30. Serial determination of the _____ is a means of monitoring immune compromise in AIDS and assessing the effects of treatment, and decline of this count below 200 cells/mm^3 [0.2 x 10^9 cells/L] or of the relative proportion below _____ indicates severe immune compromise and the need for prophylaxis against opportunistic infections.

31. Atypical lymphocytes (also called _____) occur in lymphatic leukemia, brucellosis, viral hepatitis, and various other viral infections.

32. The platelet count may be increased in _____.

33. The platelet count is decreased in _____.

34. _____ is a test used to assess the clumping characteristic of platelets, which helps to control bleeding by forming a mechanical plug at the site of vascular injury.

35. The _____, a modification of the prothrombin time test in which a phospholipid preparation is substituted for thromboplastin, is a more sensitive indicator of deficiency of plasma coagulation factors.

36. Bone marrow may be obtained by _____ from the sternum or by _____ from the iliac crest or, in infants and small children, the anterior tibia.

37. _____ is of paramount importance in blood transfusion and in the diagnosis and treatment of certain conditions associated with pregnancy.

38. An Rh positive child born to a previously sensitized Rh negative mother develops jaundice at birth or shortly thereafter because of extensive hemolysis, and nucleated (immature) red blood cells appear in the fetal circulation, a condition known as _____ or _____.

39. Testing for Duffy (Fy), Kell (K), Kidd (Jk), Lewis (Le), and Lutheran (Lu) finds its principal application in _____, but DNA testing is more conclusive.

40. In crossmatching for transfusion purposes, donor cells are mixed with recipient serum (major crossmatch) and recipient cells are mixed with donor serum (minor crossmatch). Any agglutination or hemolysis in either major or minor crossmatch is evidence of _____ and a _____ to transfusion.

Exercises

Multiple Choice: Circle the letter of the best answer from the choices given.

1. Introducing into the patient's body a measured quantity of a substance as a challenge to an organ such as the liver or kidney to incorporate or excrete the substance is performed in which kind of laboratory testing?
   A. Chemical.
   B. Qualitative.
   C. Quantitative.
   D. Function.
   E. Culture.

2. Which of the following types of cells are unique among body cells in having no nuclei throughout the entire course of their functional existence?
   A. White blood cells.
   B. Platelets.
   C. Red blood cells.
   D. Erythroblasts.
   E. Leukocytes.

3. Which of the following types of cells function to carry oxygen from the capillaries of the lungs to the capillaries of the rest of the body, and carbon dioxide from the tissues to the lungs for excretion?
   A. Granulocytes.
   B. White blood cells.
   C. Erythroblasts.
   D. Platelets.
   E. Erythrocytes.

4. What is the iron-containing substance, which is responsible for the red color of blood, forms a loose chemical union with oxygen in the lungs and releases it in the tissues?
   A. Hemoglobin.
   B. Serum.
   C. Globulin.
   D. Albumin.
   E. Protein.

5. Which of the following terms does NOT apply to granulocytes?
   A. Polymorphonuclear leukocytes.
   B. Monocytes.
   C. Neutrophils.
   D. Eosinophils.
   E. Basophils.

Exercises

6. _____ are leukocytes with large, kidney- or horseshoe-shaped, and eccentrically placed nuclei that function as phagocytes.
   A. Neutrophils.
   B. B lymphocytes.
   C. T lymphocytes.
   D. Monocytes.
   E. Eosinophils.

7. _____, the most numerous of all white blood cells, have granules that show approximately equal affinity for acidic and basic stains.
   A. Polymorphonuclear leukocytes.
   B. Monocytes.
   C. Neutrophils.
   D. Eosinophils.
   E. Basophils.

8. Which of the following types of leukocytes increase in number in parasitic infestation and allergic disorders, and decrease after administration of adrenocortical steroid drugs?
   A. Eosinophils.
   B. Neutrophils.
   C. Basophils.
   D. Stab cells
   E. Polymorphonuclear leukocytes.

9. Which of the following leukocytes have granules that stain with basic dyes and produce histamine, serotonin, and other biochemically active substances?
   A. Eosinophils.
   B. Neutrophils.
   C. Basophils.
   D. Stab cells
   E. Polymorphonuclear leukocytes.

10. Which cell type develops from precursor cells in bone marrow, migrates to other tissues before maturing, produces antibodies, modulates immune processes, and performs other protective functions?
    A. Polymorphonuclear leukocytes.
    B. Lymphocytes.
    C. Monocytes.
    D. Neutrophils.
    E. Erythrocytes.

Exercises

11. _____ curb the production of antibody by B cells and plasma cells.
    A. Cytotoxic (killer) T cells.
    B. Helper (or inducer) T cells.
    C. Natural killer cells.
    D. Null cells.
    E. Suppressor T cells.

12. _____ stimulate or augment the production of antibody by B cells and plasma cells.
    A. Cytotoxic (killer) T cells.
    B. Helper (or inducer) T cells.
    C. Natural killer cells.
    D. Null cells.
    E. Suppressor T cells.

13. _____ are specialized lymphocytes that produce antibodies and release them into the circulation.
    A. Platelets.
    B. Erythrocytes.
    C. Leukocytes.
    D. Plasma cells.
    E. Neutrophils.

14. Which of the following are very small round or oval bodies found in circulating blood that are not cells and do not have nuclei but function in blood clotting?
    A. Eosinophils.
    B. Neutrophils.
    C. Platelets.
    D. Stabs.
    E. Bands.

15. An elevation of the red blood cell count is known as
    A. Polycythemia.
    B. Erythrocytopenia.
    C. Erythrocytosis.
    D. Leukocytosis.
    E. A & C.

Exercises

16. Iron, protein, or vitamins deficiencies, disease or destruction of bone marrow, increased hemolysis, or acute or chronic hemorrhage may all be causes of which of the following conditions?
    A. Reduced hemoglobin.
    B. Erythrocytopenia.
    C. Anemia.
    D. Reduced hematocrit.
    E. All of the above.

17. An increase in the mean corpuscular volume means red blood cells are larger than normal and is called
    A. Macrocytosis.
    B. Leukocytosis.
    C. Erythrocytosis.
    D. Polycythemia.
    E. Erythrocytopenia.

18. Increased mean corpuscular volume accompanied by reduction in the red blood cell count results in a condition known as
    A. Polycythemia.
    B. Erythrocytopenia.
    C. Macrocytic anemia.
    D. Microcytic anemia.
    E. Leukocytosis.

19. Reduction in mean corpuscular volume is referred to as
    A. Macrocytosis.
    B. Microcytosis.
    C. Spherocytosis.
    D. Erythrocytosis.
    E. Anisocytosis.

20. Greater variation in red cell size (_____) occurs in many disorders associated with abnormal erythro-poiesis, including congenital hemolytic anemias and anemias occurring in deficiency states or chronic disease.
    A. Macrocytosis.
    B. Erythrocytosis.
    C. Spherocytosis.
    D. Anisocytosis.
    E. Microcytosis.

Exercises

21. Which of the following refers to erythrocytes with a bull's-eye appearance due to flattening of the cell with a prominent spot of hemoglobin in the center?
    A. Target cells.
    B. Burr cells.
    C. Ovalocytes.
    D. Spherocytes.
    E. Sickle cells.

22. Recently formed erythrocytes may contain remnants of nuclear chromatin called _____ and are found in increased numbers in some hemolytic anemias and after splenectomy.
    A. Nucleated red blood cells.
    B. Howell-Jolly bodies.
    C. Spherocytes.
    D. Sickle cells.
    E. Siderocytes.

23. In older children and adults _____ may indicate hemolytic anemia, pernicious anemia, or lead poisoning.
    A. Nucleated red blood cells.
    B. Howell-Jolly bodies.
    C. Spherocytes.
    D. Sickle cells.
    E. Siderocytes.

24. _____ must be used to confirm the diagnosis of most hereditary disorders in the synthesis of hemoglobin and the formation of red blood cells.
    A. Hemoglobin electrophoresis.
    B. Red cell indices.
    C. Red cell morphology.
    D. White cell differential.
    E. Hematocrit.

25. The most commonly encountered abnormal hemoglobin is hemoglobin S, which is characteristic of
    A. Macrocytic anemia.
    B. Microcytic anemia.
    C. Sickle cell anemia.
    D. Hemolytic anemia.
    E. Pernicious anemia.

Exercises

26. A condition common in persons of Mediterranean or Far Eastern ancestry associated with abnormal structure of the red blood cell (target cells) and with varying amounts of hemoglobin C, E, and F is
    A. Sickle cell anemia.
    B. Elliptocytosis.
    C. Spherocytosis.
    D. Thalassemia.
    E. Dresbach syndrome.

27. Hereditary deficiency of glucose-6-phosphate dehydrogenase (G-6-PD) in red blood cells, also called _____, is a type of hemolytic anemia in which red cells are subject to hemolysis after exposure to certain drugs, chemicals, and foods.
    A. Favism.
    B. Sickle cell anemia.
    C. Thalassemia minor.
    D. Dresbach syndrome.
    E. Hemolysis.

28. The breakdown of red blood cells with release of hemoglobin into the plasma occurs in many congenital hemoglobinopathies, in transfusion reactions, and in certain toxic states is referred to as
    A. Granulocytopenia.
    B. Leukemia.
    C. Erythropenia.
    D. Anemia.
    E. Hemolysis.

29. Determining the concentration of _____, an alpha2-globulin normally present in circulating blood that binds any free hemoglobin released by hemolysis, is an indirect measure of hemolysis.
    A. Carboxyhemoglobin.
    B. Methemoglobin.
    C. Glucose-6-phosphate dehydrogenase.
    D. Haptoglobin.
    E. Sulfhemoglobin.

30. The level of _____ is increased in rare hereditary metabolic errors and after absorption of certain oxidizing agents.
    A. Carboxyhemoglobin.
    B. Methemoglobin.
    C. Glucose-6-phosphate dehydrogenase.
    D. Haptoglobin.
    E. Sulfhemoglobin.

Exercises

31. Measuring the concentration in the blood of _____ provides evidence of carbon monoxide intoxication and permits assessment of its severity.
    A. Cyanmethemoglobin
    B. Methemoglobin.
    C. Carboxyhemoglobin.
    D. Haptoglobin.
    E. Sulfhemoglobin.

32. Osmotic fragility is reduced—that is, hemolysis occurs at lower osmolalities than with normal red blood cells—in all of the following conditions except
    A. Congenital and acquired hemolytic anemias.
    B. Sickle cell anemia.
    C. Thalassemia.
    D. Iron deficiency anemia.
    E. Microcytic anemias.

33. The _____ is increased in many acute and chronic inflammatory conditions, acute myocardial infarction, various toxic states, and various malignancies including particularly those accompanied by production of abnormal globulins.
    A. Sedimentation rate.
    B. Erythrocyte sedimentation rate.
    C. Erythrocyte survival time.
    D. Osmotic fragility.
    E. Reticulocyte count.

34. Elevation of the white blood cell count, or _____, occurs in acute or chronic inflammation of any cause and in leukemia and some lymphomas.
    A. Erythropenia.
    B. Leukopenia.
    C. Erythrocytosis.
    D. Monocytosis.
    E. Leukocytosis.

35. Depression of the white blood cell count, or _____, results from suppression of their production by toxic substances, chemotherapy, radiation, or disease of hematopoietic tissue.
    A. Erythropenia.
    B. Leukocytosis.
    C. Erythrocytosis.
    D. Leukopenia.
    E. Monocytosis.

Exercises

36. When atypical lymphocytes (also called Downey cells or virocytes) exceed 10% of all white blood cells they are virtually diagnostic of
    A. Lymphatic leukemia.
    B. Brucellosis.
    C. Infectious mononucleosis.
    D. Viral hepatitis.
    E. Multiple myeloma.

37. Hemophilia A, a sex-linked recessive trait carried by females but expressed only in males, is due to a congenital deficiency of the clotting factor, _____.
    A. Factor V.
    B. Factor VIII.
    C. Prothrombin.
    D. Fibrinogen.
    E. Thrombin.

38. _____, which results from imbalance between the mechanisms of coagulation and of fibrinolysis, can be induced by infection, trauma, shock, complications of pregnancy and parturition, and myelocytic leukemia.
    A. Disseminated intravascular coagulation.
    B. Von Willebrand disease.
    C. Osler-Weber-Rendu disease.
    D. Glanzmann disease.
    E. Idiopathic thrombocytopenic purpura.

39. The Duke and Ivy methods are used to test for
    A. Platelet function.
    B. Clotting time.
    C. Bleeding time.
    D. Tourniquet time.
    E. Capillary fragility.

40. The Lee-White method is the standard test for _____.
    A. Platelet function.
    B. Clotting time.
    C. Bleeding time.
    D. Tourniquet time.
    E. Capillary fragility.

Exercises

41. The test used to assesses capillary fragility and platelet function is the _____.
    A. Rumpel-Leede test.
    B. Lee-White method.
    C. Ivy method.
    D. Duke method.
    E. Factor VIII assay.

42. The _____ finds the time required for a clot to form by adding a combination of calcium and thromboplastin to a specimen of plasma previously treated with an anticoagulant to bind the calcium that is naturally present.
    A. Lee-White method.
    B. Thrombin time test.
    C. Rumpel-Leede test.
    D. Factor VIII assay.
    E. Prothrombin time test.

43. The _____ determines the speed with which a clot forms in a specimen of the patient's blood to which thrombin has been added.
    A. Lee-White method.
    B. Thrombin time test.
    C. Rumpel-Leede test.
    D. Factor VIII assay.
    E. Prothrombin time test.

44. A disturbance of plasmin function can lead to excessive plasmin activity and a rise of _____ in the circulating blood, with both abnormal bleeding and abnormal clotting (disseminated intravascular coagulation, DIC).
    A. Thrombin.
    B. Prothrombin.
    C. Factor VIII.
    D. Fibrin degradation products.
    E. Plasminogen.

45. _____ is a specific fibrin degradation product whose level in the blood is elevated in about 95% of patients with pulmonary embolism.
    A. Plasminogen.
    B. Prothrombin.
    C. D-dimer.
    D. Antithrombin.
    E. Cryofibrinogen.

Exercises

46. The _____ is positive in a newborn with erythroblastosis fetalis and in persons with acquired hemolytic disease due to production of abnormal globulins, as in leukemia, lymphoma, and collagen diseases.
    A. Direct Coombs test.
    B. D-dimer.
    C. Indirect Coombs test.
    D. Cryofibrinogen.
    E. Fibrin degradation products.

47. The _____ is positive in the mother of an infant with erythroblastosis fetalis and in any person with anti-Rh antiglobulins or other acquired hemolyzing antibodies, as in hematopoietic malignancies and collagen diseases.
    A. Direct Coombs test.
    B. D-dimer.
    C. Indirect Coombs test.
    D. Cryofibrinogen.
    E. Fibrin degradation products.

Short Answers

1. Briefly explain the scope of the following branches of clinical pathology:
    a. hematology _____
        _____
    b. clinical chemistry _____
        _____
    c. urinology _____
        _____
    d. microbiology _____
        _____
    e. serology _____
        _____

2. What is meant by quantitative data? Give examples of the difference between qualitative and quantitative data. (See introduction to Section VI.)

    _____
    _____
    _____

Exercises

3. How is "normal" defined in practice?

    _____

    _____

    _____

    _____

4. What factors govern the physician's choice of a laboratory procedure when several similar methods are available?

    _____

    _____

    _____

    _____

5. What examinations make up the complete blood count?

    _____

    _____

    _____

    _____

6. What is the significance of the reticulocyte count?

    _____

    _____

    _____

    _____

7. List some basic tests that are included in a coagulation panel.

    _____

    _____

    _____

    _____

Exercises

8. List blood groups and explain their clinical significance.

_____

_____

_____

_____

9. Sickle cell disease differs from sickle cell trait in what ways?

a. _____

b. _____

10. Describe the procedure performed to test for erythrocyte survival time.

_____

_____

_____

_____

11. List the six different types of white cells and the significance of each.

a. _____

b. _____

c. _____

d. _____

e. _____

f. _____

12. The myeloid/erythroid ratio, that is, the ratio of leukocyte to erythrocyte precursors in the marrow, is useful for evaluating what kinds of conditions?

_____

_____

_____

_____

Exercises

Activities for Application and Further Study

1. Illustrate the interaction of clotting factors in the process of coagulation using a drawing, graph, chart, or some other pictorial method.

2. What is meant by saying that "disease is life under altered conditions"? Find several other definitions of disease from ancient and contemporary sources. Compare and contrast the definitions. Write your own definition of disease.

Chemical Examination of the Blood

20

LEARNING OBJECTIVES

Upon completion of this chapter, the student should be able to

- Give a general description of the role of electrolytes, minerals, and blood gases in health and disease;

- Explain the diagnostic application of various tests for enzymes, hormones, proteins, lipids, and glucose in circulating blood;

- Describe the use of testing for tumor markers and waste products in diagnosis.

Chapter Outline

Osmolality

Electrolytes and Acid-Base Balance

Minerals

Arterial Blood Gases

Enzymes

Hormones

Proteins, Peptides, and Amino Acids

Lipids and Lipoproteins

Blood Sugar

Tumor Markers

Waste Products

Drug Monitoring, Detection of Poisons

Panels

Thousands of test procedures are currently available to the clinical laboratory technician to identify and measure hundreds of chemical substances in the blood. Some of these procedures are rarely performed because they are expensive, require special equipment, pertain to rare diseases or conditions, or have been superseded by tests that are cheaper, simpler, faster, more sensitive, or more specific. Others are performed by the tens of thousands every day in laboratories throughout the world. Most of the tests discussed in this chapter are within the standard repertory of virtually all clinical chemistry laboratories.

Although every chemical test of the blood starts with a specimen of whole blood, the initial processing of this specimen varies depending on the type of test to be done. Most chemical tests of the blood seek to determine the concentration of substances (analytes) in the plasma by quantitative analysis. Because the concentration of some of these substances (for example, potassium, phosphorus, and some enzymes) is much higher in normal red blood cells than in normal plasma, the cellular elements of the blood must be removed before chemical testing begins.

Although this could be done by allowing the blood to coagulate naturally and waiting for the clot to separate from the serum, this method involves considerable delay and does not yield consistent serum fractions. In practice, the cells are separated from the plasma as soon as possible in a centrifuge, which spins the specimen at high speed so that the cells are caused to sediment rapidly and completely. One type of centrifuge tube, called a separator tube, contains a plug of semisolid material whose specific gravity lies midway between that of cells and that of plasma. The settling cells fall below this plug and the plasma remains above it. Keeping cells and plasma completely segregated in this manner is important; otherwise some red blood cells may leak or burst (hemolyze) and release their contents into the plasma while the specimen is awaiting analysis.

Hemolysis in a blood specimen is one of the commonest reasons for false elevations of plasma chemistry levels.

Some tests are done directly on plasma, others on serum (that is, blood with both cells and fibrinogen removed), still others on a protein-free filtrate of plasma. This is prepared by adding to plasma a reagent such as phosphotungstic acid which coagulates all protein so that it can be removed from the specimen by filtration.

Modern clinical chemistry makes use of a wide variety of analytic techniques to identify and measure substances in the blood. Older and more cumbersome gravimetric techniques, requiring precise weighing, and volumetric techniques, requiring drop-by-drop titration, have been replaced by quantitative analytic methods that use electronic equipment. This equipment measures the concentration of various analytes indirectly but very precisely by determining various physical properties of a test solution, such as its capacity to transmit light (spectrophotometry), or the wave length of a color change (colorimetry). Other analytic methods include electrophoresis, based on the differing behavior of various solutes in an electric field; gas, liquid, and thin-layer chromatography; radioimmunoassay, which measures specific proteins by observing their reaction with isotopically labeled monoclonal antibodies; and molecular biology methods, which detect DNA sequences that are unique to certain proteins and enzymes.

Automated analytic devices can perform twenty or more tests on blood samples at a rate of one sample or more a minute. Despite their great expense, these analyzers reduce the cost of chemical testing because they are capable of processing a much higher volume of material than a human technician. In addition, they permit better standardization of results and eliminate many potential sources of human error.

Routine tests performed in all clinical laboratories on venous blood include quantitative analyses for electrolytes, carbohydrates, lipids, proteins, enzymes, hormones, vitamins, nitrogenous wastes, bile pigments, prescribed drugs, and toxic substances including drugs of abuse. Important examples of each of these classes of test material will be surveyed in the following pages, and their clinicopathologic significance outlined.

Osmolality

The maintenance of osmotic balance between plasma and intercellular fluid depends on the concentration of solute (dissolved materials such as electrolytes and proteins) in the plasma. The osmotic activity (osmolality) of serum is determined by a physical (nonchemical) measurement. Pure water freezes at 0°C. Adding solute to water lowers its freezing point in proportion to the osmotic activity of the solute. Serum osmolality, as determined by the freezing point depression method, is normally 280 to 295 mOsm/kg (milliosmoles per kilogram). Increase of serum osmolality (hyperosmolality) occurs in diabetes mellitus, diabetes insipidus, dehydration, and hypercalcemia. Reduction (hyposmolality) is noted in congestive heart failure, cirrhosis, Addison disease, hyponatremia, and inappropriate secretion of antidiuretic hormone.

Electrolytes and Acid-Base Balance

An electrolyte is a substance capable of conducting an electric current when dissolved in water. In chemical parlance, the term electrolyte refers to any substance that ionizes in water, that is, that breaks down into ions. An ion is an atom or group of atoms having a positive or negative charge. A cation is an ion that has a positive charge because it has lost one or more electrons, while an anion has a negative charge because it has gained one or more electrons. The principal cations of the plasma are sodium and potassium, and the principal anions are chloride and bicarbonate.

The concentrations and ratios of these substances are held within fairly narrow limits in the normal body, principally by the kidneys, which excrete (or retain) sodium, potassium, chloride, and water, and by the lungs, whose excretion (or retention) of carbon dioxide dissolved in the blood controls the concentration of bicarbonate ion.

The cortex of each kidney contains more than a million renal corpuscles, each consisting of a tuft or tangle of capillaries called the glomerulus and a two-layered envelope surrounding it called the Bowman capsule (*see Fig. 20.1, p. 358*). As blood passes through the capillaries making up the glomerulus, water and dissolved substances diffuse from it into the space between the two layers of the Bowman capsule.

The normal glomerular membrane is permeable not only to water but also to electrolytes, simple sugars, amino acids, waste products such as urea and creatinine, and indeed nearly all substances carried in the blood except large protein molecules, red and white blood cells, and platelets. The fluid formed in the Bowman capsule thus has essentially the same composition as blood minus the cells and proteins. The glomerular filtration rate (GFR) depends on systemic blood pressure, the resistance of glomerular capillaries to blood flow, and the integrity of the glomerular basement membrane, which is subject to damage by a variety of inflammatory, degenerative, and toxic factors.

What takes place in the glomerulus is only the beginning of the process of urine formation. Each Bowman capsule gives origin to a tubule, which after following a somewhat tortuous course through the renal cortex and medulla discharges its urine from one of the renal papillae into the pelvis of the kidney. The tubules play an active role in determining the eventual volume and composition of urine by simultaneously performing three distinct operations on the glomerular filtrate: passively reabsorbing most of the water and dissolved electrolytes, actively reabsorbing certain substances (sodium, chloride), and

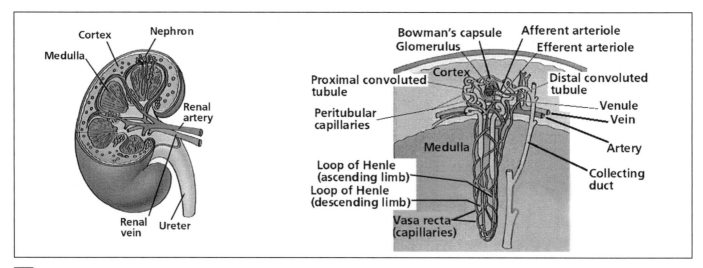

Fig. 20.1. Gross and microscopic anatomy of kidney.

Reference: http://mcdb.colorado.edu/courses/3280/lectures/class08.html

actively secreting other substances (potassium, hydrogen ions, urea).

Each section of a renal tubule performs different reabsorptive and excretory functions. Numerous congenital disorders have been identified in which specific excretory or reabsorptive functions of the renal tubules are impaired or lacking. Some of these can cause severe developmental failure, mental retardation, or death.

The concentrations of sodium, potassium, and chloride in the blood depend to a large extent on the renal retention or excretion of these ions. These processes in turn are regulated by aldosterone and related hormones produced by the adrenal glands. Aldosterone promotes the renal tubular retention (that is, the reabsorption from glomerular filtrate) of sodium, the principal cation (positively charged ion) of the blood and extracellular fluid, and of chloride, the principal anion (negatively charged ion). It also promotes the tubular excretion of potassium, the principal cation of intracellular fluid.

Disorders of the kidney or of the respiratory system, as well as other conditions causing abnormal loss or retention of body water or dissolved ions, can profoundly alter the levels of serum electrolytes. Determination of serum electrolytes (often abbreviated in speech to *lytes*) is a sensitive indicator of a broad range of metabolic disorders, and can also supply valuable indirect information about water balance and acid-base balance.

Sodium, potassium, chloride, and bicarbonate are almost invariably measured together. To facilitate calculations involving these electrolytes, their concentrations are all reported in milliequivalents per liter (mEq/L) or millimoles per liter (mmol/L).

Sodium (Na) is an important constituent of all body fluids, being concerned in maintenance of osmotic pressure, water balance, membrane permeability, and the irritability of nerve cells. The principal source of sodium in the diet is table salt (sodium chloride). Sodium is filtered from the blood by the renal glomeruli, and, under the control of adrenal mineralocorticoids (principally aldosterone), partially reabsorbed in the renal tubules. Most sodium loss occurs through the kidneys, but appreciable losses also occur in sweat and stools.

Sodium is the principal cation of plasma, being present in a concentration of 136 to 145 mEq/L [136–145 mmol/L]. The commonest cause for an increase of sodium concentration (hypernatremia) is excessive loss of water due to sweating, vomiting, or diuresis (increased renal excretion of water). Diuresis may be induced by diuretic drugs and also occurs in diabetes mellitus, diabetes insipidus, and various renal disorders. Reduction in serum sodium concentration (hyponatremia) may reflect either an increase in serum water content (dilutional hyponatremia), as in congestive heart failure or hepatic or renal disease; or true depletion of sodium, as by vomiting, sweating, or excessive renal excretion of sodium in renal disease, adrenal cortical deficiency (Addison disease), or as an effect of certain diuretics.

Although present in much higher concentration within cells, **potassium** (K) is an important cation of plasma, with a normal concentration between 3.5 and 5.0 mEq/L [3.5–5.0 mmol/L]. Potassium functions to maintain acid-base balance and osmotic pressure within cells and is essential to normal activity of muscle tissue, especially cardiac muscle. The principal dietary sources of potassium are meats and fruits. It is both filtered from the blood by the glomeruli and secreted (under the influence of mineralocorticoids) by the renal tubules.

Elevation of potassium concentration (hyperkalemia or hyperpotassemia) can result from diminished excretion of potassium ions (as in renal disease or adrenal failure) or from additional amounts of potassium in the serum (as from breakdown of muscle tissue or red blood cells). Reduction of serum potassium (hypokalemia or hypopotassemia) is most often due to loss of potassium from the body in gastrointestinal secretions (as from vomiting, diarrhea, or prolonged suction drainage from the stomach or intestine). Potassium loss can also occur from the kidney in acute or chronic renal disease, Cushing syndrome, primary aldosteronism, or (very often) as an effect of some diuretic drugs.

Chloride (Cl), the principal anion of intercellular fluid, is also present in significant concentration within cells. Particularly high concentrations are found in cerebrospinal fluid and gastric juice. Chloride helps to maintain acid-base, osmotic, and water balance. A principal dietary source is table salt. Renal excretion of chloride ion tends to parallel that of sodium.

The normal range of serum chloride concentrations is 100 to 106 mEq/L [100–106 mmol/L]. Increase in the concentration of this ion (hyperchloremia) may result from dehydration or from reduced excretion of chloride ions in acute renal failure or other renal disease. Decrease of chloride concentration (hypochloremia) can be either dilutional (as with excessive fluid retention in congestive heart failure or renal or hepatic disease) or due to depletion by loss from the gastrointestinal tract (particularly by vomiting), from the kidney as a consequence of diuretic therapy or adrenal failure, or from the sweat glands.

The **bicarbonate** (HCO_3^-) ion is measured indirectly, being first converted to carbon dioxide. Hence this electrolyte is often referred to as carbon dioxide (CO_2). The normal serum concentration of bicarbonate is 24 to 30 mEq/L [24–30 mmol/L]. Unlike the other serum electrolytes, whose concentration is determined principally by the kidneys, bicarbonate level depends on excretion or retention of carbon dioxide gas by the lungs. Moreover, this concentration can change very rapidly with shifts in the equilibrium between bicarbonate ion and carbon dioxide.

A principal function of the bicarbonate ion is the regulation of acid-base balance. The acidity or alkalinity of a solution depends on its hydrogen ion concentration. This is measured in pH units derived from the logarithm of the hydrogen ion concentration. A pH of 7.0 indicates perfect neutrality. A pH higher than 7.0 indicates alkalinity, and a pH lower than 7.0 indicates acidity. The pH of serum is maintained between 7.35 and 7.45 by a complex set of chemical checks and balances involving renal excretion of hydrogen ions and others, and the buffering effect of cations in the serum. A buffer is a substance that resists changes in pH by combining with or releasing hydrogen ions so as to keep their concentration constant in a solution. The principal buffer of the serum is bicarbonate ion. Phosphate ion and the serum proteins (albumin and globulin) also act as buffers, but to a much lesser extent.

A rise in serum pH is called alkalosis and a fall in pH is called acidosis. Either of these conditions can be respiratory in origin, resulting from a disturbance in the excretion of carbon dioxide by the lungs, or metabolic in origin, reflecting abnormalities in the levels of other ions. Respiratory alkalosis is due to excessive loss of carbon dioxide via the lungs, as from hyperventilation, while respiratory acidosis indicates abnormal retention of carbon dioxide, as from disease of the respiratory or circulatory system that impairs pulmonary gas exchange. The causes of metabolic alkalosis include loss of hydrogen ions from the gastrointestinal tract through vomiting and loss of hydrogen ions from the kidneys as a result of diuretic administration, hyperaldosteronism, or Cushing syndrome.

Metabolic acidosis is divided into two types on the basis of the anion gap of the serum. If the sum of the cation concentrations of serum (sodium plus potassium) is compared to the sum of the anion concentrations (chloride plus bicarbonate), it will be found that the cation concentration is higher. This is because the calculation takes into account only the principal cations and anions, and the anions not included (phosphate, sulfate, protein, and various organic anions) exceed the cations not included (calcium, magnesium, and others). The difference between cation and anion concentrations when only the four principal ions are included in the calculation is called the anion gap, which is normally 12 to 20 mEq/L [12–20 mmol/L].

Metabolic acidosis with a normal anion gap may be due to loss of bicarbonate ion from the bowel through diarrhea, or from the kidney as a result of renal disease (renal tubular acidosis). When metabolic acidosis is accompanied by an increased anion gap, the difference in unmea-

sured anion is usually due to the presence of excessive anions derived from organic acids. These may be normal anions abnormally retained by a diseased kidney; anions abnormally produced in certain conditions (lactic acidosis, diabetic ketoacidosis); or extraneous substances (salicylate, methanol).

Any shift in serum pH tends to be compensated by whatever mechanism remains unimpaired. Hence, for example, metabolic acidosis leads to increased pulmonary excretion of carbon dioxide, with a resulting tendency towards respiratory alkalosis. Consequently, electrolyte imbalances are frequently complex and difficult to diagnose.

Minerals

Calcium (Ca) is the principal mineral of bones and teeth and also plays an essential role in nerve and muscle function and blood coagulation. The main dietary sources of calcium are milk and dairy products. The absorption, distribution, and excretion of calcium are controlled by vitamin D, parathyroid hormone, and calcitonin. Most of the excretion of calcium occurs in the stool.

The normal calcium concentration of serum is 8.2–10.2 mg/dL [2–2.5 mmol/L]. This level tends to vary inversely with that of phosphorus. About one-half of the calcium in the serum is bound to protein and the other half is in free (unionized) form. Elevation of serum calcium (hypercalcemia) occurs in hyperparathyroidism (usually due to a benign adenoma), vitamin D intoxication, sarcoidosis, various malignancies including particularly those of hematopoietic tissue and bone, and any condition favoring bone resorption (such as immobilization). Hypercalcemia causes muscular weakness, anorexia, increased urinary output, metastatic calcification in blood vessels and kidneys, and urolithiasis.

Serum calcium is reduced (hypocalcemia) in hypoparathyroidism, in disorders characterized by low serum albumin (nephrotic syndrome, cachexia), in acute pancreatitis with fat necrosis, and in chronic renal failure with retention of phosphorus. A significant fall in serum calcium causes heightening of neuromuscular excitability, with tetany (sustained spasm of voluntary muscles), twitching, and seizures.

Phosphorus (P) is widely distributed throughout the cells and fluids of the body, most of it being in chemical combination with calcium in bones and teeth. Phosphorus is abundant in most foods. Its metabolism closely follows that of calcium, and is therefore under the influence of vitamin D, parathyroid hormone, and calcitonin. Phosphate is a minor anion of serum but contributes some buffering effect.

The normal phosphorus concentration of serum is 2.5–4.5 mg/dL [0.8–1.5 mmol/L]. Phosphorus is increased (hyperphosphatemia) in hypoparathyroidism, vitamin D intoxication, hematologic malignancies, chronic renal failure, and various disorders of bone (healing fractures, Paget disease, multiple myeloma, metastatic neoplasm). A reduction of phosphorus level (hypophosphatemia) occurs in hyperparathyroidism, renal tubular disorders, osteomalacia, rickets, severe metabolic acidosis, malabsorption syndromes (sprue, celiac disease), and other abnormal nutritional states.

The role of **iron** (Fe) in body chemistry is limited almost entirely to the transport and utilization of oxygen. Iron occurs as a component of hemoglobin, the oxygen-carrying material of red blood cells; myoglobin, a similar compound in muscle; and several substances involved in intracellular metabolism (cytochromes, peroxidase). Under normal conditions, most of the iron in the body is recycled, but intestinal absorption of small amounts from meats and vegetables is needed to offset small losses in urine and stool and to meet needs created by menstruation, normal growth and development, and abnormal blood loss. Acid gastric juice is necessary for proper absorption of dietary iron, most of which occurs in the duodenum. In tissues other than the blood, iron is found in a storage form in combination with the protein ferritin.

The normal serum iron level is 50–160 mcg/dL [9.0–28.8 mcmol/L] for males and about 10% less for females. Most of the iron in the serum is bound to the protein transferrin. Serum iron is increased (hyperferremia) in hemochromatosis, hemosiderosis due to excessive intake of iron, hemolytic anemia (due to breakdown of red blood cells), and pernicious anemia (due to decreased incorporation of iron in red blood cells). Reduction of serum iron (hypoferremia) is observed in iron deficiency anemia due to malnutrition or to various malabsorptive states (achlorhydria, steatorrhea, surgical absence of stomach or duodenum) as well as after severe hemorrhage.

In order to distinguish among various causes of abnormal serum iron levels it is helpful to determine the **iron-binding capacity** of the blood. The amount of transferrin in normal serum is capable of binding iron to the extent of 250–350 mcg/dL [45–63 mcmol/L]. Comparison with the normal iron level shows that only 20 to 55% of this binding capacity is normally used (saturated). The iron-binding capacity is increased in anemia due to hemorrhage or dietary deficiency of iron, and decreased in hemochromatosis and in disease states associated with reduction of serum proteins (nephrotic syndrome, chronic infection, hepatic cirrhosis). The saturation of the serum iron-binding capacity is increased in hemochromatosis and hemosiderosis and reduced in anemias associated with iron deficiency and chronic disease.

Most of the **magnesium** (Mg) in the body is combined with calcium and phosphorus in bones and teeth. The normal serum level is 1.5–2.3 mg/dL [0.6–1.0 mmol/L]. Increase in this level (hypermagnesemia) occurs in renal failure and in deficiency of thyroid or adrenal cortical hormones. Reduction in magnesium (hypomagnesemia) is seen in malabsorption states, alcoholism, hyperthyroidism, and Cushing syndrome.

Copper, zinc, and certain other metallic elements are called trace elements because they occur in only small concentrations in body fluids and tissues. They are nonetheless essential components of many enzyme systems and other metabolic processes, and deficiencies of them due to inadequate dietary intake or congenital disorders can cause severe, even life-threatening metabolic imbalances.

Copper (Cu) is an essential component of enzymes and other proteins concerned in hemoglobin synthesis and bone formation. The normal serum level of copper, most of which is bound to the protein ceruloplasmin, is 0.7–1.5 mcg/mL [11–24 mmol/L]. The serum copper level is increased in acute and chronic infections, various anemias, leukemia, collagen diseases, and hemochromatosis, and decreased in Wilson's disease. (The diagnosis of Wilson disease is established by finding a low level of ceruloplasmin in serum and an increased amount of copper in the urine.)

Zinc (Zn) occurs in white blood cells and other tissues and is essential to the function of many enzyme systems. The normal concentration of zinc in serum is 0.75-1.4 mcg/mL [11.5-21.6 mcmol/L]. The level may be reduced in renal failure, leukemia, and chronic nutritional deficiency such as occurs in alcoholism. The zinc level may be increased after occupational exposure to toxic amounts of zinc dust or fumes.

Arterial Blood Gases

Chemical measurement of arterial blood gases (oxygen and carbon dioxide) is used to assess the adequacy of pulmonary gas exchange in persons with respiratory or circulatory disease and those receiving oxygen therapy, with or without ventilatory assistance. Ordinarily the pH of the specimen is also determined to identify acidosis or alkalosis and to permit indirect calculation of the bicarbonate ion concentration. The specimen for blood gas determination is drawn from an artery, not a vein. All room air is excluded from the specimen, heparin is added to prevent coagulation, and the specimen is stored in ice until testing is performed. Blood gases are measured in millimeters of mercury (mmHg or torr).

The normal partial pressure of **oxygen** (PO_2) in arterial blood is 75 to 100 torr. This level normally declines with age. The arterial oxygen may be increased in hyperventilation due to anxiety. Reduction of oxygen tension (hypoxemia) can result from any condition that depresses or inhibits respiratory movements (paralysis, chest injury, pneumothorax, massive obesity, central nervous system depression by drugs, trauma, or disease); any condition that prevents normal oxygen exchange in lung tissue (pneumonia, bronchitis, pulmonary edema, asthma, airway obstruction); or reduction of available oxygen in the atmosphere.

Oxygen saturation, which can be measured by pulse oximetry as described in Chapter 4, can also be calculated from the PO_2 and the concentration of hemoglobin. The normal oxygen saturation is 95-100%. A reduction below this level has essentially the same significance as a reduction in the partial pressure of oxygen.

The normal partial pressure of **carbon dioxide** (PCO_2) is 35 to 45 torr. Increase in carbon dioxide tension (hypercapnia) may be caused by most of the same conditions that reduce oxygen (except reduction in available oxygen). Increase in carbon dioxide and bicarbonate ion also occurs in response to metabolic alkalosis. Reduction of carbon dioxide (hypocapnia) occurs in hyperventilation and in response to metabolic acidosis.

Serum pH and bicarbonate ion concentration were discussed earlier in this chapter in connection with electrolyte studies on venous blood.

Enzymes

An enzyme is a protein that catalyzes a biochemical reaction—that is, that accelerates or facilitates that reaction without being permanently altered or consumed in the process. Digestive enzymes in saliva, gastric juice, pancreatic juice, and small intestinal secretions break down carbohydrates, lipids, and proteins to simpler compounds as a preliminary to absorption and utilization. A large number of intracellular enzymes have been identified as being essential to various phases of cell chemistry including energy metabolism and synthesis of cell products such as hormones and other enzymes.

Although only a few enzymes (such as those concerned in blood clotting) perform any function in circulating blood, a number of them can be detected in the serum, at least under certain conditions. Many kinds of cells, when damaged by injury, infarction, or inflammation, leak their cytoplasmic enzymes into the circulation. An elevation of an enzyme level in the serum may therefore indicate disease in its tissue of origin. Because most enzymes are found in a variety of tissues, it is seldom possible to make a specific diagnosis on the basis of a single enzyme level. Typically a group or panel of enzyme tests are done and diagnostic inferences drawn from a consideration of all the information thus gained. Enzyme assays are ordinarily carried out by measuring enzyme activity, which is reported in arbitrarily established units per volume (U/L) rather than by weight per volume.

A group of two or more enzymes having the same action but differing in chemical structure are called isoenzymes (or isozymes). Often each isoenzyme can be linked to a specific tissue of origin. Hence, when a rise in the serum level of a certain enzyme is detected, it may be possible to gain more precise information about its source by determining the relative proportions of the various isoenzymes present. Isoenzymes can be separated by electrophoresis, ion exchange chromatography, and other techniques.

An important group of serum enzymes are often found elevated to varying degrees in hepatic disease and in injury or infarction of muscle, particularly cardiac muscle. This group includes alanine aminotransferase, aspartate aminotransferase, creatine phosphokinase, lactic dehydrogenase, and gamma-glutamyl transpeptidase.

Aspartate aminotransferase (AST), also called serum glutamic-oxaloacetic transaminase (SGOT), has a normal level below 35 U/L. AST is elevated in active liver disease, pancreatitis, degenerative disease or extensive trauma of skeletal muscle; also in most cases of myocardial infarction and in some cases of cerebral or pulmonary infarction. In myocardial infarction the elevation begins at 6 to 12 hours and peaks at 24 to 48 hours.

Lactic dehydrogenase (LDH), normally below 110 U/L, is elevated in hepatitis, hemolytic anemia, carcinoma (especially metastatic), pulmonary embolism and infarction, and in nearly all cases of myocardial infarction. The rise in myocardial infarction begins at 12 hours and peaks at 72 hours. Five LDH isoenzymes, designated I through V, have been identified. Elevation of I predominates in myocardial infarction, of II in hemolytic disease and other infarctions, of III and IV in disseminated lupus erythematosus and malignant lymphoma, and of V in hepatic disease.

Serum **gamma-glutamyl transpeptidase** (or transferase) (SGGT), whose normal level is below 65 U/L, is elevated in biliary obstruction, hepatitis, cirrhosis, pancreatitis, alcoholism, and in 50% of cases of myocardial infarction. Elevation in myocardial infarction begins on the fourth or fifth day and peaks at 8 to 12 days.

Alanine aminotransferase (ALT), also called serum glutamic-pyruvate transaminase (SGPT), is elevated in hepatocellular disease and in traumatic and degenerative disorders of skeletal muscle. The normal range is 8–45 U/L.

The alkaline and acid phosphatases are highly useful markers of disease. Serum **alkaline phosphatase**, with a normal level of 20 to 120 U/L, is elevated in hyperparathyroidism, Paget disease, rickets, biliary obstruction, and hepatic disease, particularly malignant. It is also normally higher in children than in adults. The level of alkaline phosphatase may be depressed in hypothyroidism, malnutrition, and malabsorption. Two other enzymes, serum **leucine aminopeptidase** (SLAP), normally below 40 U/L, and **5′-nucleotidase**, normally below 12.5 U/L, are useful in interpreting elevation of alkaline phosphatase. These typically rise in hepatic disease but not in bone disease. **Acid phosphatase** is found in high concentration in prostatic tissue. The serum level of this enzyme, normally below 0.6 U/L, is usually elevated in carcinoma or infarction of the prostate. It may also be elevated in hepatic disease or metastatic bone disease.

Serum enzyme studies are routinely performed for the early diagnosis of myocardial infarction in patients with acute chest pain. In addition to AST and LDH, determination of **creatine kinase** (CK) level may be helpful in confirming myocardial damage during the first 24 hours after infarction. Creatine kinase, also called creatine phosphokinase (CPK), varies from 12 to 80 U/L when the specimen is incubated at 30°C and from 55 to 170 U/L when it is incubated at 37°. The level is elevated in degenerative disease or injury of skeletal muscle, cerebral thrombosis with infarction, and in nearly all cases of myocardial infarction. Elevation in myocardial infarction begins in 4 to 8 hours and peaks at 24 hours. Three isoenzymes of CPK have been identified. Of these, the MB isoenzyme rises in myocardial infarction, the MM isoenzyme in cerebral infarction, and the BB isoenzyme (rarely) in uremia, Reye syndrome, and necrosis of the colon.

Numerous congenital disorders consist in the lack of genes that encode specific enzymes. Tests that show deficiency or absence of these enzymes are therefore valuable in the diagnosis of these disorders. An inborn metabolic disorder that results in the accumulation in tissues of excessive amounts of a normal or abnormal substance is called a storage disease.

In Gaucher disease, congenital deficiency of **beta-glucosidase** (also called glucocerebrosidase and glucosylceramidase) causes accumulation of a lipid material, glucocerebroside, in the liver, spleen, lymph nodes, and bone marrow. The diagnosis of the disease is confirmed by the finding of a deficiency of the enzyme in white blood cells (or in fibroblasts obtained by skin biopsy). Tay-Sachs disease, due to congenital deficiency of **hexosaminidase A**, causes accumulation in the brain and other tissues of gangliosides. The serum level of hexosaminidase A is normally 2.5-9 U/L.

Acetylcholinesterase is an enzyme that breaks down the neurotransmitter acetylcholine and is therefore important in the regulation of neural function. Persons with a congenital deficiency of acetylcholinesterase are abnormally sensitive to the muscle relaxant succinylcholine, which is used in general anesthesia. Tests performed on the blood actually detect **pseudocholinesterase** (serum cholinesterase), a related substance that is also depressed in congenital acetylcholinesterase deficiency. The level of this enzyme in the serum, normally 8-18 U/L, is lower in persons with congenital deficiency and also in poisoning due to organophosphate insecticides.

Hereditary deficiency of glucose-6-phosphate dehydrogenase (G-6-PD) in red blood cells was mentioned in Chapter 19 as a cause of hemolytic anemia after exposure to certain drugs, chemicals, and foods. Testing for this disorder is performed by determining the concentration of G-6-PD in red blood cells.

Digestive enzymes may appear in the serum when their tissues of origin are diseased. The serum **amylase** level (normally below 125 U/L) rises in acute pancreatitis, obstruction of the pancreatic duct, and perforation or penetration of a peptic ulcer with pancreatic involvement. It is also elevated in mumps, with or without pancreatic involvement, and in alcoholism. The serum **lipase** (normally below 1.5 U/L) also rises in pancreatic disease, including ductal obstruction and malignancy, but usually remains normal in mumps.

Pepsinogen is a precursor of the proteolytic (protein-digesting) enzyme pepsin, which is produced by the gastric mucosa. The normal level of pepsinogen in serum is 124-142 ng/mL [124-142 mcg/L]. The level is abnormally low in patients with achlorhydria (lack of hydrochloric acid in gastric juice), atrophic gastritis, pernicious anemia, and gastric carcinoma. Elevation occurs in peptic ulcer disease and particularly in Zollinger-Ellison syndrome, in which a neoplasm (usually of the pancreas) produces excessive amounts of gastrin, a hormone that stimulates gastric acid production.

Aldolase is a muscle enzyme whose level in the serum (normally 2-5 U/L) is elevated in various disorders of muscle, including muscular dystrophy, dermatomyositis (an autoimmune disorder causing chronic inflammation in muscles and skin), trichinosis (infestation of muscle with *Trichinella*, a parasitic worm), and myocardial infarction.

Renin is an enzyme, produced by the juxtaglomerular apparatus of the kidney, whose levels rise as serum sodium, fluid volume, and renal perfusion decline. Renin catalyzes the conversion of angiotensinogen to angiotensin I, which is then converted by ACE (angiotensin converting enzyme) to angiotensin II. This substance raises blood pressure by constricting blood vessels and conserves sodium by promoting release of aldosterone by the adrenal cortex. Plasma renin levels depend on body position. In the supine (recumbent) subject, the normal level is 0.2-2.3 ng/mL [4.7-54.5 pmol/L]. When the subject has been upright for at least 2 hours, the normal level is 1.6-4.3 ng/mL [38-102 pmol/L]. A specimen may be obtained directly from a renal vein with a catheter threaded through a femoral vein under fluoroscopic monitoring. The renin concentration in blood from a renal vein is normally no more than 1.5 times as much as the concentration in blood from the vena cava.

The renin level is elevated in severe or accelerated (malignant) hypertension, Addison disease, chronic renal failure, cirrhosis, and Bartter syndrome (due to a functioning tumor arising in a kidney). Levels also rise in subjects on restricted sodium diets. Abnormally low renin levels occur in Cushing syndrome and primary aldosteronism. Renin levels also decline on a high-sodium diet, after corticosteroid treatment, and with advancing age.

Angiotensin converting enzyme (ACE), produced chiefly by pulmonary endothelial cells, is elevated in sarcoidosis. The test is not sensitive or specific enough for diagnostic use but is helpful in assessing the severity of disease and the response to treatment. Elevations also occur in sarcoidosis and Gaucher disease.

The concentration of **terminal deoxynucleotidyl transferase** in lymphocytes is increased in acute lymphatic leukemia and in other leukemias and lymphomas.

Hormones

A hormone is a chemical messenger or mediator secreted by an endocrine gland or a group of specialized endocrine cells and released directly into the blood stream. Hormones are therefore normally found in the blood, and their concentrations there correlate closely with the condition of their glands or tissues of origin. Arrived at its target (or end) organ, a hormone exerts some stimulant (occasionally suppressant) action on a specific type of cell or tissue.

The chief importance of diseases of endocrine glands and tissues lies in the effect they can have on circulating hormone levels and hence on the function of the tissues and organs normally maintained, stimulated, or inhibited by them. Degenerative or destructive lesions of a gland may lead to a deficiency of its hormone, while functioning neoplasms of glandular tissue often produce excessive levels of hormone. Disease in one endocrine gland can alter the function of another. For example, a reduction in pituitary thyroid-stimulating hormone (TSH) due to disease of the pituitary gland leads to a decline in the production of thyroxine by the thyroid gland.

Conversely, a decline in thyroxine production for any reason other than this stimulates a rise in the level of TSH.

Hormones are produced by a wide variety of organs and tissues. Besides the five anatomically discrete endocrine (ductless) glands (pituitary, thyroid gland, parathyroids, adrenals, and pineal) zones of specialized tissue in the pancreas, ovary, testicle, liver, lung, kidney, digestive tract, and nervous system also contain secretory cells that send chemical products directly into the blood.

The blood levels of virtually all known hormones can be determined by radioimmunoassay (RIA). In this technique, a serum specimen is incubated with a known quantity of monoclonal antibody to the hormone under study. By using both radioisotopically tagged and untagged hormone, this method makes possible precise and specific measurement of hormone levels in the serum. Such tests supply invaluable information for the diagnosis of most endocrine disorders. Other analytic methods are also in use for many hormones. The levels of most hormones vary with the age and gender of the subject. They may also be affected by pregnancy, certain medicines, and chronic systemic diseases.

Standard tests are available to measure hormones of the anterior pituitary gland (follicle-stimulating hormone, luteinizing hormone, prolactin, thyroid-stimulating hormone, adrenocorticotropic hormone, and somatostatin), the posterior pituitary gland (vasopressin), the thyroid gland (thyroxine or T_4, triiodothyronine or T_3, calcitonin), the parathyroid glands (parathormone), the adrenal glands (cortisol, deoxycortisol, aldosterone), the testis (testosterone), the ovary (estradiol, estriol, progesterone), the placenta (chorionic gonadotropin, human placental lactogen, estriol), the kidney (renin and the product of its action, angiotensin II), the pancreas (insulin, glucagon), and the stomach (gastrin).

The pituitary gland, also called the hypophysis, is situated beneath the brain in a bony receptacle on the floor of the skull called the sella turcica. In the anterior lobe of the pituitary gland, or adenohypophysis, acidophil cells produce growth hormone and prolactin, a hormone involved in lactation, while basophil cells produce hormones that regulate the function of the thyroid gland (thyroid stimulating hormone, TSH), the adrenal cortex (adrenocorticotropic hormone, ACTH), and the gonads (follicle-stimulating hormone, FSH; luteinizing hormone, LH). The smaller posterior lobe or neurohypophysis, an extension of the part of the brain known as the hypothalamus, produces two simple polypeptide hormones: oxytocin, which stimulates the contraction of the uterine muscle during labor; and vasopressin or antidiuretic hormone (ADH), which promotes reabsorption of water in the renal tubules.

Somatotropin (growth hormone) promotes normal body growth and fat mobilization and inhibits the mobilization of carbohydrate. The normal level of somatotropin is 5-10 ng/mL [232-465 pmol/L] in children and half of that or less in adults. Deficiency of somatotropin, which can occur in inherited forms of dwarfism, results in failure to attain adult stature. Functioning pituitary tumors derived from acidophil cells produce abnormally high levels of somatotropin. When this occurs in childhood it causes gigantism (excessive length of long bones). After closure of growth centers in bone, excessive somatotropin causes acromegaly (enlargement and deformity of hands, feet, and skull and facial bones). Besides affecting bone growth, excess somatotropin causes macroglossia (enlargement of the tongue), cardiomegaly (enlargement of the heart), splanchnomegaly (enlargement of abdominal viscera), and diabetes mellitus.

Prolactin stimulates the secretion of milk in pregnancy. Normal prolactin levels are 2.5-19 ng/mL [1.1-8.6 nmol/L] in non-pregnant women. Levels are slightly lower in men, in whom the function of prolactin is unknown. Production by the anterior lobe of the pituitary gland is normally increased during pregnancy and nursing, when the level may reach 500 ng/mL [220 nmol/L]. Elevation of prolactin (hyperprolactinemia) outside of pregnancy can be due to severe stress, strenuous exercise, marked weight loss, chronic renal or hepatic disease, hypothyroidism, or (rarely) to a functioning pituitary tumor. In women, hyperprolactinemia causes amenorrhea (cessation of menses) due to suppression of ovulation and sometimes galactorrhea (flow of milk from breasts). In men it can cause infertility and erectile dysfunction. Depression of prolactin level can result from tumor, injury, infection, or degenerative disease of the pituitary. When prolactin deficiency occurs as an isolated pituitary malfunction, its only symptom is failure of milk production in pregnancy.

Thyrotropin, also called thyroid-stimulating hormone (TSH), promotes the growth and regulates the function of the thyroid gland. The normal level of TSH in serum is 0.4-4.2 mcU/mL [0.4-4.2 mU/L]. Because this level is part of a feedback loop, it is depressed by elevation of thyroxine (thyroid hormone) and elevated when circulating levels of thyroid hormone are deficient. Hence testing the TSH level is a sensitive indicator of thyroid disease. The level of TSH can also be depressed by disease or injury of the pituitary gland.

Adrenocorticotropic hormone (ACTH) controls the nutrition, growth, and function of the adrenal cortices. The normal level of ACTH is 10-50 pg/mL [2.2-11.1 pmol/L]. An excess of adrenocorticotropic hormone due to a functioning tumor derived from basophil cells (basophilic adenoma) induces a condition called Cushing disease, which is due to overactivity of the adrenal cortices. Cushing disease is discussed below among disorders of the adrenal glands. Deficiency of ACTH causes secondary adrenal failure (Addison disease), also discussed below.

Two anterior pituitary hormones—follicle-stimulating hormone (FSH), also called follitropin, and luteinizing hormone (LH), also called *lutropin*—are known as gonadotropins because they control the nutritional status and function of the gonads (ovaries and testicles). In women these hormones play a crucial role in regulating the menstrual cycle and the hormonal events associated with pregnancy. The amounts of both hormones that are released by the anterior lobe of the pituitary are controlled by a hypothalamic substance called gonadoliberin or gonadotropin-releasing hormone (GnRH).

In women, **follicle-stimulating hormone** (FSH) stimulates the ovary to produce estrogen, which is responsible for the development of secondary sexual characteristics at puberty (pubic and axillary hair, nipple and breast development, broadening of hips, feminine distribution of body fat). FSH also controls the monthly development or maturation of an ovarian (graafian) follicle, one of hundreds of immature microscopic units, each of which contains an oocyte or female sex cell. In men, FSH stimulates formation of spermatozoa (male sex cells). Normal levels of FSH are 1.1-24 ng/mL [5.0-108 U/L] in the adult female and 0.5-4.5 ng/mL [2.2-20.0 U/L] in the adult male.

Luteinizing hormone (LH) or lutropin also affects the development and function of reproductive organs in both sexes. In women it promotes maturation of the developing oocyte. A surge of LH induces ovulation (release of the oocyte from the ovary) and stimulates promotes the development of a corpus luteum from the follicle that released the oocyte. The corpus luteum produces the hormone progesterone, which prepares the lining of the uterus for implantation of a fertilized ovum. In men, LH stimulates production of testosterone by the interstitial cells of the testes (Leydig cells), with resulting development of secondary sexual characteristics (pubic and axillary hair, beard growth, deepening of voice). Normal levels of LH are LH are 0.5-2.7 mcg/mL [4.5-24.3 U/L] in women and 0.4-1.9 mcg/mL [3.6-17.1 U/L] in men.

These levels are elevated in primary gonadal failure (disease arising in ovaries or testes and making them unresponsive to gonadotropin stimulation) and reduced by estrogen or testosterone treatment. Gonadotropin (FSH or LH) deficiency in either sex can cause failure or regression of secondary sexual characteristics and infertility or sterility. Deficiency of FSH and LH can result from failure of the pituitary gland to produce these hormones, as in Prader-Willi syndrome (also featuring obesity and mental retardation) or from deficiency of gonadotropin releasing hormone, as in Kallmann syndrome (also featuring red-green colorblindness, deafness, cleft palate, and other abnormalities).

Panhypopituitarism (Simmonds disease) denotes a deficiency of all hormones produced by the anterior lobe of the pituitary gland. Withdrawal of normal stimulation to the thyroid gland, the adrenal cortices, and the gonads results in a general decline in the function of these glands, with ensuing cachexia, reduction of body hair and skin pigment, and impairment of response to stress and resistance to infection. Total pituitary failure occurring in infancy or childhood also results in dwarfism. Panhypopituitarism may be caused by infarction of the pituitary, destruction by a neoplasm, or surgical removal. Panhypopituitarism coming on in the postpartum period as a sequel to obstetrical shock is called Sheehan syndrome.

Vasopressin (antidiuretic hormone, ADH), produced by the posterior pituitary gland, promotes reabsorption in the renal tubules of water filtered by the glomeruli. The normal serum level of this hormone is 2-12 pg/mL [1.85-11.1 pmol.L]. Deficiency of ADH, which can be caused by trauma, tumor, or degenerative disease of the posterior lobe of the pituitary or its neural connections with the hypothalamus, leads to diabetes insipidus, a condition of excessive diuresis with severe water loss.

The thyroid gland is a flattened, shield-shaped structure incompletely divided into right and left lobes and situated in the front of the neck just above the sternum. The principal secretory cells of the thyroid produce thyroxine, which has complex effects on the regulation of tissue metabolism. The C cells of the thyroid gland produce calcitonin, which affects calcium balance by acting as an antagonist to parathyroid hormone (discussed in the next section).

The primary function of **thyroxine** (also called tetraiodothyronine or T_4) is to regulate the rate of cellular metabolism, but it also has other important actions. After being absorbed into tissues from the blood stream, thyroxine breaks down to triiodothyronine (T_3), which is its metabolically active form. Some T_3 also appears in the serum. The normal serum level of T_4 is 4.5-12.0 mcg/dL [58-154 nmol/L], and that of T_3 70-190 ng/dL [1.1-2.9 nmol/L].

These levels are increased in hyperthyroidism of any cause (including Graves disease, a relatively common disorder of young and middle-aged women due to circulating autoantibodies that simulate the effects of TSH on the thyroid gland) and often in acute thyroiditis (inflammation of the thyroid gland causing increased leakage of hormone into the circulation). They are decreased in hypothyroidism of any cause (including deficiency of dietary iodine) and may also be low in malnutrition and other chronic disease states.

The symptoms of hyperthyroidism (thyrotoxicosis) are tachycardia, flushing, sweating, weight loss, and emotional instability. Deficiency of thyroxine (hypothyroidism) beginning before or shortly after birth causes cretinism, a syndrome of physical and mental retardation associated with coarseness of the skin, macroglossia, and skeletal malformations. When thyroid deficiency begins later in life, the result is myxedema. In this condition the pulse and blood pressure are low, the skin coarse and dry, the hair thinned, the face and hands puffy, speech hoarse, slow, and slurred, mental functioning retarded, gonadal function impaired, and serum cholesterol elevated. In adulthood the commonest causes of myxedema are surgical removal of the thyroid gland and drug treatment of an overactive thyroid gland.

Most of the thyroxine in the circulation is combined chemically with a plasma protein called thyroxine binding globulin (TBG). Only the small amount of free (unbound) thyroxine in the blood is responsible for the metabolic effects of the hormone. Radioimmunoassays of T_4 and T_3 measure only bound fractions of the hormones. Hence they may underestimate or overestimate the levels of active hormone in conditions that alter thyroid binding (such as pregnancy, liver or kidney disease, and chronic systemic disease) and in persons taking certain medicines, including oral contraceptives and corticosteroids.

Other tests may therefore be used to obtain a more accurate estimate of the amount of available thyroid hormone. The **T_3 uptake test** indirectly measures the amount of TBG in the circulation that is unsaturated (not attached to T_4). A specimen of the patient's serum is incubated with radioactively labeled T_3, which is taken up by binding sites on TBG that are unoccupied by T_4. Unbound T_3 is then removed by a resin and measured. The normal range of T_3 uptake is 25-38% [0.25-0.38]. Higher values occur in hyperthyroidism, metastatic malignancy, and severe hepatic disease. Lower values are seen in hypothyroidism and pregnancy.

The **free T_4 index**, calculated from the T_4 level and the T_3 uptake ratio (and hence sometimes also called the T_7), adjusts the measured level of thyroxine in proportion to the amount of unsaturated TBG present. The rationale for this procedure lies in the fact that conditions that falsely elevate the serum level of T_4 by increasing TBG also lower the T_3 uptake, and vice versa, while conditions that falsely lower the T_4 by lowering TBG also elevate the T_3 uptake. Free (unbound) T_4 can also be measured directly, but that test is more expensive. The normal level is 0.9-2.1 ng/dL [12-27 pmol/L].

In practice, measurement of thyroid-stimulating hormone (TSH), discussed above among hormones produced by the pituitary gland, is widely used as a screening procedure to detect thyroid disease. The level of TSH is elevated in primary hypothyroidism and reduced in primary hyperthyroidism. Acute and chronic disorders not affecting the thyroid gland have little effect on TSH level.

Attached to the thyroid capsule but structurally distinct from the thyroid gland are the four parathyroid glands. The secretion of the parathyroid gland, parathyroid hormone (PTH) or parathormone, regulates calcium and phosphorus metabolism by increasing the reabsorption of calcium in the renal tubules, decreasing the reabsorption of phosphorus, and mobilizing calcium from bone.

The normal level of **parathyroid hormone** is 11-54 pg/mL [1.2-56 pmol/L]. The most common cause of deficiency of parathyroid hormone is inadvertent surgical removal of the glands in the course of thyroidectomy. Rarely, all parathyroid glands may be destroyed by degenerative disease. When parathyroid hormone is deficient, serum calcium falls, with resultant heightening of neuromuscular excitability. This can lead to tetany, twitching, and seizures. An increase of parathyroid hormone may stem from benign or malignant tumors of the parathyroid glands or from diffuse hyperplasia of the glands, either as a primary disorder or in response to chronic hypocalcemia of any cause, including renal failure, rickets, and multiple myeloma. The rise in serum calcium occurs at the expense of bones, which undergo fibrosis, cyst formation, and deformity, a condition called osteitis fibrosa cystica.

Calcitonin, a hormone produced by various organs including the thyroid and parathyroid glands and the lungs, functions as a check on the action of parathyroid hormone by suppressing the mobilization of calcium from bone when the serum level of calcium rises. It also promotes reabsorption of calcium and phosphorus from renal tubules. The normal level of calcitonin in the adult male is 0-15 pg/mL [0-4.20 pmol/L]. Levels are somewhat lower in women.

The adrenal glands are paired, one being situated atop each kidney. As in the pituitary, each adrenal gland consists of two distinct tissue types that have fused into an anatomically unified structure. The cortex contains cells that produce glucocorticoids for the regulation of carbohydrate and protein metabolism, mineralocorticoids for the control of electrolyte (sodium and potassium) balance, and androgen, which affects protein metabolism.

Adrenal **glucocorticoids** have a broad range of metabolic regulatory functions, including increased breakdown of protein, increased conversion of protein to glucose in the liver, and a complex series of biochemical responses that constitute a stereotyped response to physical stress. The principal glucocorticoid is cortisol. The serum cortisol level is subject to diurnal variation, being highest in the morning and lowest at night. At 8:00 a.m. the normal range is 5-23 mcg/dL [138-635 nmol/L]. By 4:00 p.m. the level has fallen to 3-16 mcg/dL [83-441 nmol/L]. At 10:00 p.m. the level is normally less than 50% [<0.5] of the 8:00 a.m. level.

Mineralocorticoids, as discussed earlier in this chapter, reduce the renal excretion of sodium and increase the excretion of potassium. The level of aldosterone, the principal adrenal mineralocorticoid, varies with body position. The normal serum level in the supine (recumbent) subject is 3-16 ng/dL [0.08-0.44 nmol/L], while a specimen obtained after the subject has been standing for several minutes shows a level of 7-30 ng/dL [0.19-0.83 nmol/L].

Adrenal androgens are adrenal cortical hormones with masculinizing effects similar to testosterone. However, normal levels of adrenal androgens are roughly equal in men and women, and androgenic effects are observed only when the levels of these hormones are abnormally increased. Adrenal androgen secretion is promoted by ACTH but not by pituitary gonadotropins (FSH and LH). These hormones function primarily to maintain normal protein synthesis and muscle development.

Chronic deficiency of adrenal cortical hormones, resulting from atrophy, tuberculosis, amyloidosis, or metastatic malignancy of both adrenal glands, is called Addison disease. The principal features of this syndrome are weakness, weight loss, increased pigmentation of the skin (especially over the knees, elbows, and knuckles), elevation of serum potassium and nitrogen, and depression of serum sodium and glucose. The heart size decreases and there is a tendency to acute vascular collapse (addisonian crisis). Waterhouse-Friderichsen syndrome is a more acute adrenal cortical deficiency, often fatal, occurring usually in children with meningococcal septicemia (occasionally other infections) and resulting from bilateral massive hemorrhage of the adrenal glands. In adrenocortical hypofunction due to deficiency of pituitary ACTH, the pigmentation seen in Addison disease does not occur.

Cushing syndrome is a constellation of symptoms and signs resulting from excessive levels of adrenal cortical hormones in the circulation. The commonest cause is treatment with adrenocortical steroids. The condition may also result from bilateral adrenocortical hyperplasia or from overstimulation of the adrenals by a basophil adenoma of the pituitary gland (in which case it is called Cushing disease). The principal features of Cushing syndrome are obesity, focal edema (moon face, buffalo hump), atrophy and fatty degeneration of muscle, osteoporosis, hypertension, diabetes mellitus, facial hirsutism, and acne. Administration of dexamethasone, a synthetic analogue of cortisol, normally suppresses ACTH secretion by the pituitary and thus leads to a drop in serum cortisol. In the dexamethasone suppression test, serum levels of cortisol are determined before and one day after a dose of dexamethasone. Failure of cortisol levels to drop is noted in Cushing syndrome and in clinical depression.

Conn syndrome (primary aldosteronism), manifested by retention of sodium and excessive loss of potassium by the kidney, is due to adenoma (occasionally, adenocarcinoma) of the adrenal cortex producing excessive amounts of aldosterone. The symptoms include hypertension, alkalosis, and muscular weakness or paralysis. Secondary aldosteronism, with similar symptoms, occurs in response to certain metabolic imbalances of hydration such as those of nephrotic syndrome, hepatic cirrhosis, and congestive cardiac failure.

Congenital adrenal hyperplasia (adrenogenital syndrome) results from a hereditary inability of the cells of the adrenal cortex to produce cortisol. Pituitary ACTH levels accordingly rise and the overstimulated adrenal glands form excessive amounts of androgen. In female children this androgen produces virilization of the genitalia (clitoral hypertrophy and labial fusion) and often polycystic ovaries. Virilization can result at any age from functioning benign or malignant tumors of the adrenal cortex.

The adrenal medulla produces a group of hormones characterized chemically as catecholamines—epinephrine (adrenalin), norepinephrine (noradrenalin), and dopamine—which serve as chemical mediators in acute stress ("flight or fight") responses. The net effect of these hormones is to dilate the pupils, increase the rate and force of cardiac contractions, dilate the bronchi, increase the circulation to skeletal muscle, and shunt blood away from the digestive organs. Basal serum levels of these hormones are low, and when they are released to meet a crisis they are quickly metabolized and disappear from the circulation.

Pheochromocytoma (chromaffinoma) is a tumor of the adrenal medulla that produces excessive amounts of norepinephrine, causing palpitations, tremors, and paroxysmal or sustained hypertension. Diagnosis is usually con-

firmed by the finding of an elevated level of catecholamine breakdown products in a 24-hour urine specimen, as discussed in Chapter 24.

The pineal gland is a cone-shaped body less than 1 cm in greatest dimension, which is attached by a stalk to the roof of the third ventricle of the brain. The pineal gland undergoes regression after age 7. Its principal secretion, the hormone **melatonin** (N -acetyl-5-methoxytryptamine), plays a role in sexual maturation and in maintenance of diurnal bodily rhythms. Melatonin production is linked to both sleep-wakefulness and light-dark cycles. Serum levels rise just before sleep and reach a peak around midnight. Twenty-four-hour secretion is higher in winter than in summer and declines with age. The normal melatonin level at 8:00 a.m. is 0.8-7.7 pg/mL [3.5-33 pmol/L]. At midnight the normal range is 3.7-23.3 pg.mL [16-100 pmol/L].

The pancreas is a flat, tongue-shaped, fleshy organ lying against the posterior abdominal wall in the left upper quadrant, between the duodenum and the spleen. As a digestive gland, the pancreas produces a secretion that contains enzymes for the breakdown of carbohydrates, fats, and proteins. This secretion flows into the duodenum by the duct of Wirsung. In addition, the pancreas contains spherical masses of specialized endocrine cells, the islets of Langerhans, that produce the hormones insulin, glucagon, and somatostatin.

Insulin, produced by pancreatic beta cells, regulates carbohydrate metabolism by mediating the rapid transport of glucose and amino acids from the circulation into muscle and other tissue cells, by promoting the storage of glucose in liver cells as glycogen, and by inhibiting the conversion of protein to glucose. The normal stimulus for the release of insulin from the pancreas is an elevation in blood glucose following a meal. The fasting level of insulin is 5-25 mcU/mL [34-172 pmol/L].

Diabetes mellitus is a chronic metabolic disorder caused by a reduction in the availability or efficacy of insulin. This disorder is characterized by elevation of blood glucose (hyperglycemia) and appearance of glucose in the urine (glycosuria). About 95% of persons with diabetes have type 2, in which pancreatic production of insulin may be normal or only slightly reduced but peripheral tissues resist its effects on glucose transport. In the less common type 1 diabetes mellitus, insulin production is diminished or absent, so that treatment with exogenous insulin is required for long-term survival. Untreated type 1 diabetes can lead to severe water and electrolyte loss, ketoacidosis (accumulation of waste products of abnormal metabolism), coma, and death. Long-term complications of both type 1 and type 2 diabetes mellitus include degenerative changes of small blood vessels, particularly those of the retina and the kidney, as well as heightened risk of atherosclerosis of larger arteries leading to stroke, heart attack, and peripheral circulatory impairment. Diabetes mellitus affects at least 16 million Americans and ranks seventh as a cause of death. The diagnosis and monitoring of diabetes mellitus are based on determinations of plasma glucose level, as discussed below.

Glucagon, produced by alpha cells in the pancreatic islets of Langerhans, promotes glucose production from protein by the liver and storage of glucose as glycogen, thus in effect reversing the effects of insulin. The normal stimulus for glucagon release is a drop in blood sugar. The normal fasting glucagon level is 50-200 pg/mL [14-57 pmol/L]. Elevation occurs in glucagonoma (a functioning tumor originating from pancreatic alpha cells), diabetes mellitus, and acute pancreatitis. The level of glucagon may be low in chronic pancreatitis or in congenital disorders characterized by failure of glucagon secretion.

Somatostatin is produced by the pancreas as well as by other tissues, particularly in the digestive and central nervous systems. Its principal known functions are the inhibition of other hormones, particularly somatotropin (pituitary growth hormone), the pancreatic hormones insulin and glucagon, and the digestive tract hormones gastrin, cholecystokinin, secretin and vasoactive intestinal peptide (VIP).

Gastrin is a digestive hormone produced in the mucosa of the stomach as well as in the pancreas and other sites. Gastrin promotes secretion of hydrochloric acid and the digestive enzyme pepsin by the stomach and other proteolytic enzymes by the pancreas, stimulates bile flow, and increases gastrointestinal motility. The normal level of gastrin is 21-125 pg/mL [10-59.3 pmol/L]. Abnormally high levels occur in Zollinger-Ellison syndrome (due to a pancreatic tumor producing excessive gastrin) and in some patients with peptic ulcer disease. In patients with Zollinger-Ellison syndrome, gastrin levels rise markedly after intravenous injection of calcium gluconate or the hormone secretin. In patients with peptic ulcer, gastrin levels rise markedly after a meal rich in protein.

Sex hormones are produced, under the influence of pituitary FSH and LH, by specific endocrine tissue found alongside the sex-cell-forming tissues in the gonads (ovaries in women, testicles in men). These hormones are responsible for the development and maintenance of the reproductive organs in both sexes as well as for the appearance of secondary sexual characteristics (pubic and axillary hair, breast development in women, deep voice and facial hair in men) at puberty.

In women the serum level of **estrogens**, particularly estradiol and estrone, increases gradually during the menstrual cycle, being lowest at the end of menses (24-68 pg/mL [90-250 pmol/L] and highest just before the beginning of the next menstrual period (73-149 pg/mL [270-550 pmol/L]. The levels are low in ovarian failure of any cause, including congenital disorders and pituitary disease, and after menopause. Estrogen levels are elevated in functional ovarian tumors, in severe hepatic disease, and in women taking hormones for birth control or for estrogen replacement after menopause.

After ovulation, the follicle from which the mature oocyte has been released evolves into a corpus luteum, which produces the hormone **progesterone**. This substance promotes development of the endometrium (the lining of the uterus) to prepare it for implantation of a fertilized ovum. Progesterone levels are therefore higher after ovulation (2-28 ng/mL [6.4-89 nmol/L] than before ovulation (0.1-0.5 ng/mL) [0.3-1.6 nmol/L]. If conception occurs, the placenta also produces progesterone to maintain endometrial development, the level eventually reaching 50-250 ng/mL [159-795 nmol/L]. Elevation of progesterone level can also be due to functioning ovarian tumors or consumption of birth control pills. Abnormally low levels can be due to primary or secondary ovarian failure, toxemia of pregnancy, or fetal death. Very low levels are found in males and after menopause.

Besides progesterone, the normal placenta produces other hormones that function in the maintenance of pregnancy. **Human chorionic gonadotropin** (hCG) appears in the serum by the ninth day of pregnancy. This hormone supplements the effects of pituitary LH in promoting development of the corpus luteum until placental production of progesterone is sufficient to maintain endometrial proliferation. Tests for the beta subunit of human chorionic gonadotropin (ßhCG) in urine are the basis of most rapid pregnancy tests, including self-administered or "home" tests. Quantitative assays of hCG in serum or urine may be useful in diagnosing certain disorders of pregnancy. Levels are abnormally high in functioning tumors of placental tissue (hydatidiform mole, choriocarcinoma) and are low in fetal death and ectopic pregnancy.

Estriol is an estrogenic hormone produced by the placenta in mid- to late pregnancy. Serial testing of the serum level of this hormone may be used to monitor placental health in toxemia of pregnancy, maternal diabetes mellitus, and other conditions that threaten fetal viability. Serial assays of **human placental lactogen** (hPL), another hormone of placental origin, can also be used to monitor placental well-being.

Testosterone, the principal androgenic hormone of the testicle, is produced by Leydig cells in response to pituitary LH. Testosterone supports spermatogenesis (formation of spermatozoa, male sex cells), is responsible for the development and maintenance of male secondary sexual characteristics, and also promotes growth and protein synthesis. The normal level in the adult male is 300-1200 ng/dL [10.5-42 nmol/L]. The level is low in primary or secondary gonadal failure and after orchidectomy. It is elevated in certain functioning tumors arising in a testicle or adrenal gland.

Erythropoietin (EPO), a hormone produced by the kidney, stimulates the growth and differentiation of primitive cells in bone marrow that are destined to become red blood cells. The synthesis and release of EPO occur in response to hypoxia (a drop in oxygen tension) of the blood passing through the kidney. The normal range is 5-30 mU/mL [5-30 U/L]. The level is reduced in chronic renal disease, with resulting so-called renal anemia, and may be much increased in anemia of any other cause.

Proteins, Peptides, and Amino Acids

Proteins are polypeptides—that is, large molecules consisting of straight or branching chains of amino acids. Proteins serve as essential components of cells, connective tissue fibers, and muscle. Many are enzymes, hormones, or other biologically active substances. Because the molecular structures of many large proteins is unknown, their serum concentrations cannot be given in molar equivalents, but are expressed as mass (grams or a submultiple of grams) per liter.

The plasma proteins vary greatly in structure and molecular weight. The principal plasma proteins are albumin, globulin, and fibrinogen. **Albumin**, which is produced in the liver, has a molecular weight around 69 000 and functions principally in water balance by maintaining the osmotic pressure of the blood. It also acts as a plasma buffer. The normal level of albumin in the serum is 3.5–5.0 g/dL [35–50 g/L]. The level is reduced in liver disease, malnutrition, and chronic infections.

Globulins are a complex mixture of related proteins varying in molecular weight from 150 000 to 1 300 000. On the basis of their stratification in the ultracentrifuge, globulins have been classified as alpha, beta, and gamma globulins. The globulins include the metal-binding proteins transferrin and ceruloplasmin and the lipoproteins, all formed in the liver, which are discussed earlier in this chapter.

The gamma globulins or immunoglobulins (Ig), produced by lymphocytes and plasma cells, include all known circulating antibodies. They are divided on the basis of ultracentrifugation and electrophoresis patterns into five classes: IgG (more than 75% of the total globulin fraction), IgA (15%), IgM (10%), IgD (less than 1%), and IgE (less than 0.1%). Study of the electrophoretic pattern of the first three of these can supply clues to a variety of disorders characterized by disturbances in gamma globulin levels (gammopathies), including chronic infection, collagen disease, lymphoma, leukemia, multiple myeloma, immunodeficiency disorders, sarcoidosis, and cystic fibrosis.

The **total globulin** fraction of serum is normally between 1.5 and 3.0 g/dL [15-30 g/L]. The quotient obtained by dividing albumin level by globulin level is known as the A/G ratio. Normally this ratio is between 1.5 and 3.0. In a number of disorders (collagen diseases, nephrotic syndrome, Hodgkin disease, multiple myeloma, chronic infection, metastatic malignancy), a reduction of serum albumin combined with elevation of one or more globulins causes the A/G ratio to be less than 1.0, a condition loosely referred to as "reversal" or "inversion" of the ratio.

Fibrinogen, prothrombin, and other serum proteins concerned in blood coagulation are discussed in Chapter 19.

Many inherited disorders of growth and metabolism are due to the lack of genes that encode specific proteins. Determining the level of these proteins is often the most direct means of diagnosing congenital deficiency. **Alpha₁ antitrypsin** (AAT), a protein produced in the liver, normally inhibits the action of trypsin, neutrophil elastase, and other tissue enzymes. Persons with congenital deficiency of alpha₁ antitrypsin are at risk of developing emphysema early in life. The normal level of AAT is 100-300 mg/mL [20-60 mmol/L].

Ceruloplasmin is a serum globulin that is involved in the storage and transport of copper and also participates in the regulation of iron metabolism. The normal serum level of ceruloplasmin is 23-44 mg/dL [230-440 mg/L]. The levels are low in Wilson disease (also called hepatolenticular degeneration, an inherited metabolic defect in which deposition of copper in the liver, brain, and eyes cause severe, progressive degenerative changes), Menkes syndrome (in which hair is kinky and brittle and cerebral degeneration leads to early death), and sometimes in chronic renal disease.

Two proteins, ferritin and transferrin, are involved in the storage and transport of iron. Measurement of their levels, particularly that of ferritin, can provide valuable information about the nature and prognosis of anemias and other disorders involving iron. Iron is stored in the liver and other tissues in chemical combination with ferritin. The normal serum level of **ferritin** is 20-200 ng/mL [20-200 mcg/L]. Somewhat higher levels occur in men, somewhat lower levels in children. The serum level of ferritin closely parallels total iron stores. Low levels indicate depletion of body iron due to chronic deficiency. Ferritin is elevated in hemolytic anemias, hepatic disease, hemochromatosis (inherited or acquired disorder in which excess iron is absorbed and stored in tissues, particularly the liver and pancreas), and in some leukemias and lymphomas.

Iron is transported in the blood stream by a second protein, **transferrin** (siderophilin). The normal serum level of transferrin is 250-430 mg/dL [2.5-4.3 g/L]. Depression of this level occurs in chronic liver or kidney disease, protein deficiency, or malignancy. Elevation of transferrin is noted in iron deficiency anemia.

An amino acid is any organic acid containing an amino ($-NH^2$) group. Amino acids are arranged in peptide chains to form proteins. Twenty amino acids are recognized as components of proteins in human metabolism, 9 of them essential (that is, not synthesized by the human body and hence essential nutrients). Normally the serum level of the amino acid **phenylalanine** is 2-4 mg/dL [121-242 mcmol/L]. More than a tenfold rise may be seen in patients with phenylketonuria (PKU), a hereditary disorder of phenylalanine metabolism that causes mental retardation if not detected and treated early. Testing for this disorder by measuring serum phenylalanine within the first few days of life is a routine procedure in well-baby care, and is required by law in most jurisdictions. A drop of blood, obtained from the infant by heelstick, is soaked into each of three circles on a form printed on filter (highly absorptive) paper. The form is then mailed to the health department for testing.

Numerous other genetic disorders are characterized either by deficiency or by impaired excretion and abnormal accumulation of amino acids. Determination of the blood levels of the various amino acids may be performed as a screening test in an infant suspected of having a congenital disturbance of amino acid metabolism. Urine screening may indicate excess of certain amino acids that do not normally appear in the urine.

Measurement of the serum level of some vitamins is useful in the diagnosis of certain deficiency states. Quantitative tests are available in most laboratories for vitamins A, B_1, B_{12}, C, and D, carotene, folic acid, and others.

Extensive hemolysis of red blood cells within the circulation releases hemoglobin into the serum. Measurement of the **hemoglobin** level in the serum, of which it is not a normal component, therefore gives information about recent or current hemolysis, as in hemolytic anemia or transfusion reaction. Further information can be obtained by measurement of the level of **haptoglobin** in the serum. As mentioned in Chapter 19, haptoglobin is an alpha$_2$-globulin, normally present in circulating blood, that binds any free hemoglobin released by hemolysis. The concentration of haptoglobin is thus an indirect measure of hemolysis. The normal hemoglobin-binding capacity of the serum haptoglobins is 40 to 180 mg/dL [0.4-1.8 g/L]. This level is increased in the presence of acute or chronic inflammation and reduced in hemolysis and liver disease—in the latter case, because of reduced synthesis of haptoglobin.

Myoglobin is an iron-containing protein, similar to hemoglobin, that is found in skeletal and cardiac muscle, where its functions include the storage, transport, and release of oxygen. The normal level of myoglobin in serum is 14-51 mcg/L [0.8-2.9 nmol/L]. This level is increased after extensive injury to skeletal muscle and in myocardial infarction, generalized disorders of muscle such as polymyositis and dermatomyositis, shock, and renal failure.

Troponins C, I, and T are proteins that play a role in muscle contraction. Myocardial infarction causes release of these proteins into the circulation, where they can often be detected earlier than enzymes used in the diagnosis of myocardial infarction, such as AST and CK. The level of **troponin I** (TnI), which occurs only in cardiac muscle, is normally less than 1.5 ng/mL [1.5 mcg/L]. Rises in the level of troponin T (TnT), although not specific to cardiac muscle, may be more sensitive indicators of myocardial necrosis. The normal level of troponin T is less than 0.029 ng/mL [0.029 mcg/L].

Homocysteine, a homologue of the essential amino acid cysteine, is normally found in the serum at a level less than 1.6 mg/L [12 mcmol/L]. The level is higher in men and tends to rise with advancing age and particularly after menopause. Elevation of homocysteine above 2.0 mg/L [15 mcmol/L] is associated with premature development of atherosclerosis and heightened risk of myocardial infarction, stroke, and thromboembolic disease. During pregnancy, elevation of maternal homocysteine increases the risk of fetal neural tube defects including spina bifida and anencephaly. Elevation of homocysteine occurs in various inherited enzyme deficiencies; in dietary deficiency of folic acid, vitamin B_6 (pyridoxine), or vitamin B_{12}; and in chronic renal failure, hypothyroidism, and some malignancies.

Natriuretic peptides are a class of biologically active substances that participate in the regulation of blood volume, blood pressure, and electrolyte balance by opposing the release or action of aldosterone and renin and thus favoring the renal excretion of sodium (natriuresis) and the retention of potassium. **Atrial natriuretic peptide** (ANP) is produced and stored in the atrial myocardium. Increased synthesis occurs in response to distention of the atria, increased levels of angiotensin II, and activation of adrenergic (sympathetic) receptors. Serum levels are elevated in congestive heart failure and other conditions associated with increased blood volume (hypervolemia). **Brain natriuretic peptide** (BNP) is produced and stored principally in ventricular myocardium and to a lesser extent in the brain. The normal level of BNP is less than 50 pg/mL [50 ng/L]. The level is increased in ventricular dilatation and congestive heart failure, and serum levels correlate with the degree of failure. BNP levels are also increased in coronary artery disease (unstable angina, acute myocardial infarction). The principal clinical use of BNP testing is to rule out congestive failure in patients with dyspnea of unknown origin.

Complement is a generic term for a family of more than 20 proteins that are involved in immune function. Measurement of complement levels can be performed by various methods and units and reference ranges vary with the method. Complement levels are reduced in various congenital and acquired disorders of immunity, in systemic lupus erythematosus, chronic liver disease, and some malignancies. Elevation of complement can occur in a broad variety of disorders, including myocardial infarction, ulcerative colitis, diabetes mellitus, and rheumatoid arthritis.

Certain plasma proteins, including fibrinogen and ceruloplasmin, are called acute phase reactants because their levels rise within a few hours in the presence of acute inflammation. Because some acute phase reactants are not normally present, their detection provides objective evidence of organic disease. But although they are sensitive indicators of inflammation, they are also highly nonspecific. Their production can be triggered by a wide range of abnormal conditions, including systemic or localized infection, myocardial infarction, autoimmune disorders such as lupus erythematosus and rheumatoid arthritis, and extensive or metastatic malignancy. Testing for one such substance, called C-reactive protein (CRP), is widely used to identify patients with significant organic illness. Serial determinations of CRP can be used to monitor the progress of a disease or the effects of treatment.

Lipids and Lipoproteins

A lipid is a fat or fatlike organic compound, composed largely of straight-chain fatty acids, that is soluble in volatile solvents but not in water. Lipids are an important constituent of all tissues, particularly cell membranes and nerve tissue, and fatty acids are essential nutrients.

Cholesterol is a complex organic compound synthesized in the liver and other tissues, widely distributed throughout the body, especially in nerve tissue, and serving as a building block for steroid hormones (cortisol, aldosterone, testosterone, progesterone). Dietary cholesterol from animal fats (including butter fat and egg yolk) is absorbed from the intestine and transported in the serum in combination with lipoproteins. Persons whose diet is high in cholesterol or who have genetic disorders of lipoproteins may show marked elevation of serum cholesterol. Such persons are at increased risk of atherosclerosis, an inflammatory and degenerative disorder of arteries in which plaques of lipid material reduce caliber and obstruct blood flow.

The normal fasting serum level of cholesterol is below 200 mg/dL [520 mmol/L]. Higher levels (hypercholesterolemia) occur in biliary obstruction, nephrotic syndrome, hypothyroidism, and pancreatic disease as well as in dietary and familial disorders of cholesterol metabolism. In addition, the cholesterol level tends to rise with age. Very low levels (below 50 mg/dL [130 mmol/L]) suggest severe malnutrition or hepatic disease.

A lipoprotein is any of several protein-lipid complexes in which lipids are transported in the blood. Lipoproteins are classified on the basis of their behavior under ultracentrifugation as high density lipoproteins (HDL), low density lipoproteins (LDL), and very low density lipoproteins (VLDL). Lipoprotein assay provides additional diagnostic information in cases of hypercholesterolemia. The normal level of HDL cholesterol is 35-80 mg/dL [1-2 mmol/L], and the normal level of LDL cholesterol is 40-130 mg/dL [1-3 mmol/L]. A relative preponderance of HDL, which carry cholesterol away from tissues, is associated with lower risk of atherosclerosis, while a preponderance of LDL, which deposit cholesterol in tissues, implies increased risk of atherosclerosis.

The term **triglyceride** is a chemical designation for animal fats—compounds of glycerol with fatty acid radicals. The normal fasting triglyceride level is below 160 mg/dL [1.80 mmol/L]. Significant elevation of serum triglycerides (hypertriglyceridemia), which is a risk factor for atherosclerosis and pancreatitis, occurs in hyperlipidemias, liver disease, nephrotic syndrome, hypothyroidism, and diabetes mellitus. Very low levels (below 10 mg/dL [0.12 mmol/L]) suggest severe malnutrition.

Free (nonesterified) fatty acids (FFA) are transported in serum in combination with albumin. The level of free fatty acids, normally 8-20 mg/dL [0.2-0.7 mmol/L], rises in diabetes mellitus, hyperthyroidism, some hepatic and renal diseases, chronic nutritional deficiency, and pheochromocytoma.

Blood Sugar

Glucose is a simple sugar (monosaccharide) that is derived from digestion of dietary carbohydrate (starches and more complex sugars), stored in the liver and muscle tissue as glycogen, and used by body cells as their principal source of energy. The uptake of glucose by cells depends on the hormone insulin. Glucose filtered by the glomeruli from the plasma is normally reabsorbed completely by the renal tubules.

Plasma glucose is usually measured in the fasting state to eliminate the variations caused by absorption of dietary carbohydrate. The fasting plasma glucose (fasting blood sugar) is normally between 60-115 mg/dL [3.3-6.4 mmol/L]. Abnormally low serum glucose (hypoglycemia) is seen in starvation, insulin reaction, and hyperinsulinism due to tumors of the pancreatic islet cells. Elevation of serum glucose (hyperglycemia) is a cardinal feature of diabetes mellitus, which was described above in the section on the pancreatic hormone insulin. The diagnosis of diabetes mellitus is confirmed when any two measurements of plasma glucose performed on different days yield levels at or above established thresholds: in the fasting state, 126 mg/dL [7.0 mmol/L]; 2-hours postprandially (after a 75-g oral glucose load), or at random, 200 mg/dL [11.1 mmol/L].

More useful information about glucose metabolism can be obtained by testing the blood glucose at one or several precisely timed intervals after ingestion of a meal or (preferably) after ingestion of exactly 75 mg of carbohydrate. When blood is drawn for testing at several intervals (for example, 30, 60, 90, 120, and 180 minutes), the results can be plotted as a **glucose tolerance curve**. The curve is elevated, with a slow fall towards normal, in diabetes mellitus. A low or flat curve occurs in hyperinsulinism or in decreased digestive absorption of glucose. Variations due to absorption can be avoided by giving the carbohydrate load intravenously.

The most important single value in the glucose tolerance curve is the **two-hour postprandial** level. Normally this is below 140 mg/dL [7.7 mmol/L]. A two-hour postprandial blood sugar between 140 and 200 mg/dL [7.7 and 11.1 mmol/L] indicates impaired glucose tolerance and a level over 200 mg/dL [11.1 mmol/L] is diagnostic of diabetes mellitus.

Current standards of medical care call for persons with diabetes to monitor their blood sugar levels frequently—often several times a day. Various portable electronic meters are available for this purpose. Testing is performed on fingerstick blood, which is obtained by the patient with a spring-loaded device that automatically punctures the finger to the correct depth with a disposable lancet.

One disadvantage of using the blood sugar level as a means of monitoring long-term control of diabetes mellitus is that this level fluctuates constantly. A valuable technique for assessing diabetic control over a period of weeks is the measurement of **glycosylated hemoglobin**, a chemical compound of glucose and the A_{1c} fraction of red blood cell hemoglobin; thus, the test is sometimes referred to as a hemoglobin A_{1c}. In nondiabetics, glycosylated hemoglobin constitutes less than 6% of total hemoglobin. When diabetic control has been satisfactory during the 8 weeks preceding the test, glycosylated hemoglobin constitutes less than 8% of total hemoglobin.

Tumor Markers

High levels of certain proteins, glycoproteins, and carbohydrates appear in the serum of some patients with certain malignant neoplasms. Tests to measure these tumor markers are used to diagnose neoplastic disease, to distinguish between benign and malignant tumors, to stage malignancies after diagnosis, and to detect recurrences after treatment. Although testing for these substances is usually carried out by immunologic or molecular biology methods, they are described here for the sake of completeness. The use of these tests to screen asymptomatic persons is not recommended.

Carcinoembryonic antigen (CEA) is present in many cases of carcinoma, particularly of the lung, digestive tract, and pancreas. Because it is also elevated in other malignancies and in nonmalignant inflammatory diseases of the bowel, as well as in many heavy smokers, it is not of much use in screening or diagnosis. It is valuable, however, in testing treated cancer patients for recurrence or metastases. **Alpha-fetoprotein** (AFP) is a globulin produced by the liver and other tissues of the fetus and newborn. Its level normally declines after one year of age. The serum level in nonpregnant women and adults of either sex is normally less than 15 ng/mL [15 mcg/L]. Elevation of alpha-fetoprotein occurs in hepatocellular carcinoma, viral hepatitis, hepatic cirrhosis, and various teratocarcinomas and embryonal carcinomas of gonadal origin. Elevation also occurs in pregnancy, but extremely high levels in maternal serum may indicate fetal neural tube defects (anencephaly, spina bifida) or fetal death.

The normal serum level of **prostate specific antigen** (PSA), a proteolytic enzyme produced by cells of the prostate gland, is less than 4 ng/mL [4 mcg/L]. Elevation of serum PSA can occur in both cancer (adenocarcinoma) of the prostate and in benign disorders such as prostatitis and benign prostatic hyperplasia. A level above 10 ng/mL [10 mcg/L] usually indicates carcinoma.

Measurement of both free PSA and PSA that is complexed with the protease inhibitor α1 anti-chymotrypsin (PSA-ACT) enhances the sensitivity of testing for carcinoma in men with total PSA levels between 4 and 10 ng/dL. A free PSA that is less than 10% of total PSA has a positive predictive value of more than 50% for malignant disease, but only an 8% predictive value when more than 25% is free. An annual increase of more than 0.75 ng/mL [0.75 mcg/L] is also highly suggestive of prostate cancer.

CA (cancer antigen) 19-9 is elevated in some patients with malignant tumors of the stomach, bowel, liver and pancreas. Elevations of **CA 125** occur with a majority of ovarian cancers, but also in digestive tract neoplasms, in some benign tumors of the reproductive tract, and in normal pregnancy. **CA 27.29** is elevated in one-third of early breast cancers and in two-thirds of later-stage breast cancers. **HER-2** protein is expressed in many breast cancers and its presence indicates a poorer prognosis and the need for more aggressive treatment. Other important tumor markers are p53 protein, vascular endothelial growth factor, CAK1, and LK26.

Waste Products

The normal daily breakdown of protein in the body produces about 15 g of nitrogen, most of which is excreted by the kidneys. The principal form in which nitrogen is excreted is **urea**, which is synthesized in the liver. Urea is filtered through the renal glomeruli and neither reabsorbed nor secreted by the renal tubules. Hence the level of urea in the serum, measured as blood urea nitrogen (BUN), reflects principally glomerular function. The normal BUN is 5-20 mg/dL [1.8-7.1 mcmol/L]. An increase in this level (azotemia) occurs in renal disease, particularly glomerular disease; in conditions causing increased protein breakdown or impairing renal blood flow (prerenal azotemia); and in urinary tract obstruction (postrenal azotemia). The BUN may be reduced in severe liver disease and severe protein deficiency.

Creatinine, also a nitrogenous waste, is a breakdown product formed in muscle tissue from creatine. It is both filtered at the renal glomeruli and actively secreted by the renal tubules. The normal serum level of creatinine is 0.6-1.2 mg/dL [50-100 mcmol/L]. Elevation occurs in the same conditions as elevation of BUN, as well as in pituitary gigantism and acromegaly. The ratio of BUN to creatinine is normally about 10:1, but creatinine is considered a more sensitive indicator of renal functional impairment.

A renal clearance test, which compares the concentration of a substance in the serum with the total amount of that substance excreted in the urine during 24 hours, provides an estimate of kidney function. **Creatinine clearance** can be used to determine the glomerular filtration rate (GFR), which, for optimum precision, is expressed in milliliters of filtrate per minute per standard body surface area of 1.73 m^2. The normal GFR is 90-135 mL/min/1.73 m^2 [0.86-1.3 mL/sec/m^2]. Normal levels are somewhat higher for men. Creatinine clearance is reduced in acute and chronic kidney disease, shock, congestive heart failure, and dehydration.

Ammonia, yet another nitrogenous waste, is produced in tissues by the normal breakdown of protein, in the intestine by the action of bacteria on dietary protein, and to a lesser extent by the kidneys as part of their regulation of acid-base balance. Ammonia is normally converted by the liver to urea and other products, which are then cleared from the blood by the kidneys. In a healthy person the level of serum ammonia is only 15–45 mcg/dL [11–32 mcmol/L]. This level rises in hepatic failure of any cause. Ammonia is toxic to the central nervous system, causing tremors, coma, and death.

Uric acid is the ultimate breakdown product of purines (guanine and xanthine), which are components of nucleoproteins in both body cells and food. Uric acid is filtered at the renal glomeruli and both reabsorbed and secreted by the renal tubules. The normal level of uric acid in the serum is 3.4-7 mg/dL [202-416 mcmol/L]. An increase in this level (hyperuricemia) occurs in gout, renal disease, and many disorders causing increased breakdown of nucleoproteins, such as hemolytic anemia, hematologic malignancies, and psoriasis. Nonspecific increases occur in many other conditions and in some normal persons, including relatives of persons with gout. Measurement of the uric acid level is used primarily to diagnose and monitor gout. It is not a sensitive indicator of renal disease.

Approximately 6 g of hemoglobin are turned over each day in the normal breakdown of red blood cells. The heme fraction of this hemoglobin is converted in reticuloendothelial cells to the yellow pigment **bilirubin**, of which about 0.3 g is formed daily. Bilirubin, which is nearly insoluble in plasma, is transported in the blood bound to protein. It is taken up in this form by the liver and conjugated with glucuronic acid, which renders it water-soluble. It is then excreted in the bile. In the intestine, bilirubin is further broken down to urobilinogen. Most of this urobilinogen is eliminated in the stool, but a fraction of it is reabsorbed and re-excreted by the liver.

Both conjugated and unconjugated bilirubin are normally present in the serum. Significant elevation of either or both forms (hyperbilirubinemia) results in the temporary yellow staining of the tissues, including the skin, known as jaundice. Conjugated bilirubin is also called direct-reacting bilirubin because it is water-soluble and therefore reacts directly with analytic reagents. The normal level of direct-reacting bilirubin in serum in 0.1 to 0.4 mg/dL [1.7–6.8 mcmol/L]. Elevation of this level occurs when bilirubin that has been conjugated by the liver enters the circulation as a result of biliary tract obstruction or disease of the intrahepatic biliary duct system. Because conjugated bilirubin is water-soluble, excessive amounts of it in the blood spill into the urine, where it can be chemically detected and may intensify or alter the color of the urine.

Unconjugated bilirubin is also called indirect-reacting bilirubin because it is insoluble in water and must be treated with methanol before quantitative analysis can be carried out. Unconjugated bilirubin does not appear in the urine. In practice, direct and total bilirubin are determined by quantitative analysis, and the indirect bilirubin is calculated as the difference between them. The normal total bilirubin level is 0.1 to 0.9 mg/dL [1.7-15.3 mcmol/L] and the normal indirect-reacting bilirubin level is 0.1 to 0.5 mg/dL [1.7–8.5 mcmol/L]. Elevation of indirect-reacting bilirubin occurs in acute or chronic liver disease (viral hepatitis, cirrhosis, hepatic necrosis) and after massive hemolysis. The combination of hemolysis in the neonatal period with immaturity of liver function often produces transient "physiologic" jaundice in newborns.

Organic compounds containing a carbonyl group (C=O) within a carbon chain are called ketones. **Ketones** (ketone bodies) produced in human metabolism include various products (acetone, acetoacetic acid, beta-hydroxybutyric acid) of the abnormal breakdown of fatty acids that accumulate in the blood in uncontrolled type 1 diabetes mellitus and in starvation, causing a condition called ketoacidosis. The diagnosis of ketoacidosis is usually made clinically and by chemical detection of ketone bodies in the urine.

The normal serum level of **lactic acid**, a product of anaerobic glycolysis (carbohydrate metabolism in the absence of oxygen), is 4.5-19.8 mg/dL [0.5-2.2 mmol/L]. The level is increased after strenuous exercise and in diabetes mellitus, shock, nutritional deficiency, inflammatory and malignant disease, and in congenital deficiency of enzymes catalyzing the conversion of lactic to pyruvic acid.

Drug Monitoring, Detection of Poisons

Monitoring blood levels of certain prescribed medicines is currently standard practice in establishing and maintaining optimum dosage. Analytic methods are available for most drugs in regular use. The therapeutic range of a drug is the range of concentrations in serum below which the therapeutic effect is inadequate or absent, and above which toxic effects may occur. Monitoring of drug levels is particularly important with drugs having narrow margins between therapeutic and toxic effects (gentamicin, lithium, theophylline, tobramycin), drugs used to control cardiac arrhythmias (digitoxin, digoxin, procainamide, quinidine), and drugs used to prevent seizures (carbamazepine, phenobarbital, phenytoin, valproic acid).

For some drugs, determination of both peak (maximum) and trough (minimum) levels in the serum is necessary to monitor drug metabolism so as to avoid levels above or below the therapeutic range.

Quantitative analysis of serum for toxic materials such as drugs of abuse and chemical poisons may provide an explanation for various abnormal conditions, including dementia, coma, and shock. Toxicologic screening by thin-layer chromatography can isolate and identify virtually any extraneous chemical substance, provided that it is present in sufficient concentration in the specimen. Specific quantitative methods are available for alcohol, cannabis, amphetamines, barbiturates, hypnotics, narcotics, salicylate, tranquilizers, and industrial poisons.

Laboratory determination of serum or urine levels of certain substances may be performed as diagnostic procedures that assess the function of certain organs or tissues. When taken orally, **D-xylose**, a metabolically inert sugar of plant origin, is normally absorbed from the small intestine and excreted unchanged in the urine. Testing blood and urine levels at standard intervals (blood, 1 or 2 hours; urine, 5 hours) after consumption of a standard dose (25 g) of D-xylose can therefore be used as a test of intestinal absorption. At 2 hours the adult serum concentration should be 25-40 mg/dL [1.7-2.7 mmol/L] and at 5 hours at least 3.5 g should have been excreted in the urine. Lower levels of absorption and excretion occur in various malabsorption syndromes (sprue, celiac disease) as well as in regional enteritis, Whipple disease (intestinal infection with *Tropheryma whippelii*), and other disorders of the intestinal mucosa.

Lactose, the sugar of milk, is normally broken down to glucose and galactose in the intestine by the enzyme lactase. Deficiency of lactase, which can be congenital or acquired, results in lactose intolerance, that is, cramping and diarrhea after consumption of milk and unfermented dairy products. In the **lactose tolerance test**, blood levels of glucose are determined in the fasting state and 30, 60, and 120 minutes after oral administration of a standard dose (50 g) of lactose. If adequate lactase activity is present, the plasma glucose level rises at least 200 mg/dL [11 mmol/L] above the fasting level by 60 minutes.

Panels

The following are representative examples of standard automated serum chemistry panels:

- Basic metabolic panel (8 tests): Sodium, potassium, chloride, CO_2, calcium, glucose, BUN, creatinine.
- Comprehensive metabolic panel (14 tests): All of the above plus total protein, albumin, total bilirubin, alkaline phosphatase, aspartate aminotransferase, alanine aminotransferase.
- Hepatic function panel (10 tests): Total protein, albumin, total bilirubin, direct bilirubin, ammonia, cholesterol, alkaline phosphatase, aspartate aminotransferase, alanine aminotransferase, lactic dehydrogenase.
- Renal function panel (10 tests): Sodium, potassium, chloride, CO_2, calcium, phosphorus, albumin, glucose, BUN, creatinine.

- Lipid panel (3 tests): Total cholesterol, high-density lipoprotein cholesterol, (low-density lipoprotein cholesterol calculated from above figures), triglycerides.

Exercises

Fill in the Blanks

1. Rather than allowing a blood specimen to coagulate naturally, it is placed in a _____ which spins the specimen rapidly to separate the cells from _____.

2. One of the commonest reasons for false elevations of plasma chemistry levels in a blood specimen is _____.

3. The substance left when both cells and fibrinogen are removed from blood is _____.

4. Older and more cumbersome analytic techniques, such as _____ techniques, requiring precise weighing, and _____ techniques, requiring drop-by-drop titration, have been replaced by _____ analytic methods that use electronic equipment.

5. An _____ is a substance capable of conducting an electric current when dissolved in water, but in chemical parlance, the term refers to any substance that _____ in water.

6. _____ are the principal cations of the plasma, and _____ are the principal anions.

7. The electrolyte _____ is an important constituent of all body fluids, being concerned in maintenance of osmotic pressure, water balance, membrane permeability, and the irritability of nerve cells.

8. _____ is increase of sodium concentration, while _____ is a decrease in sodium concentration.

9. _____ refers to the increased renal excretion of water.

10. Two terms that mean elevation of potassium concentration are _____ or _____.

11. Two terms that mean decreased potassium concentration are _____ or _____.

12. _____ (increased chloride concentration) may result from dehydration or from reduced excretion of chloride ions in acute renal failure or other renal disease.

13. _____ (decreased chloride concentration) can be either dilutional (as with excessive fluid retention in congestive heart failure or renal or hepatic disease) or due to depletion by loss from the gastrointestinal tract (particularly by vomiting), from the kidney as a consequence of diuretic therapy or adrenal failure, or from the sweat glands.

14. The _____ level depends on excretion or retention of carbon dioxide gas by the lungs.

15. The pH of serum is maintained between 7.35 and 7.45 or slightly _____.

Exercises

16. A rise in serum pH is called _____ and a fall in pH is called _____.

17. Any shift in serum pH tends to be compensated by whatever mechanism remains unimpaired. Hence, for example, metabolic acidosis leads to increased pulmonary excretion of carbon dioxide, with a resulting tendency towards _____.

18. The level of calcium tends to vary inversely with that of _____.

19. Hypocalcemia occurs in _____ with a corresponding hyperphosphatemia.

20. In order to distinguish among various causes of abnormal serum iron levels it is helpful to determine the _____ of the blood.

21. The two minerals combined with calcium in the bones and teeth are _____ and _____.

22. The partial pressures of oxygen and carbon dioxide are measured by _____.

23. An _____ is a protein that accelerates or facilitates a biochemical reaction without being permanently altered or consumed in the process.

24. The significance of an elevation of an enzyme level in the serum is that it may _____.

25. An older name for aspartate aminotransferase (AST) is _____.

26. An older name for alanine aminotransferase (ALT), is _____.

27. Another name for creatine kinase (CK) is _____.

28. An inborn metabolic disorder that results in the accumulation in tissues of excessive amounts of a normal or abnormal substance is called a _____.

29. A _____ is a chemical messenger or mediator secreted by an endocrine gland or a group of specialized endocrine cells and released directly into the blood stream.

30. The concentrations of _____ in the blood correlate closely with the condition of their glands or tissues of origin.

31. The blood levels of virtually all known hormones can be determined by _____.

32. Another name for the pituitary gland is the _____.

Exercises

33. Another name for vasopressin is _____.

34. Two anterior pituitary hormones—follicle-stimulating hormone (FSH), also called follitropin, and luteinizing hormone (LH), also called lutropin—are known as _____ because they control the nutritional status and function of the gonads (ovaries and testicles).

35. The _____ is a cone-shaped body less than 1 cm in greatest dimension, attached by a stalk to the roof of the third ventricle of the brain, which undergoes regression after age 7.

36. The principal plasma proteins are _____, _____, and _____.

37. Twenty _____ are recognized as components of proteins in human metabolism, nine of them essential (that is, not synthesized by the human body and hence essential nutrients).

38. A rise in the level of _____ can be more diagnostic than AST or CK of myocardial infarction, while rises in the level of troponin T (TnT), although not specific to cardiac muscle, may be more sensitive indicators of _____.

39. The principal clinical use of brain natriuretic peptide (BNP) testing is to rule out _____ in patients with dyspnea of unknown origin.

40. Certain plasma proteins, including fibrinogen and ceruloplasmin, are called _____ because their levels rise within a few hours in the presence of acute inflammation.

41. The _____ of a drug is the range of concentrations in serum below which the therapeutic effect is inadequate or absent, and above which toxic effects may occur.

Multiple Choice: Circle the letter of the best answer from the choices given.

1. Which of the following is a chemical analytic method based on the differing behavior of various solutes in an electric field?
   A. Chromatography.
   B. Gravimetric method.
   C. Electrophoresis.
   D. Molecular biology method.
   E. Radioimmunoassay.

Exercises

2. Which of the following chemical analytic methods measures specific proteins by observing their reaction with isotopically labeled monoclonal antibodies?
   A. Radioimmunoassay.
   B. Electrophoresis.
   C. Gravimetric method.
   D. Volumetric method.
   E. Chromatography.

3. DNA sequences that are unique to certain proteins and enzymes are detected using which of the following laboratory methods?
   A. Chromatography.
   B. Gravimetric method.
   C. Electrophoresis.
   D. Molecular biology method.
   E. Radioimmunoassay.

4. One method for determining serum osmolality is the
   A. Gravimetric method.
   B. Volumetric method.
   C. Quantitative method.
   D. Molecular biology method.
   E. Freezing point depression method.

5. Serum osmolality (hyperosmolality) is increased in all of the following conditions except
   A. Diabetes mellitus.
   B. Inappropriate secretion of antidiuretic hormone.
   C. Dehydration.
   D. Hypercalcemia.
   E. Diabetes insipidus.

6. Serum osmolality is decreased in which of the following conditions?
   A. Congestive heart failure.
   B. Cirrhosis.
   C. Addison disease.
   D. All of the above.
   E. None of the above.

Exercises

7. Which of the following terms applies to an atom or group of atoms having a positive or negative charge?
   A. Ion.
   B. Anion.
   C. Cation.
   D. Electrolyte.
   E. Osmole.

8. Which of the following terms applies to an atom or group of atoms having a negative charge because it has gained one or more electrons?
   A. Ion.
   B. Anion.
   C. Cation.
   D. Electrolyte.
   E. Osmole.

9. Which of the following terms applies to an atom or group of atoms having a positive charge because it has lost one or more electrons?
   A. Osmole
   B. Electrolyte
   C. Cation.
   D. Anion.
   E. Ion.

10. Which organ is principally responsible for maintaining the concentrations and ratios of sodium, potassium, and chloride within fairly narrow limits?
    A. The heart.
    B. The brain.
    C. The lungs.
    D. The stomach and intestines.
    E. The kidneys.

11. Which organ through excretion (or retention) of carbon dioxide dissolved in the blood controls the concentration of bicarbonate ion?
    A. The brain.
    B. The heart.
    C. The lungs.
    D. The kidneys.
    E. The stomach and intestines.

Exercises

12. Which of the following electrolytes is responsible for maintaining acid-base balance and osmotic pressure within cells and is essential to normal activity of muscle tissue, especially cardiac muscle?
    A. Sodium.
    B. Potassium.
    C. Chloride.
    D. Nitrogen.
    E. Bicarbonate.

13. Which of the following ions is measured indirectly, being first converted to carbon dioxide and, in fact, often referred to as carbon dioxide (CO_2)?
    A. Bicarbonate.
    B. Chloride.
    C. Nitrogen.
    D. Potassium.
    E. Sodium.

14. Which of the following conditions can be respiratory in origin, resulting from a disturbance in the excretion of carbon dioxide by the lungs?
    A. Alkalosis.
    B. Phosphatemia.
    C. Acidosis.
    D. A & C.
    E. A & B.

15. What is the difference between cation and anion concentrations called when only the four principal ions are included in the calculation?
    A. Metabolic acidosis.
    B. Respiratory acidosis.
    C. Cation concentration.
    D. Anion concentration.
    E. Anion gap.

16. Which of the following minerals is the principal mineral of bones and teeth and also plays an essential role in nerve and muscle function and blood coagulation?
    A. Iron.
    B. Calcium.
    C. Phosphorus.
    D. Magnesium.
    E. Copper.

Exercises

17. The presence of hypercalcemia and hypophosphatemia may be an indication of which of the following conditions?
    A. Hyperthyroidism.
    B. Hypoparathyroidism.
    C. Hyperparathyroidism.
    D. Hypothyroidism.
    E. Pernicious anemia.

18. The role of which of the following minerals in body chemistry is limited almost entirely to the transport and utilization of oxygen?
    A. Magnesium.
    B. Phosphorus.
    C. Calcium.
    D. Iron.
    E. Copper.

19. Which of the following minerals is an essential component of enzymes and other proteins concerned in hemoglobin synthesis and bone formation?
    A. Copper.
    B. Phosphorus.
    C. Calcium.
    D. Magnesium.
    E. Zinc.

20. Which of the following studies is used to assess the adequacy of pulmonary gas exchange in persons with respiratory or circulatory disease and those receiving oxygen therapy, with or without ventilatory assistance?
    A. Anion gap.
    B. The pH.
    C. Cation concentration.
    D. Anion concentration.
    E. Arterial blood gases.

21. Which of the following tests is performed on a blood specimen drawn from the artery rather than a vein to identify acidosis or alkalosis and to permit indirect calculation of the bicarbonate ion concentration?
    A. Anion gap.
    B. The pH.
    C. Cation concentration.
    D. Anion concentration.
    E. Arterial blood gases.

Exercises

22. Which of the following serum enzymes was not indicated in the text to be elevated to varying degrees in myocardial infarction?
    A. Alanine aminotransferase (ALT).
    B. Lactic dehydrogenase (LDH).
    C. Creatine phosphokinase (CPK).
    D. Aspartate aminotransferase (AST).
    E. Serum gamma-glutamyl transpeptidase (SGGT).

23. Which of the following serum enzymes was not indicated in the text to be elevated in liver disease or hepatic abnormalities?
    A. Alanine aminotransferase (ALT).
    B. Lactic dehydrogenase (LDH).
    C. Creatine phosphokinase (CPK).
    D. Aspartate aminotransferase (AST).
    E. Serum gamma-glutamyl transpeptidase (SGGT).

24. Which of the LDH isoenzymes predominates in cases of myocardial infarction?
    A. I
    B. II
    C. III
    D. IV
    E. V

25. Which of the following enzymes is more diagnostic of traumatic and degenerative disorders of skeletal muscle?
    A. Aspartate aminotransferase (AST).
    B. Lactic dehydrogenase (LDH).
    C. Serum gamma-glutamyl transpeptidase (SGGT).
    D. Alanine aminotransferase (ALT).
    E. Creatine phosphokinase (CPK).

26. Which of the following isoenzymes is elevated in myocardial infarction?
    A. CPK BB.
    B. LDH II.
    C. CPK MM.
    D. LDH V.
    E. CPK MB.

Exercises

27. Elevation of LDH I and CPK MB would be most indicative of which of the following conditions?
    A. Cerebral infarction.
    B. Myocardial infarction.
    C. Hepatic injury.
    D. Disseminated lupus erythematosus.
    E. Severe trauma of skeletal muscle.

28. Which of the following serum enzymes is usually elevated in infection or carcinoma of the prostate?
    A. Alkaline phosphatase.
    B. Acid phosphatase.
    C. Creatine kinase.
    D. Beta-glucosidase.
    E. Hexosaminidase A.

29. Elevation of the digestive enzymes serum amylase and lipase might be an indication of which of the following conditions?
    A. Gaucher disease.
    B. Cancer of the colon.
    C. Pancreatic disease.
    D. Gastric carcinoma.
    E. Addison disease.

30. Which of the following enzymes raises blood pressure by constricting blood vessels and conserves sodium by promoting release of aldosterone by the adrenal cortex?
    A. Creatine kinase.
    B. Renin.
    C. Angiotensin converting enzyme.
    D. Amylase.
    E. Lipase.

31. Which of the following hormones promotes normal body growth and fat mobilization and inhibits the mobilization of carbohydrate?
    A. Somatotropin.
    B. Vasopressin.
    C. Thyroxine.
    D. Cortisol.
    E. Oxytocin.

Exercises

32. Which of the following is a chronic metabolic disorder caused by a reduction in the availability or efficacy of insulin?
    A. Addison disease.
    B. Pheochromocytoma.
    C. Diabetes insipidus.
    D. Diabetes mellitus.
    E. Hyperparathyroidism.

33. Which of the following is a protein that functions principally in water balance by maintaining the osmotic pressure of the blood? It also acts as a plasma buffer.
    A. Globulin.
    B. Fibrinogen.
    C. Insulin.
    D. Cortisol.
    E. Albumin.

34. Which are the two proteins that are involved in the storage and transport of iron?
    A. Albumin and globulin.
    B. Fibrinogen and prothrombin.
    C. Ferritin and transferrin.
    D. Cortisol and ACTH.
    E. Trypsin and antitrypsin.

35. Measuring this amino acid within the first few days of life is a routine procedure in well-baby care and required by law in most jurisdictions because it can prevent a hereditary disorder that causes mental retardation if not detected and treated early.
    A. Alanine.
    B. Phenylalanine.
    C. Cysteine.
    D. Taurine.
    E. Methionine.

36. Elevation of all of the following can be diagnostic of myocardial infarction except
    A. Homocysteine.
    B. AST.
    C. CK.
    D. Troponin I.
    E. Troponin T.

Exercises

37. Elevation of which of the following is associated with premature development of atherosclerosis and heightened risk of myocardial infarction, stroke, and thromboembolic disease?
    A. Troponin T.
    B. CK.
    C. AST.
    D. Troponin I.
    E. Homocysteine.

38. Serum levels of this substance are elevated in congestive heart failure.
    A. Atrial natriuretic peptide (ANP).
    B. Sodium.
    C. Homocysteine.
    D. Aldosterone.
    E. C-reactive protein (CRP).

39. Acute phase reactants, while sensitive indicators of inflammation, are also highly nonspecific and can be triggered by a wide range of abnormal conditions, including systemic or localized infection, myocardial infarction, autoimmune disorders such as lupus erythematosus and rheumatoid arthritis, and extensive or metastatic malignancy. One such substance is _____.
    A. Atrial natriuretic peptide (ANP).
    B. Homocysteine.
    C. Sodium.
    D. C-reactive protein (CRP).
    E. Aldosterone.

40. Which of the following is a valuable technique for assessing diabetic control over a period of weeks.
    A. Fasting serum glucose.
    B. Glucose tolerance test.
    C. Glycosylated hemoglobin.
    D. Two-hour postprandial blood sugar.
    E. Serum insulin.

41. Which of the following serum blood tests is not a test of renal function?
    A. Creatinine clearance test.
    B. Blood urea nitrogen (BUN).
    C. BUN-creatinine ratio.
    D. Creatinine.
    E. Ammonia.

Exercises

42. Which of the following is elevated in a condition known as gout?
    A. Creatine.
    B. Blood urea nitrogen (BUN).
    C. Ammonia.
    D. Creatinine.
    E. Uric acid.

43. Both the conjugated and unconjugated forms of this substance are normally present in the serum, and significant elevation of either or both forms results in the temporary yellow staining of the tissues, including the skin, known as jaundice.
    A. Creatinine.
    B. Ammonia.
    C. Bilirubin.
    D. Blood urea nitrogen.
    E. Uric acid.

44. Which of the following is a result of the abnormal breakdown of fatty acids that accumulate in the blood in uncontrolled type 1 diabetes mellitus and in starvation?
    A. Ketones (ketone bodies).
    B. Uric acid.
    C. Lactic acid.
    D. Ammonia.
    E. Bilirubin.

45. This substance, a product of anaerobic glycolysis (carbohydrate metabolism in the absence of oxygen), is elevated after strenuous exercise.
    A. Bilirubin.
    B. Ammonia.
    C. Uric acid.
    D. Lactic acid.
    A. Ketones.

Exercises

Short Answers

1. Define or explain.

   a. A/G ratio _____

   _____

   b. anion _____

   _____

   c. buffer _____

   _____

   d. cation _____

   _____

   e. hypercapnia _____

   _____

   f. hypokalemia _____

   _____

   g. isoenzyme _____

   _____

   h. pH _____

   _____

   i. trace elements _____

   _____

2. List some reasons why several tests are often done together in a group or "panel."

   _____

   _____

   _____

   _____

   _____

   _____

   _____

   _____

   _____

Exercises

3. Give an example of a laboratory value derived by calculation from other laboratory values.

_____

_____

_____

_____

4. Why is it usually important to separate red blood cells from plasma promptly and completely in a blood specimen intended for chemical testing?

_____

_____

_____

_____

5. What are some advantages of automated chemical testing of blood?

_____

_____

_____

_____

6. What are the principal serum electrolytes?

_____

_____

_____

_____

7. What is the point of determining the cholesterol level in an apparently healthy person?

_____

_____

_____

_____

Exercises

8. What important class of substances is included in the gamma globulin fraction of plasma?

   _____

   _____

   _____

   _____

9. What is the principal nitrogenous waste product excreted in urine?

   _____

   _____

   _____

   _____

10. List three factors affecting the glomerular filtration rate.

    a. _____

    b. _____

    c. _____

11. List the three distinct operations performed on the glomerular filtrate by the tubules of the kidney that determine the eventual volume and composition of urine.

    a. _____

    b. _____

    c. _____

12. List two ways in which aldosterone affects tubular function.

    a. _____

    _____

    b. _____

    _____

13. Hyponatremia may be a reflection of two different factors. What are these two factors?

    a. _____

    _____

    b. _____

    _____

Exercises

14. List the components of an arterial blood gas study and the importance of each.

    a. _____

    _____

    b. _____

    _____

    c. _____

    _____

    d. _____

    _____

15. List the serum enzymes often found elevated to varying degrees in hepatic disease and in injury or infarction of muscle, particularly cardiac muscle.

    a. _____

    b. _____

    c. _____

    d. _____

    e. _____

16. If the serum leucine aminopeptidase (SLAP) and the 5´-nucleotidase are elevated in conjunction with an elevated alkaline phosphatase, what is the most likely diagnosis? If they are normal in the presence of an elevated alkaline phosphatase, what is the most likely diagnosis?

    _____

    _____

    _____

    _____

17. Numerous congenital disorders consist in the lack of genes that encode specific enzymes. List four of these enzymes and the diseases associated with their deficiency.

    a. _____

    _____

    b. _____

    _____

    c. _____

    _____

Exercises

d. _____

_____

18. List the five anatomically discrete endocrine (ductless) glands and the hormones they produce.

a. _____

b. _____

c. _____

d. _____

e. _____

19. List the areas, other than the endocrine glands, where zones of specialized tissue contain secretory cells and the chemical products they send directly into the blood.

_____

_____

_____

_____

_____

20. List the fractions of cholesterol and their significance.

_____

_____

_____

_____

_____

_____

21. List six tumor markers and their significance.

a. _____

_____

b. _____

_____

c. _____

_____

Exercises

d. _____

_____

e. _____

_____

f. _____

_____

22. Discuss the importance of monitoring drug levels.

_____

_____

_____

_____

_____

_____

_____

Activities for Application and Further Study

1. Diagram or illustrate pictorially the creation of urine in the kidneys. Label the areas where the excretion or reuptake of important electrolytes occurs.

2. Using a dictionary or the Internet, research and list several storage diseases not mentioned in the text that result from an inborn error of metabolism. In a separate column, list the deficiency causing the disease, and in a third column list the major signs or symptoms associated with the disease. In a fourth column, you might indicate whether these diseases are treatable or fatal.

3. On an outline of the human body, identify the organs and tissues that produce hormones and name the hormones they produce. Draw lines ending in arrows to show the organs/tissues upon which the hormones act.

4. In a reference book or on the Internet, find a list of the nine essential amino acids. Summarize the importance of each.

Medical Microbiology

21

Virtually all of the procedures performed in a medical microbiology laboratory pertain to infectious disease—confirming the presence of infection, identifying the causative organisms, selecting antibiotics effective against them, and verifying microbiologic cure after treatment. In medical microbiology, diagnostic focus is of paramount importance. No laboratory procedure or group of procedures can isolate or identify all possible pathogens. The source of a specimen provides some clues as to which pathogens are likely to be found and hence some direction as to the choice of culture techniques. Ideally, however, the patient's medical history and physical findings, the results of other laboratory tests, the response to treatment, and the clinician's tentative diagnosis are all taken into account in processing a microbiologic specimen.

Much of the routine work is in bacteriology, whose two principal diagnostic methods are the microscopic examination of stained smears and the culture of microorganisms. A smear is a translucent layer of fluid or semisolid material thinly spread over a microscope slide. A smear can be prepared from any natural body fluid, waste product, or abnormal secretion. Standard procedures are in use for making smears from throat, nasopharyngeal, vaginal, and anal swabs and from sputum, stool, wound drainage, and pus. Clear fluids such as spinal fluid, urine, and serous exudates may be centrifuged or filtered, as described in Chapter 17 under cytologic techniques, to improve the yield of bacteria.

Bacteriologic smears are routinely stained by the **Gram method**. In this technique, crystal violet is first applied, along with a mordant (an agent that causes the stain to react chemically with some components of the smear) that contains iodine. Certain bacteria, called gram-positive, take up this stain and resist decolorization with alcohol. Other organisms, called gram-negative, do not retain the stain after washing with alcohol. These are counterstained red with safranin in the final step of the technique. The technician examining the smear notes whether one or several kinds of organism are present and, by considering their size, shape, grouping, and Gram-staining characteristics, forms a judgment as to whether the smear contains only normal flora (nonpathogenic organisms normally found in the source material or bodily region in question) or whether infection is present, and if so what kind.

Specimens of sputum or other material may also be stained by the **acid-fast method**, which is used to detect mycobacteria, including the organisms that cause tuberculosis and leprosy. In this technique a carbolfuchsin stain is applied and the specimen is then washed in acidified alcohol. Only mycobacteria take up the red stain and retain it after acid decolorization—hence, "acid-fast." Acid-fast organisms cannot be satisfactorily stained by the Gram method. A number of other special stains are used to identify specific organisms.

A **culture** is a growth of microorganisms under controlled artificial conditions in the laboratory. Culturing offers several advantages over the simple smear for diagnostic purposes. When only a few organisms are present in a specimen, they may be missed in a smear. Theoretically, in a culture every viable organism in the specimen will generate a separate, pure colony. Hence culturing permits isolation of various organisms from a mixture for individual study. Observation of the growth characteristics of organisms in a culture supplies additional identifying data, and pure colonies from the culture can be studied in stained smears. Smears or suspensions made from pure cultures are also more suitable for study with serologic reagents such as agglutinins applied to detect the presence of specific organisms.

By the addition of nutrients and inhibitors to a culture medium, certain types of organisms can be favored while others are suppressed. Reagents and indicators added to the culture medium allow prompt detection of distinctive products of bacterial growth through color change. For more precise identification, organisms from a culture can be subcultured in one or more special media. For antibiotic sensitivity testing, disks impregnated with known concentrations of various antibiotics are incorporated in the culture medium. Zones of inhibition of bacterial growth around certain disks indicate sensitivity of the organism to those antibiotics.

Several kinds of bacteriologic media are in regular use, each with its specific purpose. Fluid media, usually called broths, are placed in sterile glass test tubes stoppered with cotton wool, which allows entry and exit of gases but prevents contamination of the culture by bacteria and molds from the air. Many media contain a vegetable gum called agar which gives them a stiff gel-like consistency below 45°C. Organisms grown on agar present more distinctive cultural characteristics than those grown in broth, and individual colonies can be observed and sampled. In addition, the use of sensitivity disks requires a solid medium. When an agar medium is placed in tubes, the tubes are usually allowed to cool in a slanted position so as to provide a larger surface area ("agar slants"). More often, agar media are placed in shallow transparent glass or plastic plates called Petri dishes. Each Petri dish has a loosely fitting cover which allows entry of oxygen and escape of gases but prevents contamination of the medium.

Introduction of infectious material into a culture medium is called inoculation (not "innoculation"). A minute amount (inoculum) of the specimen may be picked up with a sterile wire or wire loop and immersed in broth or streaked across the surface of an agar plate or slant. Streaking can also be done with a cotton swab, as in the case of a throat culture. Blood cultures are inoculated by adding freshly drawn whole blood to a nutrient broth in a culture flask.

After inoculation, cultures are ordinarily incubated at human body temperature (98.6°F, 37°C) for 48 to 72 hours and observed periodically for growth. Growth of certain microorganisms is favored by incubation in an atmosphere with little or no oxygen or with increased carbon dioxide. Organisms that grow best at very low oxygen tension are called anaerobes. Cultures for acid-fast organisms (mycobacteria) require six to eight weeks of incubation.

Throat cultures are performed on **blood agar**, a medium containing whole blood of animal origin, to facilitate identification of streptococci. Alpha-hemolytic streptococci and some other organisms cause greenish discoloration of the medium due to partial hemolysis. Beta-hemolytic streptococci and some other organisms cause the medium to become perfectly transparent around each colony by more complete chemical breakdown of blood. A disk impregnated with bacitracin may be included in the medium to distinguish Group A beta-hemolytic streptococci, whose growth is inhibited by bacitracin, from other beta-hemolytic organisms, which are resistant to bacitracin.

Chocolate agar, so called because of its color, contains blood that has been chemically altered by heating. Chocolate agar is a preferred medium for certain organisms, such as *Neisseria* and *Haemophilus*. Thayer-Martin medium is chocolate agar containing various antibiotics to inhibit the growth of organisms other than *Neisseria*. Differentiation among similar colon bacilli is achieved by simultaneous incubation in media containing various sugars (glucose, maltose, lactose, sucrose) ("differential sugars") and observation of growth patterns. Identification of organisms in a culture may depend on chemical detection of biochemical products such as hydrogen sulfide, indole, or nitrites from nitrates.

Quantitative techniques have been developed for culturing some specimens, notably urine. The standard urine colony count, requiring precise dilution of the specimen before inoculation, is reported in colonies per cubic millimeter of urine. A colony count over 100 000/mm³ is regarded as evidence of urinary tract infection, but lower counts may also be significant for some organisms or in some patients.

In procuring a "clean-catch" urine specimen for microbiologic study, the patient is instructed to follow procedures that ensure that the specimen is representative of bladder urine and that reduce the risk of contamination by extraneous bacteria and other materials. To obtain a midstream specimen the patient begins voiding into the toilet, catches 1-2 ounces (30-60 mL) of urine in a container, and then finishes voiding into the toilet. (In contrast, when the urine will be tested by DNA probe or other methods for detection of microorganisms in urethral cells, the first portion of urine passed must be preserved.) Women patients are instructed to cleanse around the urethral meatus with cotton balls saturated with antiseptic to remove any vaginal secretions, including menstrual blood.

Medical **mycology**, the study of pathogenic fungi, employs techniques similar to those of bacteriology. However, most fungi cannot be stained by the Gram method or others routinely used in bacteriologic work. Because fungal material is more resistant than human cells to digestion by potassium hydroxide (KOH) solution, treatment of material such as sputum or wound drainage with this alkali often leaves fungal hyphae or spores clearly visible on microscopic examination. Special culture media are required for fungi. Sabouraud agar, containing peptone and dextrose, is the most widely used. Incubation, usually at room temperature, must be continued for several weeks.

The basic techniques of diagnostic **virology** differ markedly from those of bacteriology and mycology. Viruses cannot be seen by light microscopy, and cannot be cultured in artificial media. Many viruses can, however, be cultured in living cells, and standard procedures are available to isolate and identify herpes simplex virus, cytomegalovirus, influenza viruses A and B, varicella-zoster virus, and others by culture.

A specimen for viral culture (nasopharyngeal secretions, sputum, blister fluid, stool, urine, or tissue) is placed in a liquid transport medium containing an antibiotic to prevent growth of contaminants and refrigerated until it is inoculated into a cell culture. The choice of cell line depends on the anatomic origin of the specimen and the probable or suspected diagnosis. Because viruses are harder to culture in the laboratory than most bacteria, viral cultures are less sensitive and false negatives occur more frequently. Culture techniques are not available for the hepatitis viruses, human papillomavirus, rotavirus, and many others.

Because of the limitations of viral culturing and because viruses cannot be visualized with a standard microscope, immunologic methods (discussed in the next chapter) are extensively used to diagnose viral infections.

Many kinds of **parasite** are visible to the naked eye or are so distinctive in smears or tissue sections as to leave no doubt about their identity. Standard procedures are in use for examination of stool, urine, and sputum for protozoan parasites, worms, cysts, and ova. Malarial parasites, trypanosomes, and leishmaniae are detectable in appropriately stained blood smears. Pinworm infestation (enterobiasis) can sometimes be diagnosed by finding ova on a Scotch tape swab taken from the perianal region in the morning upon arising. Vaginal trichomoniasis can be diagnosed by finding motile trichomonads in a wet mount or hanging drop preparation of vaginal secretions.

Exercises

Fill in the Blanks

1. The _____ provides some clues as to which pathogens are likely to be found and hence some direction as to the choice of culture techniques.

2. The two principal diagnostic methods in _____ are the microscopic examination of stained smears and the culture of microorganisms.

3. A _____ is a translucent layer of fluid or semisolid material thinly spread over a microscope slide.

4. Organisms that take up crystal violet stain and resist decolorization with alcohol in a Gram stain are called _____.

5. A urine colony count over 100 000/mm3 is regarded as evidence of _____.

6. Culture techniques are not available for the _____, _____, _____, viruses, and many others.

Multiple Choice: Circle the letter of the best answer from the choices given.

1. Which of the following is an agent that causes the stain to react chemically with some components of the smear?
   A. Agar.
   B. Mordant.
   C. Counterstain.
   D. Carbolfuchsin.
   E. Culture medium.

2. Which of the following terms refers to nonpathogenic organisms normally found in the source material or bodily region in question?
   A. Gram-positive organism.
   B. Gram-negative organism.
   C. Normal flora.
   D. Acid-fast organism.
   E. Alpha-hemolytic streptococci.

Exercises

3. Which of the following is an organism that cannot be detected by the Gram method but can be detected when a carbolfuchsin stain is applied and the specimen is then washed in acidified alcohol, retaining the stain after acid decolorization?
   A. Aerobic bacteria.
   B. Anaerobic bacteria.
   C. Fungi.
   D. Viruses.
   E. Mycobacteria.

4. In order to determine which antibiotic will most effectively treat the bacteria in question, this test is performed.
   A. Sensitivity testing.
   B. Acid-fast testing.
   C. Gram stain.
   D. Culture.
   E. Chromatography.

5. Which of the following refers to fluid media are placed in sterile glass test tubes stoppered with cotton wool, which allows entry and exit of gases but prevents contamination of the culture by bacteria and molds from the air?
   A. Broths.
   B. Agar.
   C. Chocolate agar.
   D. Inoculation media.
   E. Blood.

6. Introduction of infectious material into a culture medium is called
   A. Sensitivity testing.
   B. Culturing.
   C. Gram staining.
   D. Inoculation.
   E. Acid-fast staining.

7. Organisms that growth best by incubation in an atmosphere with little or no oxygen or with increased carbon dioxide are called
   A. Aerobic organisms.
   B. Anaerobic organisms.
   C. Gram-negative organisms.
   D. Gram-positive organisms.
   E. Acid-fast organisms.

Exercises

8. Which of the following organisms cause greenish discoloration of blood agar medium due to partial hemolysis?
   A. *Neisseria*.
   B. *Haemophilus*.
   C. Alpha-hemolytic streptococci.
   D. Mycobacteria.
   E. Beta-hemolytic streptococci.

9. Treatment of material such as sputum or wound drainage with potassium hydroxide (KOH) helps to make these organisms clearly visible on microscopic examination.
   A. Bacteria.
   B. Mycobacteria.
   C. Viruses.
   D. Parasites.
   E. Fungi.

10. These organisms cannot be seen by light microscopy, and cannot be cultured in artificial media.
    A. Viruses.
    B. Fungi.
    C. Mycobacteria.
    D. Parasites.
    E. Bacteria.

11. Which of the following organisms can often be detected simply by visual examination of tissue or smears?
    A. Bacteria.
    B. Fungi.
    C. Mycobacteria.
    D. Parasites.
    E. Viruses.

Short Answers

1. Define or explain:
   a. agar _____
   _____

   b. Gram stain _____
   _____

   c. mycology _____
   _____

Exercises

  d. normal flora _____

   _____

  e. sensitivity test _____

   _____

2. What are the two basic laboratory procedures in bacteriology?

  a. _____

   _____

  b. _____

   _____

3. In what ways can culturing a pathogenic microorganism contribute to its identification?

  _____

  _____

  _____

  _____

4. What is the standard medium for throat cultures?

  _____

  _____

5. Mention two types of pathogenic microorganism that cannot be grown in cultures.

  a. _____

  b. _____

6. Mention two types of pathogenic microorganism that take several weeks to grow in cultures.

  a. _____

  b. _____

Exercises

7. Explain the procedure to ensure that the urine specimen is representative of bladder urine and to reduce the risk of contamination by extraneous bacteria and other materials.

_____

_____

_____

_____

Activities for Application and Further Study

1. Make a chart of popular culture media and the organisms for which they are used. Go beyond your text and add 5-10 media from your own research.

2. Make a chart of each of the following types of organisms. List a few features which distinguish each organism from the others. List one or more species for each organism and the body tissue affected or the disease which each causes.
   a. bacteria
   b. fungi
   c. viruses
   d. parasites

Immunology 22

Immunology is the branch of biology and medicine that is concerned with the defensive responses of living organisms to antigenic challenge—that is, to exposure to substances or organisms that are recognized as foreign and potentially harmful. Serology embraces laboratory technologies and strategies based on antigen-antibody reactions, including a number of procedures that do not involve testing of serum. Antibody formation in response to infecting organisms and allergens is discussed briefly in Chapter 18. Serologic methods are used to identify acute infections due to certain bacteria, fungi, viruses, and parasites, and also to detect immunity to certain pathogenic organisms resulting from prior infection or from administration of vaccine. In addition, serologic testing is applied to the diagnosis of some noninfectious diseases, particularly autoimmune disorders and neoplasms.

Serology

Serologic testing is often easier, less expensive, faster, and more specific than routine procedures for isolation and identification of infecting organisms, particularly viruses. The basic laboratory procedure in serology is the identification of an antibody or an antigen by bringing about an antigen-antibody reaction under controlled conditions. Antibodies are sought in serum by challenge with specific or nonspecific antigens. A specific antigen is chemically or biologically identical to the one that elicited antibody formation—for example, an extract of *Salmonella* organisms used in a serologic test for antibody stimulated by *Salmonella* infection. A nonspecific antigen reacts with one or more antibodies even though it is biologically different from the antigen that elicited antibody production—for example, sheep or horse red blood cells that react with heterophile antibodies in infectious mononucleosis.

As in clinical chemistry, several methods may be available to detect and measure a given antigen or antibody, including molecular biology methods, to be discussed in the next chapter. The choice of method depends on cost, the availability of materials, equipment, and trained personnel, the volume of testing performed by the laboratory, turnaround time, relative sensitivity and specificity of procedures, and other factors.

The reaction between antigen and antibody can take many forms in the laboratory. The antigen and antibody, separately suspended in solution or gel form, can be combined in a plate or tube in such a fashion that a turbid, opaque, or insoluble complex is formed between them. Such a reaction is called **precipitation**. When the precipitate appears to consist of irregular fleecy masses it may be called **flocculation**. The reaction between antigen and antibody can be accelerated by passing an electric current through the system, which promotes migration of proteins towards the cathode (**immunoelectrophoresis**). In an **agglutination test**, suspended particles of antigenic material are caused to clump by exposure to antibody. These particles may be killed microorganisms, red blood cells, or inert material such as latex coated with antigen.

Besides being treated with chemical stains, bacteriologic smears can also be examined by a **fluorescent antibody technique**. In this method, the smear is treated with a combination of monoclonal antibody to a suspected organism and a fluorescent dye such as rhodamine. If the anticipated antigen-antibody reaction occurs, sites of fixation of the fluorescent antibody can be observed by microscopic examination of the smear with fluorescent lighting. This method is valuable in identifying intracellular organisms, such as *Chlamydia*, which stain poorly if at all by standard staining techniques.

Sometimes antibody is more readily detected by an indirect method. In **inhibition** reactions, competition between two antibodies prevents precipitation or agglutination that would otherwise have occurred. In **complement fixation** (CF) tests, a reaction between antibody and antigen is shown to have taken place by the absorption of complement, a serum protein essential to such reactions.

Precipitation tests are generally qualitative, but most of the other tests mentioned can be made quantitative. The method of using serial dilutions to determine antibody titer was described in an earlier section. A row of test tubes are prepared in which each tube contains a higher dilution of serum or specimen material than the one before it. Test material is added to each tube, and the results of the test are reported as the highest dilution of serum in which antibody activity can still be detected. A report of 1:200 means that antibody activity occurred in all tubes up to and including the one containing the 1:200 dilution of serum, but not at 1:400 or higher dilutions.

A past history of certain infections (or of active immunization against them), and presumed protection against reinfection, is shown by finding a protective titer of antibody to the infecting organisms. In the serologic diagnosis of an acute infection, blood is drawn as soon as possible after the onset of illness and a second specimen of blood is obtained approximately two weeks later. When the suspected infection is present, simultaneous testing of the two specimens shows at least a fourfold rise in the titer of antibody to the infecting organism from the "acute serum" to the "convalescent serum."

Some serologic methods involve application of antibody to detect antigen. Fluorescent antibody (FA) testing has been mentioned already as a means of identifying certain bacteria in smears under the fluorescence microscope. This is an example of direct immunofluorescence. In indirect immunofluorescence, the antibody that reacts with the antigen in the specimen is not fluorescently tagged. After this initial reaction, a fluorescent antibody to the first antibody is applied. In **radioimmunoassay** (RIA) procedures, the antigen or antibody is radioactively tagged. In an **enzyme-linked immunosorbent assay** (ELISA), the antigen or antibody is tagged with an enzyme, whose activity, measured after addition of a suitable substrate, gives a measure of the antigen or antibody bound in the reaction.

In the **Western blot** (immunoblot) procedure (*see box*), proteins (antigens) are separated electrophoretically into bands and then blotted (transferred by direct contact) to a nitrocellulose membrane, where they retain their relative positions. One or more antibodies, tagged with radioisotopes, fluorescent dye, or an enzyme, are then applied to the membrane, where they bind to corresponding antigens, if present. For technical reasons, two antibodies may be used. The first of these, which is unlabeled, reacts with the antigen of interest. The second antibody, chemically tagged, then reacts with the first antibody.

Western Blot

The name of the Western blot is based on a pun. In the 1970s the British biologist Edwin M. Southern developed a method of locating specific DNA sequences by blotting the specimen to a membrane. A variant of this procedure, which used a similar method to isolate RNA sequences, was jocularly called Northern blotting. Inevitably, when a third blotting procedure was invented it came to be known as Western blotting.

Antibody testing using specific antigens is employed routinely in the serologic diagnosis of acute infection, or in establishing prior history of infection, with measles, rubella, mumps, herpes simplex, varicella-zoster, human immunodeficiency virus, cytomegalovirus, and various fungal and parasitic diseases, including toxoplasmosis. The **antistreptolysin O** (ASO) titer is a standard means of detecting recent streptococcal infection. A level of 500-5000 Todd units is seen in active rheumatic fever and acute glomerulonephritis. The **Widal agglutination** test for typhoid fever determines antibody to two antigens (0 and H) derived from *Salmonella* organisms. The *Treponema pallidum* immobilization (TPI) test is a specific antibody test for syphilis, as is the fluorescent treponemal antibody (FTA) test, which uses indirect immunofluorescence.

Several routine tests for the diagnosis of infectious disease use nonspecific antigens, that is, antigens that are biologically distinct from the ones that elicited formation of the antibody with which they react in the test. The serum of a patient with acute or recent infectious mononucleosis contains **heterophile antibodies** in addition to more specific antibodies directed against the causative virus (Epstein-Barr virus). Heterophile antibodies react with a variety of antigens. In the standard heterophile agglutination test, sheep or horse erythrocytes are agglutinated by the serum of a patient with infectious mononucleosis in a titer of 1:112 of higher. The serum is first treated with an extract of guinea pig kidney to adsorb nonrelevant antibodies.

The **VDRL** (Venereal Disease Research Laboratories) test for syphilis, and its modification, the **RPR** (rapid plasma reagin), use beef heart cardiolipin as an antigen. Sometimes the term serology is used in the narrow sense of "serologic test for syphilis," which may also be abbreviated STS. In the **Weil-Felix** test, antigens from various strains of *Proteus vulgaris* are used to identify antibody to various rickettsiae. High levels of antibody to *Proteus* antigens OX-19 and OX-2 are found in Rocky Mountain spotted fever and typhus, while antibody to OX-K antigen occurs in scrub typhus. Patients with mycoplasmal pneumonia form antibodies called **cold agglutinins**, which agglutinate type O human erythrocytes at 4°C but not at 20° or 37°.

Serologic tests with nonspecific antigens are often preferred to more specific tests because they are inexpensive and relatively sensitive. But for the very reason that they are less specific, they may yield a high proportion of false positive tests, and their results must be interpreted in the light of the patient's history, physical findings, and other test results.

A panel of tests for various **febrile agglutinins** is sometimes performed in cases of fever of unknown origin. A typical panel includes agglutination titers for typhoid (Widal O and H), paratyphoid, brucellosis, tularemia, leptospirosis, and rickettsiae (Weil-Felix).

Methods are available to detect viral and other antigens in serum with monoclonal antibody. Testing for three antigenic fractions of the hepatitis B virus (hepatitis B core antigen or HB_cAg, surface antigen or HB_sAg, and e antigen or HB_eAg) in serum provides information about the stage of the disease.

Blood typing (grouping), discussed in Chapter 19, makes use of type-specific antisera. In addition, serologic testing is used to identify acquired hemolytic anemias including those arising from Rh incompatibility.

Serologic testing also finds application in the diagnosis of allergy, autoimmune disease, and certain neoplasms. The **radioallergosorbent test** (RAST), a modification of radioimmunoassay, uses isotopically tagged allergens to detect IgE antibodies to these allergens in the serum of allergic persons.

Several laboratory tests have been found useful in identifying abnormal globulin activity in persons with autoimmune disease. Such studies can detect antibody to acetylcholine receptors in myasthenia gravis, to DNA in systemic lupus erythematosus, to glomerular basement membrane in glomerulonephritis, to neutrophilic cytoplasm in Wegener's granulomatosis, to mitochondria in primary biliary cirrhosis, to myocardium in rheumatic fever and myocarditis, to gastric parietal cells in pernicious anemia and chronic gastritis, to thyroid microsomes in chronic thyroiditis, to thyrotropin receptors in Graves disease, and to pancreatic beta cells or insulin receptors in diabetes mellitus.

The lupus erythematosus cell test (**LE cell prep**) is performed by incubating the patient's blood under controlled conditions and then observing a stained smear for LE cells. The LE cell is a neutrophil with a very large cytoplasmic inclusion produced by the action of the patient's abnormal antibodies on the cell nucleus. The test is positive in disseminated lupus erythematosus and in some cases of scleroderma, dermatomyositis, and rheumatoid arthritis. Immunofluorescence testing of tissue slices for antinuclear antibody (ANA) may provide differentiating information among these disorders depending on whether the fluorescence pattern noted is homogeneous, speckled, or confined to the nuclear rim or to the nucleolus.

Rheumatoid factor (RF) is an IgM antibody that is directed against the patient's own IgG. It can be detected by various tests, including a latex agglutination test in which the patient's serum is incubated with latex particles coated with human IgG. These tests are positive in about two-thirds of patients with rheumatoid arthritis and in some persons with other autoimmune disorders.

Tumor markers are substances produced in abnormal amounts by certain neoplasms. Testing for these substances is useful diagnostically to distinguish between benign and malignant tumors, and serial testing for them can be used to monitor disease progression or to detect recurrences after surgery or chemotherapy. Several of these substances (AFP, CEA, and others) were discussed among clinical chemistry procedures in Chapter 20 for the sake of completeness, even though testing for them is usually performed with immunologic or molecular biology methods. As mentioned earlier, the use of these tests to screen asymptomatic persons is not recommended.

Skin Testing

Some diagnostic procedures are performed by applying antigens or other substances to the skin, or injecting them in small quantities between layers of the skin, and noting any local reaction (redness, swelling) that occurs. Skin testing is widely used in the diagnosis of allergy, particularly respiratory allergy (allergic rhinitis and asthma), and

of certain infectious diseases, particularly tuberculosis.

A standard battery of **allergy skin tests** might include twenty or more allergens, including various dusts, dust mites, tree and grass pollens, and molds, which are applied in a grid pattern on the upper back or on one or both arms. Reactions occur within 20-30 minutes and are graded 1+ to 4+ on the basis of the size (in millimeters) and configuration of any resulting reaction. The typical positive reaction is a wheal, a zone of skin swelling and redness. Formation of pseudopods (rounded extensions from the margin of the wheal) indicates more severe sensitivity.

Allergy skin testing must be interpreted in the light of the patient's history and physical findings. Selection of pollens that are likely to be found in the patient's geographic area is essential. Allergy skin testing can confirm specific sensitivities, identify avoidable allergens in the patient's environment, and guide selection of antigens for desensitization therapy (allergy "vaccine"). Blood testing by RAST is more expensive and less sensitive than skin testing.

Skin testing is also a standard means of diagnosing prior or active infection with *Mycobacterium tuberculosis* and certain pathogenic fungi. These tests detect tissue antibodies, which cause induration (firm swelling) at the test site after an interval of days.

Candidates for **tuberculin skin testing** include persons who have had close contact with a case of active tuberculosis, persons who are HIV-positive or are subject to other forms of immune compromise, persons with chest x-ray evidence suggestive of healed tuberculosis, and persons from geographic areas having high prevalence of tuberculosis. Health-care personnel and residents of nursing homes and correctional facilities are tested annually.

The testing material used is PPD (purified protein derivative), a standardized extract of tuberculosis organisms. In the standard Mantoux test, 0.1 mL of PPD, containing 5 units of tuberculin, is injected intradermally (between layers of the skin) on the volar surface of a forearm with a fine-gauge needle. The test is read between 48 and 72 hours after it is applied. Redness at the test site does not indicate tuberculin sensitivity and is ignored. Any induration (firm swelling) at the site is noted and measured in millimeters.

Induration of 5 mm or more is interpreted as a positive tuberculin test in an HIV-positive person or an IV drug abuser of unknown HIV status, a person who has been in contact with a person with active tuberculosis, or a person who has chest x-ray evidence of an old tuberculous infection. Induration of 10 mm or more is interpreted as a positive tuberculin test in a foreign-born person from a region where prevalence of tuberculosis is high, a homeless or indigent person, a resident of a long-term care facility, nursing home, or correctional facility, a health care worker, or a person with medical risk factors (diabetes mellitus, silicosis, end-stage renal disease, immunosuppressive therapy). In persons with no risk factors, induration of 15 mm or more is interpreted as a positive tuberculin test. A positive skin test for tuberculosis is followed up with chest x-ray and other testing as appropriate for the patient's history, physical findings, and risk factors.

In an older person, tuberculin reactivity due to infection in early life may wane so that the tuberculin test yields a negative result. The testing itself may, however, boost reactivity, so that on repeat testing the patient has a positive reaction. In order to distinguish such persons from others who truly convert from negative to positive between the first and second test, the two-step tuberculin test may be administered.

In this procedure, a person who is being tested for the first time and who will continue to receive testing annually (for example, a newly hired health-care worker) is given a second tuberculin test 1-3 weeks after the first one, if the first is negative. If the second test is positive, a booster response is probable rather than recent conversion due to current infection.

Fungal skin tests are also performed to identify past or present infection with certain pathogenic fungi, most of which cause chronic pulmonary disease. These include histoplasmosis, blastomycosis, and coccidioidomycosis.

Exercises

Fill in the Blanks

1. _____ is the branch of biology and medicine that is concerned with the defensive responses of living organisms to exposure to substances or organisms that are recognized as foreign and potentially harmful.

2. _____ embraces laboratory technologies and strategies based on antigen-antibody reactions, including a number of procedures that do not involve testing of serum.

3. In _____ tests, a reaction between antibody and antigen is shown to have taken place by the absorption of complement, a serum protein essential to such reactions.

4. In _____ procedures, the antigen or antibody is radioactively tagged.

5. In _____ the antigen or antibody is tagged with an enzyme, whose activity, measured after addition of a suitable substrate, gives a measure of the antigen or antibody bound in the reaction.

6. Antigens that are biologically distinct from the ones that elicited formation of the antibody with which they react in the test are called _____.

7. Two tests used to identify syphilis are the _____ test and the _____.

8. Patients with mycoplasmal pneumonia form antibodies called _____, which agglutinate type O human erythrocytes at 4°C but not at 20° or 37°.

9. The _____ is a neutrophil with a very large cytoplasmic inclusion produced by the action of the patient's abnormal antibodies on the cell nucleus.

10. The typical positive reaction to an allergy skin test is a _____, a zone of skin swelling and redness; formation of _____ (rounded extensions from the margin of the wheal) indicates more severe sensitivity.

Multiple Choice: Circle the letter of the best answer from the choices given.

1. Which of the following terms refers to a substance that is chemically or biologically identical to the one that elicited antibody formation?
   A. Antigen-antibody formation.
   B. Specific antigen.
   C. Nonspecific antigen.
   D. Antibody titer.
   E. Serologic test.

Exercises

2. When the antigen and antibody, separately suspended in solution or gel form, are combined in a plate or tube in such a fashion that a turbid, opaque, or insoluble complex is formed between them, the reaction is called
   A. Flocculation.
   B. Agglutination.
   C. Inhibition.
   D. Precipitation.
   E. Complement fixation.

3. Which of the following refers to the process of accelerating the reaction between antigen and antibody by passing an electric current through the system, which promotes migration of proteins towards the cathode?
   A. Complement fixation.
   B. Agglutination.
   C. Immunoelectrophoresis.
   D. Inhibition.
   E. Precipitation.

4. _____ is a test in which suspended particles of killed microorganisms, red blood cells, or inert material such as latex coated with antigen are caused to clump by exposure to antibody.
   A. Agglutination.
   B. Inhibition.
   C. Precipitation.
   D. Immunoelectrophoresis.
   E. Complement fixation.

5. In this indirect method of serologic testing, competition between two antibodies prevents precipitation or agglutination that would otherwise have occurred.
   A. Agglutination.
   B. Inhibition.
   C. Precipitation.
   D. Immunoelectrophoresis.
   E. Complement fixation.

6. Which of the following is a standard means of detecting recent streptococcal infection?
   A. Widal agglutination test.
   B. *Treponema pallidum* immobilization (TPI) test.
   C. Fluorescent treponemal antibody (FTA) test.
   D. Immunoelectrophoresis.
   E. Antistreptolysin O (ASO) titer.

Exercises

7. Which of the following is a common test for allergies?
   A. Antinuclear antibody (ANA).
   B. LE cell prep.
   C. Cold agglutinins.
   D. Febrile agglutinins.
   E. Radioallergosorbent test (RAST).

8. Which of the following tests is useful in detecting rheumatoid factor (RF), an IgM antibody that is directed against the patient's own IgG?
   A. Cold agglutinins.
   B. Febrile agglutinins.
   C. Widal agglutination.
   D. Latex agglutination.
   E. Alpha fetoprotein (AFP).

9. In addition to testing for allergies, skin testing may also be used to test for which of the following conditions?
   A. Tuberculosis.
   B. Multiple sclerosis.
   C. Measles.
   D. Chickenpox.
   E. Rubella.

10. Induration of 10 mm or more is interpreted as a positive tuberculin test in which category of persons?
    A. A healthcare worker.
    B. The immunocompromised.
    C. The foreign-born.
    D. One with no known risk factors.
    E. None of the above.

Short Answers

1. Define or explain:
   a. convalescent serum _____

   _____

   b. febrile agglutinins _____

   _____

   c. STS _____

   _____

Exercises

2. What basic type of reaction is studied in a serologic test?

     _____

     _____

3. What are some reasons for preferring serologic testing to culture of pathogenic microorganisms?

     _____

     _____

     _____

     _____

4. List three purposes for serologic testing.

     a. _____

          _____

     b. _____

          _____

     c. _____

          _____

5. Give an example of a diagnostic antibody test that uses a nonspecific antigen.

     _____

     _____

     _____

     _____

6. List some serologic tests that are used to diagnose diseases or conditions that are not infections.

     _____

     _____

     _____

     _____

Exercises

7. When several methods may be available to detect and measure a given antigen or antibody, including molecular biology methods, what does the choice of method depend on?

_____

_____

_____

_____

8. What is the fluorescent antibody technique useful for? Describe the procedure.

_____

_____

_____

_____

_____

_____

_____

_____

9. Describe the method of using serial dilutions to determine antibody titer. Is this a qualitative or quantitative analysis?

_____

_____

_____

_____

_____

_____

_____

_____

10. Which test gets its named based on a pun? Explain.

_____

_____

_____

_____

Exercises

Activities for Application and Further Study

1. Monoclonal antibodies can be used for serologic testing and for therapeutic purposes. Research and identify several popular monoclonal antibodies that are used in testing as well as several others that are used therapeutically.

2. Have you or someone you know had allergy skin testing? Describe the procedure. Bring in (by requesting from the doctor) or find on the Internet photos of reactions. Identify the testing antigen and whether the reaction was positive or negative.

3. Find photos of positive tuberculin skin tests on the Internet for the three categories of positivity discussed in the text (that is, the immunocompromised patient, the foreign born or homeless patient, and in persons with no known risk factors).

Molecular Biology 23

A branch of biochemistry that focuses on biological phenomena at the molecular level, particularly with respect to DNA, RNA, and the chemistry of genes, molecular biology has important applications to microbiology and immunology as well as to medical genetics.

DNA (deoxyribonucleic acid) is a general term for a nearly infinite variety of large molecules that are concerned in the control of cellular function and in the transmission of genetic information. As the name suggests, these molecules are found in the nuclei of cells. Every DNA molecule, no matter how complex, is made up of long chains of the same four units or building blocks in various sequences. Each of these building blocks contains a five-carbon sugar (deoxyribose), a phosphate link, and one of four nucleotide bases: the purines adenine (A) and guanine (G) and the pyrimidines cytosine (C) and thymine (T). Genes, which will be discussed in the next section, are the units of heredity. Each gene is a segment of a DNA molecule.

Besides being capable of reproducing (copying) themselves, DNA molecules direct the production of intracellular proteins and enzymes through the medium of RNA (ribonucleic acid). RNA differs from DNA only in its sugar component (ribose instead of deoxyribose) and in substituting uracil (U) for thymine. In the formation of an RNA molecule, base units pair up with base units of DNA in complementary fashion, adenine always pairing with thymine or uracil and cytosine always pairing with guanine. The DNA molecule thus serves as a template for the generation of the RNA molecule.

In turn, the RNA molecule then serves as a template for the synthesis of proteins and enzymes, a process that takes place in intracellular structures called ribosomes. A codon is a sequence of three bases (for example, AAG or CUG) that conveys a distinct piece of chemical information. Most of the 64 possible codons direct the incorporation of specific amino acids into a polypeptide chain, but a few direct chain initiation or chain termination.

Every cell nucleus in a living organism carries an identical complement of DNA that is unique to that species. (In human beings, the statistical probability is that the composition of each person's DNA is unique to that individual.) This is the basis for most molecular biology techniques, which seek to identify unique sequences of DNA in specimen material. A DNA probe is a short nucleotide sequence, synthesized in the laboratory and labeled with a radioactive isotope, dye, or enzyme, that seeks out and fuses (hybridizes) with a complementary sequence on a larger DNA molecule. Theoretically, for each unique DNA sequence sought in a specimen, a probe can be fabricated that will fuse with it.

The use of DNA probes allows identification of very small concentrations of antigen or antibody in specimens. **In situ hybridization** detects unique DNA sequences in cells or tissue specimens by application of probes that have been tagged with a radioisotope or a fluorescent dye (FISH = fluorescent in situ hybridization). **Dot-blot** (or slot-blot) hybridization detects specific DNA (deoxyribonucleic acid) sequences in small spots of specimen material that have been blotted through round holes (or slots) in a template.

The **polymerase chain reaction** (PCR) (*see box*) is a method for the repeated copying of DNA in a particular gene sequence. In this process, specimen DNA is combined with specially designed primers and then enzymatically induced to replicate many times. This technique is widely used to amplify very small quantities of biological material so as to provide adequate specimens for laboratory study.

Rapid tests to identify streptococci in material obtained by throat swab in acute pharyngitis (strep screens) and urine tests to detect chlamydia and gonococcus use PCR technology and DNA probes.

Several methods are available to measure the **plasma level of viral DNA** in chronic viral infec-

What Is a Polymerase Chain Reaction?

A polymerase is an enzyme that promotes the formation of polymers— long chains of similar molecular units. The replication of DNA in living cells is facilitated by polymerases, which build up a chain by adding free nucleotides, one at a time, that are complementary to the base pairs in the strand being copied. In the laboratory, many copies of a DNA strand can be produced by setting off a polymerase chain reaction. This is done by exposing the specimen material to a mixture of free nucleotides, primers, and Taq polymerase, which is derived from a thermophilic (heat-loving) bacterium, *Thermus aquaticus*.

Replication can be triggered repeatedly by changing the temperature of the system, each cycle yielding many copies of the DNA strands produced in the previous cycle. PCR technology is highly sensitive and highly specific, and does not require prior purification of specimens. Besides its use in diagnostic immunology, it has important applications in genetic research and oncology. The American biochemist Kary Mullis won a Nobel Prize in Chemistry in 1993 for developing this technique.

tions such as HIV infection. Serial measurements of HIV viral load are routinely performed to monitor the course of AIDS. Reported as the number of copies of viral RNA per mL of plasma, viral load indicates the prognosis of persons infected with HIV and helps in deciding when to start antiretroviral therapy, and to assess the response to therapy. Therapy is usually begun when the plasma HIV RNA concentration exceeds 10-25 000 copies/mL. When the number of copies falls below the number that can be detected, viral replication is considered to have been suppressed by treatment.

Some species of virus can be divided, on the basis of variations in DNA, into several types, which may vary in infectivity and clinical behavior. In persons infected with these viruses, **viral typing** can provide valuable diagnostic, prognostic, and therapeutic guidance.

The human papillomavirus (HPV) causes warts on skin and mucous membranes. Over 70 types have been identified, variously affecting the skin of the face, hands, plantar surfaces, and mucocutaneous surfaces (genitals and perianal regions). Genital warts, due to type 6 or 11, are the most common viral sexually transmitted disease. As discussed in Chapter 17, some types of HPV induce dysplastic changes in the cervix that culminate in malignancy. At least 80% of all cervical cancers are due to HPV infection, and 25% of all irregularities seen on Pap smears probably result from the presence of the virus.

Clinical management of cervical dysplasia is based on a consideration of the extent and severity of the dysplasia as well as risk factors for malignant change, including the presence and type of HPV infection. In patients with atypical squamous cells of undetermined significance (ASC-US) and low-grade squamous intraepithelial lesion (LGSIL), HPV testing and typing permits discrimination between those with no evidence of virus, or with low-risk virus types, in whom observation and repeat Pap smear are recommended, and those with high-risk virus types, for whom colposcopy and cervical biopsy are advisable.

Invasive cervical cancer is associated with HPV types 16, 18, 31, 33, 35, and 39. HPV typing in women with atypical squamous cells of undetermined significance (ASC-US) on cervical Pap smear helps to identify those in whom more intensive surveillance for premalignant change is warranted. Women with external genital warts are not at increased risk of cervical cancer and do not need colposcopy or other special surveillance if routine Pap smears are negative.

Medical Genetics

The inheritance of physical traits such as eye and hair color depends on the transmission of genes from parents to offspring. The gene is the functional unit of heredity, each gene transmitting a single trait or function. Most genes work by directing the synthesis of peptides, proteins, or enzymes by means of RNA, as described above. The nucleus of every cell in the body contains the same complement of genes, more than 30 000 of them, which are unique to the individual. Genes are arranged in bands lying transversely along coiled strips of DNA called chromosomes.

A human cell nucleus contains 46 chromosomes, arranged in 23 pairs. One pair, the sex chromosomes, determine the sex of an individual: females have two X chromosomes (XX) and males have an X and a Y chromosome (XY). The other 22 pairs of chromosomes, which are called autosomes, are concerned with the transmission of traits not pertaining to biological gender. The autosomes are numbered from 1 to 22, in order of decreasing length. Each consists of a long arm (q) and a short arm (p), which are joined at the centromere.

Body cells other than gametes (reproductive cells) multiply by splitting into two identical daughter cells. Before cell division takes place, the nucleus divides into two identical nuclei. In this process, called mitosis, each chromosome forms a copy of itself. In the formation of gametes (female oocyte, male sperm), the chromosome pairs divide by a process called meiosis, so that each daughter cell has only 23 chromosomes instead of 23 pairs of chromosomes. When sperm and oocyte unite, the full complement of 23 pairs of chromosomes is restored, one of each pair having come from each parent.

Each gene (for example, the eye color gene) has a fixed normal position, or locus, on a specific chromosome. Each arm of each chromosome is divided into regions, bands, and subbands for the purpose of designating gene loci. The two genes that occupy corresponding loci on a pair of chromosomes are said to be homologous. These genes may be identical or not. The group of two or more variant genes (e.g., the blue eye gene and the brown eye gene) that can occupy a given locus are called alleles.

When homologous genes are identical (for example, when both genes for eye color specify blue eyes), the individual is said to be homozygous for the trait coded by that gene. When homologous genes are not identical (for example, one coding for blue eyes and the other for brown eyes), the individual is said to be heterozygous for eye color.

Some genes exert their effects only in homozygous individuals. That is, both genes at a given locus must be identical. Such a gene is said to be recessive, because if it appears on only one chromosome of a pair, the trait for which it codes is not expressed. An individual having only one recessive gene is called a carrier of that gene, because it can be transmitted to some or all offspring. A gene that has its effect even in a heterozygous individual, that is, when paired with a gene that is not identical to it, is said to be dominant.

The phenotype of an individual is the sum of features and traits that can be observed by inspection, measurement, biochemical testing, or other means. The genotype is the individual's actual genetic composition, which determines the phenotype.

Genetic Abnormalities

As already mentioned, most genes function by encoding (directing) the cellular synthesis of proteins or enzymes. The absence of a gene, or the possession of a defective copy of it, can have a broad range of effects, or no effect at all, depending on the normal function of that gene. It is estimated that human beings are subject to at least 4,000 inheritable diseases.

Genetic defects, in general, are transmitted in the same way as normal traits. Defects in autosomes are called autosomal (dominant or recessive). Defects in sex chromosomes are called sex-linked or (since they all affect the X chromosome) X-linked. Some inherited disorders, including cleft lip and palate, apparently result from abnormalities in more than one gene.

An abnormality in the genetic composition of an individual can be inherited from one or both parents or can result from some aberration in the process whereby genetic information is transferred from parents to offspring. A germline **mutation** is an accidental biochemical change in a gene that permanently alters or cancels the effect of that gene in the individual in whom it occurs, and that can be passed on to that individual's offspring, though it may not be expressed in the first generation. For example, through mutation a person with normal parents can acquire a defective form of a gene and so fail to form a protein or enzyme coded by the normal, operative form of the gene.

Usually a mutation affects only one gene. A point mutation is a change in just one of the nucleotide bases in a single codon. This can be a missense mutation (coding the wrong amino acid), a nonsense mutation (terminating an amino acid chain instead of adding to it), or a frameshift mutation (addition or deletion of a nucleotide base).

Aberrations can occur in the process by which chromosomes divide up during meiosis and then pair off after conception. These can affect large parts of chromosomes or even whole chromosomes. **Translocation** is an interchange of fragments between two chromosomes. Chronic myelogenous leukemia results from a translocation between chromosomes 9 and 22, resulting in the so-called Philadelphia chromosome. **Inversion** means that a fragment broken off from a chromosome has rotated end-for-end before re-attaching. **Deletion** is the complete loss of part of a chromosome.

Aneuploidy is an abnormal number of chromosomes (more or less than the normal 46). This results from **nondisjunction** during meiosis,

whereby both copies of a gene are carried to one daughter cell and none to the other. A person with Down syndrome (trisomy 21) has three copies of chromosome 21 and hence a total of 47 chromosomes. A person with Turner syndrome has only one X chromosome and no Y chromosome, and hence a total of only 45 chromosomes.

A gene whose possession confers an increased risk of cancer is called an **oncogene**. Oncogenes develop through mutation of proto-oncogenes, which normally encode proteins that stimulate or regulate cell growth. When mutated or influenced by certain viruses, they can trigger malignant cell proliferation. Only one copy (allele) of a proto-oncogene need undergo mutation to induce tumor formation.

Tumor suppressor genes (antioncogenes) encode proteins that normally serve to restrain cell proliferation. If both copies of a tumor suppressor gene are mutated or deleted, unrestrained cell proliferation and malignant change may occur. A familial tendency to develop certain cancers is usually due to an inherited mutation in one copy of a tumor suppressor gene, which is thus defective in every cell in the body. If the other copy is inactivated in just one of those cells, cancer may develop. The **BRCA1** and **BRCA2** genes, which predispose to familial early-onset breast cancer and ovarian cancer, are tumor suppressor genes.

Genetic Testing

Any procedure performed to assess some aspect of a person's genetic makeup (genotype or genome) can be said to pertain to the broad field of genetic testing. Such testing may be performed to establish the identity of an individual or the blood relationship of two or more individuals; to confirm biological gender; to reveal a suspected hereditary disorder in a child with evident congenital deformity, mental or physical retardation, or delayed puberty; to screen for genetic mutations (oncogenes) known to increase the risk of certain cancers; or to confirm the presence of inheritable disease in the genotype of the subject and the likelihood of its transmission to offspring. Although most genetic testing involves examination of the subject's DNA, it may also include testing of blood, urine, or other fluids or tissues to detect biochemical markers of hereditary disease.

Laboratory techniques used to identify individuals by molecular genotyping have been called **DNA fingerprinting**. These methods, more formally called DNA profiling, are based on the detection of distinctive DNA sequences in human cellular material (skin, hair, blood, semen). Their principal applications are in determining paternity and maternity, identifying human remains, and matching biological material left at a crime scene with that of a suspect.

The most distinctive features of an individual's genetic makeup are variations in the length and distribution of variable number tandem repeats (VNTRs) and short tandem repeats (STRs) between the genes. These nucleotide sequences do not transmit genetic information but are highly consistent within each person's cells and highly variable from one person to another.

Human leukocyte antigens (HLA) are surface proteins that occur on most cell surfaces and are important in cell recognition and immune responses. They vary in type from person to person on a genetic basis. They are also called histocompatibility antigens because the likelihood of successful allografting (transfer of living tissue from one person to another) is in proportion to the match between donor's and recipient's HLA types. Besides being used to test potential graft donors and recipients, HLA typing may be performed for diagnostic purposes. Certain HLA types predispose to specific diseases. For example, HLA-DR4 is associated with rheumatoid arthritis, HLA-DR2 with multiple sclerosis. The HLA-B27 is found in 90% of persons with ankylosing spondylitis.

Sex chromatin analysis is performed on a stained smear of any body cells, usually a buccal smear (from inside the cheek). For prenatal sex determination, chromatin analysis is performed on cells from amniotic fluid obtained by amniocentesis. The Barr body is a small mass lying at the periphery of about one-half of the cells of a genetic female but absent from cells of a genetic male.

Large chromosomal abnormalities such as transposition and deletion can be detected by **karyotyping**. In this procedure, lymphocytes from a blood specimen or tissue cells from a skin biopsy are grown in tissue culture. Mitosis is induced by application of chemical agent (mitogen) and then abruptly arrested with colchicine. Slides of the cells are prepared and special stains (quinacrine, Giemsa stain, acridine orange) are applied to show chromosome banding.

The slides are examined microscopically, and if chromosomes are clearly visible in several cells undergoing mitosis, these are photographed. Individual chromosomes appearing in the photograph are cut out and pasted on a form in standard order, autosomes 1 to 22 followed by sex chromosomes (X and, if one is present, Y) (*see Fig. 23.1*). The resulting karyotype confirms the number of chromosomes and identifies gross structural aberrations such as deletion and inversion.

More specific genetic studies involve seeking DNA sequences characteristic of abnormal genes by the use of DNA probes. Testing for oncogenes or for their protein products in biopsy tissue can provide important information about the type and prognosis of a malignant tumor, as well as guiding the choice of treatment. More than 150 cytogenetic abnormalities have been associated with specific neoplasms.

Indications for **prenatal genetic studies** include advanced maternal age (which increases the risk of Down syndrome), genetic disease in either parent, a history of a birth defect with a previous pregnancy, and abnormal findings on prenatal ultrasound examination. Amniotic fluid, obtained by amniocentesis (needle aspiration from the amniotic sac) at or after the four-

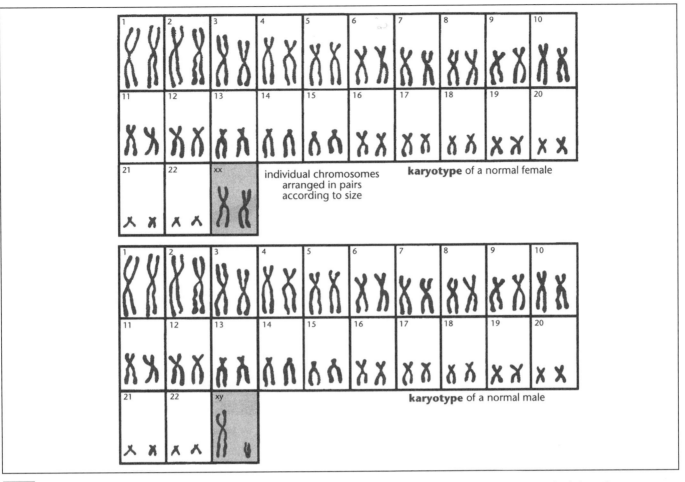

Fig. 23.1. Karyotype. Reproduced with permission from *Melloni's Illustrated Medical Dictionary*, 4th ed. (2002).

teenth week of gestation, supplies fetal cells for karyotyping, DNA analysis, and testing for biochemical markers of inherited diseases such as phenylketonuria and neural tube defects such as anencephaly and spina bifida, as discussed in Chapter 20.

Chorionic villus sampling (CVS) is a biopsy of placental (chorionic) villi performed in early pregnancy to detect genetic defects in the fetus. This biopsy can be obtained at an earlier date than amniocentesis, around 8-10 weeks' gestation, but does not provide material for detection of biochemical markers of inherited disease. A preliminary ultrasound examination of the pelvis is performed to determine the size of the gestational sac and the position of the placenta. Under further ultrasound guidance, a biopsy catheter is inserted through the cervix, or a needle is introduced into the uterine cavity through a puncture in the abdominal wall, and a small sample of material (15-20 mL) is withdrawn by suction. The risk of miscarriage after chorionic villus biopsy is 2-4%.

430 Laboratory Tests & Diagnostic Procedures in Medicine

Exercises

Fill in the Blanks

1. _____ is a branch of biochemistry that focuses on biological phenomena at the molecular level, particularly with respect to DNA, RNA, and the chemistry of genes,

2. Genes are the units of _____; each gene is a segment of a _____.

3. A _____ is a short nucleotide sequence, synthesized in the laboratory and labeled with a radioactive isotope, dye, or enzyme, that seeks out and fuses (hybridizes) with a complementary sequence on a larger DNA molecule.

4. The FISH test (or _____) detects unique DNA sequences in cells or tissue specimens by application of probes that have been tagged with a fluorescent dye.

5. _____, due to type 6 or 11, are the most common viral sexually transmitted disease.

6. At least 80% of all cervical cancers are due to _____ infection, and 25% of all irregularities seen on Pap smears probably result from the presence of the virus.

7. In patients with _____ and _____, HPV testing and typing permits discrimination between those with no evidence of virus and those with high-risk virus types.

8. Genes are arranged in bands lying transversely along coiled strips of DNA called _____.

9. Females have ____ X chromosome(s) and males have ____ X chromosome(s), ____ Y chromosome(s).

10. In body cells other than gametes, the nucleus divides into two identical nuclei by a process called _____ with each chromosome forming a copy of itself before the cell splits into two identical daughter cells.

11. The autosomes are numbered from 1 to 22, in order of decreasing length, each consisting of a _____ and _____, which are joined at the centromere.

12. _____ genes exert their effects only when both genes at a given locus on the chromosome are identical.

13. A germline _____ is an accidental biochemical change in a gene that permanently alters or cancels the effect of that gene in the individual in whom it occurs, and that can be passed on to that individual's offspring, though it may not be expressed in the first generation.

14. _____ is an abnormal number of chromosomes (more or less than the normal 46).

Exercises

15. If both copies of a _____ are mutated or deleted, unrestrained cell proliferation and malignant change may occur.

16. The _____ and _____ genes, which predispose to familial early-onset breast cancer and ovarian cancer, are tumor suppressor genes.

17. _____ at or after the fourteenth week of gestation, supplies fetal cells for karyotyping, DNA analysis, and testing for biochemical markers of inherited diseases such as phenylketonuria and neural tube defects such as anencephaly and spina bifida.

Multiple Choice: Circle the letter of the best answer from the choices given.

1. Which of the following is a general term for a nearly infinite variety of large molecules that are concerned in the control of cellular function and in the transmission of genetic information?
   A. Molecular biology.
   B. DNA (deoxyribonucleic acid).
   C. RNA (ribonucleic acid).
   D. Gene.
   E. Trait.

2. The four building blocks of DNA include all of the following except
   A. Uracil (U).
   B. Guanine (G).
   C. Cytosine (C).
   D. Thymine (T).
   E. Adenine (A).

3. The four building blocks of RNA include all of the following except
   A. Uracil (U).
   B. Guanine (G).
   C. Cytosine (C).
   D. Thymine (T).
   E. Adenine (A).

4. This test detects unique DNA sequences in cells or tissue specimens by application of probes that have been tagged with a radioisotope or a fluorescent dye.
   A. Dot-blot (or slot-blot) hybridization.
   B. Polymerase chain reaction (PCR).
   C. DNA fingerprinting.
   D. In situ hybridization.
   E. Human leukocyte antigens (HLA) testing.

Exercises

5. This test detects specific DNA (deoxyribonucleic acid) sequences in small spots of specimen material that have been blotted through round holes in a template.
   A. DNA fingerprinting.
   B. Polymerase chain reaction (PCR).
   C. Dot-blot (or slot-blot) hybridization.
   D. Fluorescent in situ hybridization (FISH).
   E. Human leukocyte antigens (HLA) testing.

6. This technique is widely used to amplify very small quantities of biological material so as to provide adequate specimens for laboratory study.
   A. Polymerase chain reaction (PCR).
   B. In situ hybridization.
   C. Dot-blot (or slot-blot) hybridization.
   D. Fluorescent in situ hybridization (FISH).
   E. Human leukocyte antigens (HLA) testing.

7. In persons infected with some species of virus which may vary in infectivity and clinical behavior on the basis of variations in DNA, this procedure can provide valuable diagnostic, prognostic, and therapeutic guidance.
   A. Viral load determination.
   B. Viral typing.
   C. Human leukocyte antigens (HLA) testing.
   D. Fluorescent in situ hybridization (FISH).
   E. Polymerase chain reaction (PCR).

8. All normal human cell nuclei contain
   A. 2 Y chromosomes.
   B. 2 X chromosomes.
   C. 1 X and 1 Y chromosome.
   D. 22 pairs of chromosomes.
   E. 23 pairs of chromosomes.

9. Which of the following terms refers to the sum of features and traits that can be observed in an individual by inspection, measurement, biochemical testing, or other means?
   A. Mitosis.
   B. Recessive
   C. Phenotype.
   D. Meiosis.
   E. Genotype.

Exercises

10. Which of the following terms refers to the individual's actual genetic composition, which determines the pheno-type?
    A. Gamete.
    B. Genotype.
    C. Dominant.
    D. Heterozygous.
    E. Meiosis.

11. Defects in the 22 pairs of chromosomes that are not sex chromosomes are called
    A. Autosomal.
    B. Dominant.
    C. Chromosomal.
    D. Recessive.
    E. X-linked.

12. Defects in sex chromosomes are called sex-linked or
    A. Autosomal.
    B. Dominant.
    C. Chromosomal.
    D. Recessive.
    E. X-linked.

13. This condition is a consequence of aneuploidy or an abnormal number of chromosomes.
    A. Chronic myelogenous leukemia.
    B. Early onset breast cancer.
    C. Ovarian cancer.
    D. Down syndrome.
    E. Type IV intersexuality.

14. The principal applications of this genotyping technique are in determining paternity and maternity, identifying human remains, and matching biological material left at a crime scene with that of a suspect.
    A. Human leukocyte antigen testing.
    B. Karyotyping.
    C. DNA profiling.
    D. Sex chromatin analysis.
    E. DNA probe testing.

Exercises

15. Besides being used to test potential graft donors and recipients, this procedure may be performed to help diagnose diseases such as rheumatoid arthritis, multiple sclerosis, and ankylosing spondylitis.
    A. Human leukocyte antigen testing.
    B. Karyotyping.
    C. DNA profiling,
    D. Sex chromatin analysis.
    E. DNA probe testing.

16. Gross structural aberrations such as deletion and inversion can be identified through a testing process called
    A. Human leukocyte antigen testing.
    B. Karyotyping.
    C. DNA profiling,
    D. Sex chromatin analysis.
    E. DNA probe testing.

17. This type of placental biopsy procedure can be performed in early pregnancy to detect genetic defects in the fetus.
    A. Amniocentesis.
    B. Chorionic villus sampling.
    C. Karyotyping.
    D. Sex chromatin analysis.
    E. Human leukocyte antigen testing.

Short Answers

1. Define or explain:
   a. codon _____

   _____

   b. gene _____

   _____

   c. karyotype _____

   _____

   d. oncogene _____

   _____

   e. polymerase chain reaction _____

   _____

Exercises

    f.   viral load _____

_____

2. List three nonmedical applications of molecular biology.

    a. _____

    b. _____

    c. _____

3. Explain the difference between a recessive gene and a dominant gene.

_____

_____

_____

_____

4. How does polymerase chain reaction technology improve the sensitivity of laboratory testing?

_____

_____

_____

_____

_____

_____

5. What are some reasons for doing prenatal genetic testing?

_____

_____

_____

_____

Exercises

6. How does cell division in gametes differ from that of non-gamete cells?

_____

_____

_____

_____

_____

_____

_____

_____

7. List and explain three aberrations that can occur in the process by which chromosomes divide up during meiosis and then pair off after conception.

a. _____

_____

b. _____

_____

c. _____

_____

Activities for Application and Further Study

1. On the Internet, find karyotypes for genetic diseases caused by aneuploidy, or an abnormal number of chromosomes. Identify the missing or extra chromosome by its location for each of the diseases you research.

2. Paternity cases are periodically in the news. Several cases have been related to the "switching" of children at birth so that infants go home with the wrong parents. Other "newsworthy" cases have been related to fathers contesting child support. Research and summarize some of these cases. Do you think the ability to use DNA testing for such purposes is a positive or negative?

Laboratory Examination of Urine, Stool, and Other Fluids and Materials

24

LEARNING OBJECTIVES

Upon completion of this chapter, the student should be able to

- Describe basic laboratory tests of urine;

- Describe basic laboratory tests of stool specimens;

- Explain the diagnostic applications of tests of other body fluids and materials.

Laboratory Examination of Urine

The history of clinical pathology began with the observation that the urine and stools of sick persons are often abnormal. Pathologic changes in the urine and stool are mentioned frequently in the works of Hippocrates and Galen. Medieval physicians often limited their diagnostic investigations to feeling the patient's pulse and holding a flask of urine up to the light.

In the modern clinical laboratory, microscopic examination and chemical analysis of urine and stool specimens can yield information not only about the excretory and digestive systems but also about other body systems, water and acid-base balance, nutrition, and the presence of toxic substances. A major advantage of urine and stool examinations is that, under ordinary circumstances, both of these materials are readily available, and obtaining specimens calls for no invasive procedures or elaborate equipment.

For most of the tests done in the urinology laboratory, the preferred specimen is 60 to 90 mL of freshly voided urine. Although a random specimen is usually suitable, a first-voided specimen (the first urine passed after arising in the morning) may be more satisfactory in testing for trace substances because it is usually more concentrated. A clean-voided specimen (clean catch) is one obtained after cleansing of the area around the urethral meatus (usually with liquid soap and cotton balls) to prevent contamination of the specimen with material from outside the urinary tract. A midstream specimen is one that contains neither the first nor the last portion of urine passed. It is obtained by introducing a specimen container into the urine stream after voiding has begun and removing it before voiding ceases. The purpose of this procedure is to obtain as pure as possible a sample of bladder urine, with minimal admixture of cells or other material from the urethra. A catheterized specimen is obtained by urethral catheter (less often by suprapubic needle puncture of the bladder), either because the patient cannot void or to prevent contamination of the specimen. A 24-hour urine specimen consists of all the urine passed by the patient during a 24-hour period.

A urine specimen is usually collected in a clean, dry bottle or cup of glass, plastic, or waxed or plasticized paper. The container need not be sterile except for bacteriologic work. Examination of urine is carried out as soon as possible after the specimen is obtained because blood cells in urine rupture early and bacterial growth in a standing specimen may alter its chemical composition. When a delay is expected, the specimen is refrigerated. A one- or two-gallon (four- or eight-liter) jug is used to collect a 24-hour urine specimen. The jug may be kept on ice during the collection period and toluene or another preservative may be placed in the jug before collection begins to inhibit the growth of bacteria in the specimen.

The principal diagnostic procedure in urinology is the **urinalysis**, a set of routine physical and chemical examinations. In most laboratories, the urinalysis includes direct observation of the specimen for color, turbidity, and other obvious characteristics; determination of specific gravity; microscopic examination of sediment for cells, crystals, and other formed elements; determination of pH; and chemical testing for glucose, protein, occult blood, and perhaps bilirubin and acetone.

Variations in color and clarity of urine usually reflect variations in concentration of solutes, including pigment. Because the daily solute load is fairly constant, changes in concentration are nearly always due to changes in volume of water excreted. Turbidity (cloudiness) may be due to the presence of phosphates, which are insoluble in alkaline urine. A smoky brown color ("Coca-Cola urine") often indicates the presence of hemolyzed blood. Color changes may be due to abnormal waste products (bilirubin, porphyrins), drugs (methylene blue, phenazopyridine), or pigments from foods (beets, blackberries). Mucus shreds, fragments of tissue, or calcareous material may be grossly evident in the specimen.

Microscopic examination of the urine is usually preceded by centrifugation of the specimen to concentrate any cells or other formed elements present. A polychrome stain such as the Sternheimer-Malbin stain (crystal violet and safranin in ethanol) may be added to the sediment to enhance the distinctive features of various cells, but is not essential. Microscopic examination is carried out on a small volume of fluid urine placed on a slide and covered with a cover slip. Dried smears of urine are not ordinarily suitable for examination.

Formed elements frequently found in urine are red blood cells, white blood cells, casts, crystals, bacteria, epithelial cells, and amorphous sediment. Cell counts are recorded as cells per high-power field (hpf), obtained as an average after examination and counting of several fields. A small number of red and white blood cells are present in normal urine. A finding of more than 1 or 2 red blood cells per high-power field (RBC/hpf), called microscopic hematuria, indicates either bleeding in some part of the excretory system or contamination of the specimen with blood, possibly menstrual. Hematuria occurs in acute glomerulonephritis, urolithiasis, hemorrhagic diseases, infarction of the kidney, tuberculosis of the kidney, benign or malignant tumors of any part of the urinary tract, and many cases of simple cystitis. The presence of more than 1 or 2 white blood cells per high-power field (WBC/hpf), known as pyuria, usually indicates infection in some part of the urinary tract.

Casts are microscopic cylindrical bodies that have been formed by concretion of cells or insoluble material within renal tubules and subsequently excreted in the urine. Casts are always abnormal. They are reported as the number counted per low-power field. Hyaline and waxy casts are homogeneous casts varying in refractivity. They consist of coagulated protein and are found in conditions associated with leakage of protein through glomeruli: nephritis, nephrotic syndrome (including lupus nephrosis and Kimmelstiel-Wilson disease), toxemia, and congestive heart failure. Granular casts are formed by aggregation of red or white blood cells or both in renal tubules and occur in many of the same conditions as hyaline and waxy casts.

A variety of **crystals** may be found on microscopic examination of the urine. Their chemical composition can usually be deduced from their shape. Crystals of uric acid, cystine, calcium oxalate, and triple phosphate may appear in the urine of persons who excrete abnormal quantities of these materials and are subject to stone formation. Bacteria in significant numbers in a freshly voided specimen (bacteriuria, bacilluria) suggest urinary tract infection. Some squamous epithelial cells (squames) are often found in urine and have little significance. Amorphous sediment is a general term for ill-defined solid material seen on microscopic examination of urine. It consists of chemical and cellular debris and is of no diagnostic importance.

Routine chemical testing of urine is usually performed with a "dipstick," a commercially produced strip of plastic or paper bearing a series of dots or squares of reagent, each designed to assess a specific chemical property of urine. The dipstick is immersed briefly in the urine and the test squares are observed for color changes. These tests are semiquantitative and are read by comparing the degree of color change in each square with an appropriate color chart. Results of dipstick tests other than pH and specific gravity are reported as either positive on a scale of 1 to 4 (1+, 2+, 3+, 4+) or negative.

The **pH** of urine (traditionally called the "reaction") is normally about 5.5. The urine may be alkaline (pH 8) in vegetarians and in persons with urinary tract infection due to urease-producing organisms such as *Proteus*, which split urinary urea to ammonia in the bladder.

The **specific gravity** of urine varies in direct proportion to the concentration of dissolved materials. It is ordinarily measured by means of a color change in the relevant square on a dipstick. A more precise measurement can be made by noting the depth to which a hydrometer, a precisely weighted float, sinks in the specimen. The normal specific gravity is 1.005 to 1.030. The specific gravity is increased in dehydration (with normal renal function), toxemia, congestive heart failure, acute glomerulonephritis, and diabetes mellitus with glycosuria. The specific gravity is decreased (hyposthenuria) after ingestion or infusion of fluid (with normal renal function), in diabetes insipidus, and in renal failure with loss of concentrating ability.

The presence of **protein** in the urine (proteinuria) is usually due to leakage of albumin from the glomeruli. Hence it is often termed albuminuria, even though routine tests for protein in urine do not distinguish which proteins are present. Protein loss from the kidney occurs in glomerulonephritis, nephrotic syndrome, renal infarction, fever, and toxemia. In addition, most chemical tests for protein are positive in the presence of hematuria or pyuria.

Normally all of the plasma glucose that appears in glomerular filtrate is reabsorbed in the renal tubules. The detection of **glucose** in the urine (glycosuria) generally indicates an abnormal elevation of plasma glucose. The renal threshold for glucose is about 180 mg/dL [10 mmol/L]. That means that, at plasma concentrations above this level, more glucose appears in glomerular filtrate than can be reabsorbed by the tubules. Glycosuria is a cardinal finding in diabetes mellitus. It also occurs after rapid absorption of dietary glucose (alimentary glycosuria) and in some persons with abnormally low renal thresholds for glucose (renal glycosuria).

Occult blood refers to blood present in insufficient quantity to alter the color of the urine. A positive test for occult blood has generally the same significance as the finding of red blood cells

in urine. Acetone and other **ketones** appear in the urine in diabetes mellitus with acidosis, in starvation, thyrotoxicosis, and high fever. As noted in the preceding chapter, only bilirubin that has been conjugated with glucuronic acid is soluble in water. Hence the appearance of **bilirubin** in the urine (bilirubinuria, choluria) is noted in obstructive jaundice, in which conjugated bilirubin enters the blood stream from bile, but not in jaundice due to hemolysis or liver disease, in which only unconjugated bilirubin is elevated in the plasma.

Qualitative testing for **hemoglobin** (not normally present in urine) is positive in disorders causing release of hemoglobin into the plasma (hemolytic anemias, burns, malaria) and in hematuria of any cause with extensive hemolysis of red blood cells in the urine. A qualitative test for **myoglobin** in urine is positive in some diseases of muscle, in crush syndrome, myocardial infarction, and various toxic states (carbon monoxide poisoning, alcoholism, diabetic acidosis).

Precise quantitative determinations of several substances in the urine are important in the diagnosis of certain conditions. Because of wide variations in urine volume and concentration due to variations in water intake and in nonrenal water losses (sweating, vomiting, diarrhea), analysis of a 24-hour urine specimen and computation of 24-hour excretion of the analyte provide much more useful information than analysis of a random specimen.

Quantitative determinations of electrolytes (sodium, potassium, chloride) in urine may help to clarify renal, adrenal, or metabolic disease in which serum electrolytes are abnormal because of inappropriate renal loss or retention. The normal 24-hour excretion of sodium varies widely (25-275 mEq/d [25-275 mmol/d]). Sodium excretion is increased in renal disease, Addison disease, hypothyroidism, and in patients treated with natriuretics (diuretics that promote excretion of sodium ions). The range for potassium is 25-125 mEq/d [25-125 mmol/d]. Urinary potassium excretion is increased in chronic renal failure, Cushing syndrome, Conn syndrome, dehydration, and starvation. Twenty-four-hour urinary excretion of chloride is 110-250 mEq/d [110-250 mmol/d]. Urinary excretion of **chloride** is increased in Cushing and Conn syndromes and decreased in metabolic alkalosis due to vomiting or diuretic therapy.

Measurement of calcium and phosphorus excretion supplies information about parathyroid function and the security of the body calcium pool. The normal range of urine **calcium** is 100-250 mg/d [2.5-6.2 mmol/d]. The level is increased in hyperparathyroidism and Paget disease of bone, reduced in hypoparathyroidism and rickets. The normal range of daily **phosphate** excretion is 0.9-1.3 g/d [29-42 mmol/d]. Phosphate excretion is increased in hyperparathyroidism, rickets, and renal tubular disease, and decreased in hypoparathyroidism and vitamin D intoxication.

Microalbuminuria (microproteinuria), a persistent excretion of protein in concentrations detectable by immunoassay but not by routine tests for urinary protein, occurs in diabetic nephropathy (glomerular disease occurring as a complication of type 1 or type 2 diabetes mellitus). Periodic testing for microalbuminuria is a routine part of the management of diabetes mellitus. Excretion of 20-200 mcg/min (30-300 mg/d) of protein, as detected by quantitative testing of a 24-hour urine specimen, indicates significant glomerular disease and strongly suggests eventual renal failure (end-stage renal disease).

An excess of one or more **amino acids** in the urine occurs in various congenital biochemical disorders. Elevation of the urinary concentration of an amino acid can result from abnormally high blood levels of the substance (e.g., phenylalanine in phenylketonuria; cystine in cystinuria; leucine, isoleucine, and others in maple syrup urine disease) or from failure of the renal tubules to reabsorb amino acids from glomerular filtrate (Fanconi syndrome). Screening of urinary amino acid concentrations by chromatography can supplement information obtained by screening serum levels in clarifying the diagnosis of various aminoacidurias.

The normal 24-hour excretion of **copper** is 15-60 mcg/d [0.22-0.9 mcmol/d]. The level of copper in the urine is increased in Wilson disease (hepatolenticular degeneration) and in some other chronic liver disorders. Excretion of **acid mucopolysaccharides** (AMP) is increased in children with Hurler syndrome, a congenital biochemical defect that causes accumulation of mucopolysaccharides in tissues.

Elevation of the 24-hour excretion of **amylase** occurs in pancreatitis and pancreatic carcinoma. The normal range depends on the method used. Urinary **urobilinogen** excretion (normally below 4 mg/d [6.8 mol/d]) is increased in hemolytic anemias, large hematomas, pulmonary infarction, and hepatic disease (viral hepatitis, cirrhosis), and reduced in biliary obstruction and starvation. Urinary excretion of **coproporphyrin** (a product of hemoglobin breakdown) is normally below 180 mcg/24h [276 nmol/d]. Increases occur in porphyria, lead poisoning, and hepatic disease (viral hepatitis, cirrhosis). Excretion of **delta-aminolevulinic acid** (normally below 7 mg/24h [53 mcmol/d]) is also increased in lead poisoning.

Identification of various products of neoplastic tissue in urine is sometimes more practical than diagnostic studies of the blood. Urine **estrogen** or **androgen** levels may be increased by functioning gonadal neoplasms. **Catecholamines** are a class of biologically active substances produced by the adrenal medulla, the brain, and other tissues and including dopamine, epinephrine, and norepinephrine. Functioning tumors derived from tissues that secrete catecholamines cause a rise of catecholamines and their breakdown products in the blood and urine. Excretion of **vanillylmandelic acid** (VMA), a breakdown product of epinephrine and norepinephrine, and of **homovanillic acid** (HVA), a breakdown product of dopamine, is increased in pheochromocytoma and neuroblastoma. In carcinoid tumor with carcinoid syndrome, urinary excretion of **5-hydroxyindoleacetic acid** (5-HIAA) is increased above the normal range of less than 9 mg/d [less than 47.1 mcmol/d].

Adrenal cortical hyperplasia or neoplasia, or increased production of cortical steroids due to excessive secretion of ACTH by the pituitary gland, is reflected in increased renal excretion of by-products of hormonal metabolism, **17-keto-steroids** (also increased in pregnancy and in certain gonadal tumors of both sexes) and **17-hydroxycorticosteroids**. Excretion of these substances is decreased in Addison disease and pituitary failure. **Bence Jones protein** in urine (as detected by electrophoresis or immunoelectrophoresis) suggests multiple myeloma but may also be found in some collagen diseases and lymphomas.

Urine pregnancy tests depend on identification of **chorionic gonadotropin** in urine. Measurement of urinary urea or creatinine is essential for determination of glomerular filtration rate as a function of urea or creatinine clearance, as mentioned in Chapter 20. One means of testing for intestinal malabsorption is to administer a test meal of **D-xylose** and measure urinary excretion, also mentioned in Chapter 20. The **Schilling test** is a radioisotope study designed to identify persons with pernicious anemia. Oral administration of vitamin B_{12} tagged with radioactive cobalt (^{57}Co or ^{60}Co) is followed by collection of a 24-hour urine specimen. Recovery of less than 3% of administered radioisotope in the urine indicates impairment of vitamin B_{12} absorption. Repetition of the test with administration of intrinsic factor shows normal absorption of vitamin B_{12} in pernicious anemia but not in intestinal malabsorption.

Analysis of urine for toxic chemicals and drugs of abuse is a routine screening procedure in many occupational settings and in competitive athletics.

Urine **osmolality** (osmotic activity of total solute content) can be measured by the freezing point depression method, as described for serum osmolality in Chapter 20. The normal range of urine osmolality is 500 to 1200 mOsm/kg. Abnormally low urine osmolality despite restriction of water intake indicates renal disease with impairment of concentrating ability. In severe renal tubular disease the osmolality of urine approximates that of plasma (isosthenuria).

For urine culture, with or without colony count and sensitivity testing, the specimen is obtained under sterile conditions in a sterile container, as described in Chapter 21. Culture is performed in the microbiology laboratory.

Laboratory Examination of Stool

Laboratory examinations of stool specimens are performed less frequently than examinations of urine. This is partly because procuring a stool specimen is esthetically objectionable to patients, but more importantly because only limited information can be gained by examining the stool. Tests that are routinely performed on stool specimens are qualitative analysis for occult blood and fat; quantitative determination of urobilinogen; smears for leukocytes, parasites, and parasite ova; Gram stain for pathogenic organisms; and culture in infectious diarrheas.

The qualitative **occult blood** test is useful in identifying gastrointestinal hemorrhage at any level and in screening for malignant disease of the colon. The test involves application of guaiac, benzidine, or ortho-toluidine to a specimen of stool. A color change indicates a positive test, but false negative results may be caused by ingestion of antacids or vitamin C and false positives by eating red meat or horseradish. For maximum sensitivity of the test, stools should be tested for occult blood on three days in succession, and for maximum specificity the patient should be on a meat-free diet for three days before collection of the first specimen and throughout the test period.

Patient-prepared specimen cards are widely used for occult blood testing of stools. A set of three cards is given to the patient, with instructions to collect a small quantity of stool from the toilet or from toilet paper on each of three successive days with a disposable wooden spatula and to apply it to the appropriate box or circle on one of the cards. Cards are then sent to the physician's office or to a clinical laboratory for testing.

A more sophisticated test for gastrointestinal bleeding involves determination of radioactivity in the stool after tagging of some of the patient's red blood cells with radioactive chromium (^{51}Cr). A finding of excessive **fat** in the stool by testing with Sudan III suggests steatorrhea (malabsorption of fat). Quantitative testing for fat normally shows less than 7 g/d. Testing for steatorrhea is more sensitive if the patient consumes at least 60 g of fat daily for three days before collection of the specimen. Stool urobilinogen (normally 40 to 280 mg/24h [68–473 mcmol/d]) is increased in hemolytic anemias and reduced in severe intrinsic liver disease and biliary obstruction.

Microscopic examination of stool normally shows undigested vegetable and muscle (meat) fibers, some fat, epithelial cells, and bacteria. A few white blood cells are also seen. Increase in white blood cells suggests inflammatory bowel disease (Crohn disease, ulcerative colitis) or bacterial infection. Bacteriologic smear and culture of the stool are performed in the microbiology laboratory. For the detection of intestinal parasites (protozoa, helminths, cysts, ova), a stool specimen is subjected to repeated concentrations (washing and centrifugation). Serologic studies may be more reliable for diagnosis of parasitism than isolation and identification of organisms from the stool.

Examination of Other Fluids and Materials

Although blood, urine, and stool are the principal objects of scrutiny in the clinical laboratory, any other body fluid or product, normal or abnormal, can be subjected to microscopic inspection, chemical analysis, and bacteriologic culture. For some fluids (cerebrospinal fluid, amniotic fluid, semen), certain examinations are routine. For others (sputum, gastric aspirate), the diagnostic focus determines what examinations are done.

Procedures for the cytologic study of transudates, exudates, and aspirates for malignant cells are discussed in Chapter 17, and microbiologic examinations are discussed in Chapter 21. Most of the other tests performed on body fluids consist of either microscopic examination of stained or unstained smears or quantitative chemical analysis for substances increased or decreased in certain diseases or conditions.

Cerebrospinal fluid is obtained by lumbar puncture ("spinal tap") (less often by cisternal puncture) in cases where central nervous system infection (meningitis, encephalitis), neoplasm, or hemorrhage is suspected, and in various other conditions. Separate specimens are routinely obtained for cell count, chemical testing, and smear and culture.

The normal **white blood cell count** of spinal fluid is less than 10 cells/mm³, and normally all cells found are mononuclear. A rise in mononuclear cells occurs in viral encephalitis and meningitis and in tuberculous meningitis. Appearance of polymorphonuclear leukocytes indicates pyogenic (bacterial) meningitis or encephalitis or brain abscess. **Red blood cells** are not normally found in spinal fluid. Their presence in a specimen may indicate intracranial hemorrhage, but is often due to a "traumatic tap," that is, puncture of a small blood vessel by the needle used to obtain the specimen. Significant hemorrhage within the preceding 2-4 weeks may impart a yellow color (xanthochromia) to the specimen. Xanthochromia can also result from the presence of bilirubin in a jaundiced patient.

The total **protein** concentration of spinal fluid (about 90% of it albumin) is normally 15 to 45 mg/dL [0.15–0.45 g/L]. Protein is increased in encephalitis, meningitis, poliomyelitis, neoplasm of the brain or spinal cord, and cerebral or subarachnoid hemorrhage. A rise in protein without a rise in cell count (albuminocytologic dissociation) is characteristic of Guillain-Barré syndrome. The glucose level of spinal fluid is normally about 20 mg/dL [0.2 g/L] less than that of the blood. Hence for proper interpretation the blood level must be tested at the same time as the spinal fluid level. Spinal fluid glucose is increased in diabetic coma and reduced in bacterial meningitis.

Spinal fluid is examined by smear (Gram stain and, if indicated, acid-fast stain or India ink preparation for *Cryptococcus*) and culture for pathogenic microorganisms, and can also be subjected to immunologic study for antigens or antibodies indicative of specific pathogens, autoimmune disorders, or certain neoplasms.

Pleural, pericardial, and peritoneal fluid obtained by needle aspiration can be tested for specific gravity and protein concentration in order to distinguish between a transudate (specific gravity less than 1.016 and protein less than 3.0 g/dL [0.03 g/L]) and an exudate (specific gravity 1.016 or more and protein 3.0 g/dL or more). A finding of polymorphonuclear leukocytes in a stained smear indicates pyogenic infection.

Synovial fluid obtained by needle aspiration from a joint in acute or chronic arthritis with effusion is subjected to cell count and examination by compensated polarized light microscopy for crystals. A white blood cell count over 200/mm³ suggests inflammation and over 2000/mm³ suggests infection. Very high counts (to 100 000/mm3) are seen in septic arthritis. Uric acid crystals are found in gout, calcium pyrophosphate crystals in pseudogout.

Gastric analysis (testing of the acid content of gastric juice obtained by nasogastric tube) is carried out both in the basal state and after stimulation with histamine. The normal basal production of acid is 2 to 5 mEq/h, and one hour after stimulation with histamine this may rise to 20 mEq/h. Gastric acid secretion is increased in duodenal ulcer and greatly increased in Zollinger-Ellison syndrome. It is decreased or absent in gastric carcinoma, achlorhydria, and pernicious anemia.

A smear of nasal secretions stained by the Wright or Giemsa method shows eosinophils in allergic rhinitis. Sweat electrolytes (concentrations of sodium and chloride in sweat) are increased in cystic fibrosis.

On semen analysis, more than 50,000,000 spermatozoa/mL should be found. More than 60% of these should be motile and fewer than 50% should show morphologic abnormalities.

Chemical analysis of urinary calculi helps to identify disorders that cause renal excretion of abnormal substances or of normal substances in abnormal amounts.

Amniotic fluid, obtained by needle aspiration from the amniotic sac at or after the fourteenth week of gestation, supplies fetal cells for karyotyping, described in Chapter 23, and can also be tested chemically. Elevation of alpha-fetoprotein (AFP) occurs in neural tube defects (anencephaly, spina bifida). The lecithin/sphingomyelin ratio, determined by thin-layer chromatography, is less than 1.0 before fetal lungs mature, more than 1.0 when lung maturity has been attained.

Exercises

Fill in the Blanks

1. A _____ (the first urine passed after arising in the morning) may be more satisfactory in testing for trace substances because it is usually more concentrated.

2. Examination of urine is carried out as soon as possible after the specimen is obtained because _____ and _____.

3. A _____ color or _____ urine often indicates the presence of hemolyzed blood.

4. Cell counts are recorded as cells per _____, obtained as an average after examination and counting of several fields.

5. Two substances found in the urine on urinalysis of little or no diagnostic significance are _____ and _____.

6. Routine chemical testing of urine is usually performed with a _____, a commercially produced strip of plastic or paper bearing a series of dots or squares of _____, each designed to assess a specific chemical property of urine.

7. Proteinuria is often termed _____, even though routine tests for protein in urine do not distinguish which proteins are present.

8. _____ is a cardinal finding in diabetes mellitus.

9. _____ is noted in obstructive jaundice but not in jaundice due to _____.

10. A 24-hour quantitative determination of electrolytes in the urine is used to the determine the amount of _____, _____, and _____ in the urine.

11. _____ is a persistent excretion of protein in concentrations detectable by immunoassay but not by routine tests for urinary protein.

12. Glomerular disease occurring as a complication of type 1 or type 2 diabetes mellitus is a condition known as _____.

13. The Schilling test, which is performed with a radioisotope of _____, is designed to identify persons with _____.

Exercises

14. In order to avoid false positive results when the stool is tested for occult blood, the patient should not consume _____ or _____ before the test nor should the patient eat _____ or _____ in order to avoid false negative results.

15. A rise in mononuclear cells in the cerebrospinal fluid occurs in _____ and _____ and in _____.

16. Appearance of polymorphonuclear leukocytes in the cerebrospinal fluid is indicative of _____ or _____ or _____.

17. The presence of red blood cells in a cerebrospinal fluid specimen may indicate _____, but is often due to a _____, that is, puncture of a small blood vessel by the needle used to obtain the specimen.

18. Spinal fluid glucose is _____ in diabetic coma and _____ in bacterial meningitis.

19. Pleural, pericardial, and peritoneal fluid obtained by needle aspiration can be tested for specific gravity and protein concentration in order to distinguish between a _____ (specific gravity less than 1.016 and protein less than 3.0 g/dL [0.03 g/L]) and an _____ (specific gravity 1.016 or more and protein 3.0 g/dL or more).

20. Very high white blood cell counts (to 100 000/mm3) in synovial fluid are seen in _____.

Multiple Choice: Circle the letter of the best answer from the choices given.

1. This finding indicates either bleeding in some part of the excretory system or contamination of the specimen with blood, possibly menstrual.
   A. Choluria.
   B. Microscopic hematuria.
   C. Pyuria.
   D. Bacteriuria.
   E. Glycosuria.

2. The presence of this in the urine usually indicates infection in some part of the urinary tract.
   A. Choluria.
   B. Microscopic hematuria.
   C. Pyuria.
   D. Bacteriuria.
   E. Glycosuria.

Exercises

3. These substances in the urine consist of coagulated protein and are found in conditions associated with leakage of protein through glomeruli: nephritis, nephrotic syndrome (including lupus nephrosis and Kimmelstiel-Wilson disease), toxemia, and congestive heart failure.
   A. Bacteria.
   B. Bile.
   C. Pus.
   D. Red blood cells.
   E. Hyaline casts.

4. These substances are formed by aggregation of red or white blood cells or both in renal tubules and occur in many of the same conditions as hyaline and waxy casts.
   A. Bacteria.
   B. Squamous epithelial cells.
   C. Amorphous sediment.
   D. Uric acid crystals.
   E. Granular casts.

5. Crystals of uric acid, cystine, calcium oxalate, and triple phosphate may appear in the urine of persons who excrete abnormal quantities of these materials and who are subject to which of the following conditions.
   A. Urinary tract or kidney stones.
   B. Urinary tract infections.
   C. Glomerular nephritis.
   D. Lupus erythematosus.
   E. Congestive heart failure.

6. Which of the following might account for an elevated urine specific gravity?
   A. Diabetes insipidus.
   B. *Proteus* urinary tract infection.
   C. Proteinuria.
   D. Diabetes mellitus.
   E. Hemoglobinuria.

7. A decreased urine specific gravity might be caused by which of the following?
   A. Drinking too much liquid.
   B. Congestive heart failure.
   C. Proteus urinary tract infection.
   D. Hemoglobinuria.
   E. Proteinuria.

Exercises

8. Which of the following findings is not likely to be associated with diabetes mellitus?
   A. Elevated urine specific gravity.
   B. Ketones in the urine.
   C. Bilirubinuria.
   D. Acetonuria.
   E. Glycosuria.

9. Hemolytic anemias, burns, malaria might be evidenced by which of the following findings?
   A. Bilirubinuria.
   B. Hemoglobinuria.
   C. Acetonuria.
   D. Myoglobinuria.
   E. Proteinuria.

10. Which of the following might be evidence of crush syndrome, myocardial infarction, or carbon monoxide poisoning?
    A. Bilirubinuria.
    B. Hemoglobinuria.
    C. Acetonuria.
    D. Myoglobinuria.
    E. Proteinuria.

11. A 24-hour urine collection is required for which of the following?
    A. Quantitative determinations of electrolytes.
    B. Quantitative determinations of red blood cells.
    C. To obtain an accurate pH.
    D. To obtain an accurate specific gravity.
    E. To determine the amount of glucose in the urine.

12. An elevated urinary calcium and phosphate might be an indication of which of the following conditions?
    A. Diabetes mellitus.
    B. Hyperparathyroidism.
    C. Congestive heart failure.
    D. Cirrhosis.
    E. Pheochromocytoma

Exercises

13. A reduced urine calcium with an increased phosphate level might be evidence of which of the following conditions?
    A. Pheochromocytoma.
    B. Viral hepatitis.
    C. Rickets.
    D. Diabetes mellitus.
    E. Phenylketonuria.

14. Because diabetic nephropathy is a common complication of type 1 or 2 diabetes mellitus, periodic testing for which of the following is a routine part of management of diabetes mellitus?
    A. Bilirubinuria.
    B. Coproporphyrins.
    C. Catecholamines.
    D. Acid mucopolysaccharides.
    E. Microalbuminuria.

15. Pancreatitis and pancreatic carcinoma are associated with elevation in the 24-hour excretion of which of the following?
    A. Bilirubin.
    B. Amino acids.
    C. Amylase.
    D. Protein.
    E. Albumin.

16. Which of the following findings in the urine is not likely to be related to a tumor or neoplasm?
    A. Estrogen.
    B. Catecholamines.
    C. Androgen.
    D. Vanillylmandelic acid (VMA).
    E. Delta-aminolevulinic acid.

17. Increased renal excretion of one or both of these substances, 17-ketosteroids and 17-hydroxycorticosteroids, may be an indication of which of the following conditions?
    A. Adrenal cortical hyperplasia or neoplasia.
    B. Pregnancy.
    C. Certain gonadal tumors.
    D. All of the above.
    E. None of the above.

Exercises

18. The presence of Bence Jones protein in urine (as detected by electrophoresis or immunoelectrophoresis) may be an indication of which of the following?
    A. Multiple myeloma.
    B. Adrenal cortical hyperplasia.
    C. Congestive heart failure.
    D. Hepatitis.
    E. Diabetic nephropathy.

19. Which of the following urine tests is used to diagnose pregnancy?
    A. Bence Jones protein.
    B. Chorionic gonadotropin.
    C. Schilling test.
    D. 17-ketosteroids.
    E. Urine osmolality.

20. A rise in protein in the cerebrospinal fluid without a rise in cell count (albuminocytologic dissociation) is characteristic of which of the following conditions?
    A. Bacterial meningitis.
    B. Subarachnoid hemorrhage.
    C. Guillain-Barré syndrome.
    D. Viral encephalitis.
    E. Brain abscess.

21. Sweat electrolytes (concentrations of sodium and chloride in sweat) are increased in which of the following conditions?
    A. Gout.
    B. Zollinger-Ellison syndrome.
    C. Allergic rhinitis.
    D. Pyogenic infection.
    E. Cystic fibrosis.

22. The lecithin/sphingomyelin ratio, determined by thin-layer chromatography, on amniotic fluid is an important determination for which of the following?
    A. Neural tube defects.
    B. Hydrocephaly.
    C. Cystic fibrosis.
    D. Fetal lung maturity.
    E. Spina bifida.

Exercises

Short Answers

1. Define or explain:

   a. choluria _____

   _____

   b. clean catch _____

   _____

   c. glycosuria _____

   d. lumbar puncture _____

   _____

   e. occult blood _____

   _____

   f. pyuria _____

   _____

   g. specific gravity _____

   _____

2. What procedures can be used to limit contamination of a urine specimen by cells or secretions from outside the urinary tract?

   _____

   _____

   _____

   _____

3. What examinations make up the standard urinalysis?

   _____

   _____

   _____

   _____

Exercises

4. What is the origin of casts in the urine?

_____

_____

_____

5. What conditions other than diabetes mellitus may account for the appearance of glucose in the urine?

_____

_____

_____

_____

6. List some constituents of urine for which analysis requires collection of a 24-hour specimen.

_____

_____

_____

_____

7. What two factors might account for an alkaline pH in the urine?

_____

_____

8. What constituent of the stool is likely to be increased in malabsorption syndromes?

_____

9. Which tests are routinely performed on stool specimens?

_____

_____

_____

_____

Exercises

10. What routine examinations are performed on cerebrospinal fluid?

_____

_____

_____

_____

11. In what conditions are abnormalities of gastric acid secretion noted?

_____

_____

_____

_____

12. What diagnostic procedures can be performed on amniotic fluid?

_____

_____

_____

_____

Activities for Application and Further Study

1. Under what circumstances might a lecithin/sphingomyelin ratio be performed on the amniotic fluid? How might this information affect the further management of a pregnancy?

2. Many test strip products (dipsticks) are available over-the-counter for testing urine and other bodily fluids. Obtain some of these products. Test yourself, your family members, friends. Summarize your findings (keeping identification of the subjects anonymous, of course).

Glossary

Terms not found in the Glossary should be looked up in the Index, and vice versa.

ABC Aspiration biopsy cytology.

abduction Movement of a body part away from the midline of the body.

acellular Without cells.

acoustical shadowing Reflection of ultrasound from the surface of structures or materials that are physically incompressible (bone, gallstones), resulting in failure to visualize structures behind them.

adduction Movement of a body part toward the midline of the body.

adhesion An abnormal fibrous connection between two structures or surfaces.

adipocere A waxy material formed by the decomposition of fatty materials in a dead body, especially one submerged in water or buried in damp ground.

aerobic Living, growing, or taking place in the presence of oxygen.

afferent Conducting towards a structure.

agminated Clustered, aggregated.

agonal Referring to the last moments of life.

air-fluid level A horizontal line representing the surface of a collection of fluid within a hollow organ or cavity, with air or gas above it.

aliquot A portion of a specimen that is some known fraction of the entire specimen. Quantitative analyses or other measurements performed on the aliquot can be multiplied by the reciprocal of this fraction to yield figures applicable to the whole specimen.

amniocentesis Removal of a quantity of amniotic fluid from the pregnant uterus for diagnostic purposes.

amorphous Without form or shape.

amphophilic Attracting stains of both acidic and basic reaction.

anaerobic Living, growing, or taking place in the absence of oxygen.

analyte The substance whose presence is tested for in a qualitative analysis or whose concentration in the specimen is determined in a quantitative analysis.

anastomosis (1) A network formed by small vessels with many interconnections. (2) A surgically created connection between two vessels or hollow structures such as parts of the digestive tract.

anencephaly Congenital absence of the cranium and of most or all of the cerebrum.

anisonucleosis Abnormal variation in the sizes of cell nuclei.

anlage The earliest discernible rudiment of a structure during embryonic development; primordium.

anorexia Loss of appetite.

anoxia Deficiency of oxygen.

antimesenteric Referring to the side of the bowel opposite the attachment of the mesentery.

apatite A calcium phosphate salt found in bones and teeth.

apoptosis Fragmentation of a worn-out cell into particles, each of which is surrounded by a membrane.

arthralgia Pain in one or more joints, with or without evidence of inflammation.

artifact Any deviation from an expected appearance or normal test result that is caused by the test procedure itself rather than reflecting an abnormality in the specimen.

asplenia Absence of the spleen.

assay Any quantitative test; applied particularly to measurement of biological activity, as of hormones.

astigmatism A visual error resulting from a cylindrical deformity of the normally spherical cornea.

atresia Congenital absence or closure of an orifice or passage.

atypia Irregularity, departure from expected appearance.

azurophilic Showing an affinity for blue aniline stains.

bacteremia The presence of bacteria in the blood circulation.

BAL Bronchoalveolar lavage.

Bard-Parker blade Proprietary name for disposable scalpel blades available in a variety of shapes and used in surgery and in performing autopsies.

baseline A test performed on an apparently healthy person, or in advance of some other test or procedure, to provide a basis for comparison with results of future tests.

beefy Having the appearance or texture of raw lean meat.

bench test A laboratory test performed manually by a technician, as opposed to one done by automated machinery.

bifurcation Division of a vessel or other structure into two branches.

bioptome A cutting instrument for obtaining biopsies.

bivalve Having two symmetric parts that are hinged together, said of instruments such as a vaginal speculum.

bland Without evidence of inflammation.

bony island A benign developmental abnormality consisting of a localized zone of increased density in a long bone.

borderline (adjective) Referring to a test result that is close to the border between normal and abnormal.

boss A rounded prominence or knob.

bosselated Marked or covered by bosses.

bridging osteophytes Osteophytes on adjacent vertebrae that meet and fuse, forming a "bridge" across the joint space.

calcinosis Deposition of calcium salts in tissue.

calibration Adjustment or correction of a testing instrument or method by means of a standard.

calvaria The top of the skull.

cancerization Malignant degeneration.

cannula A hollow tube, usually of metal, that is used to conduct materials into or out of a normal or abnormal cavity within the body. See *trocar*.

carneous degeneration Tissue change producing a fleshy texture.

carnification Same as the preceding.

cast An elongated mass formed by inspissation of semisolid material in a tubular structure.

cathode-ray tube (CRT) An electronic device that permits display on a fluorescent screen of waveforms representing rapidly shifting quantities, such as input from an ECG or other diagnostic device whose data are, or can be converted to, electrical signals.

Caves-Schultz-Stanford bioptome An instrument for obtaining a biopsy of the myocardium via a transvenous catheter.

cells and flare Turbidity of the aqueous humor of the eye due to inflammation, as observed with a slit lamp.

chancre The primary lesion of syphilis, a painless indurated ulcer.

Chiba needle An aspiration biopsy needle.

chilblain Local cutaneous inflammation caused by exposure to cold and damp.

choristoma A mass of heterotopic tissue.

chylous Containing or resembling chyle, the milky fluid containing absorbed nutrients passing from the digestive tract to the circulatory system via the thoracic duct.

circumscribed Surrounded, clearly demarcated from adjacent structures.

coagulopathy Any disorder of blood coagulation.

collateral vessels Vascular channels newly formed from existing ones to maintain the circulation of a tissue or organ whose normal blood supply has been impaired by disease or injury.

collateralization Formation of collateral vessels.

collecting system The nonexcretory portions of the kidney, which collect newly formed urine and conduct it to

the ureter; the minor and major calyces and the renal pelvis, as seen on IVP.

concretion A gritty or sandy material, usually formed by deposition of mineral salts.

coned-down view A radiographic study limited to a small area by the use of a cone that narrows and "focuses" the x-ray beam.

congenital Present from birth.

consolidative process An abnormal process that increases the density of a tissue or region.

contiguous images A series of CT scans without intervals of unexamined tissue between them.

control A specimen whose properties are already known, which is subjected to a test or measurement as a means of calibrating an instrument or verifying the accuracy of a procedure.

Cook needle An aspiration biopsy needle.

costophrenic angle The acute angle formed by the ribs (chest wall) and the periphery of the diaphragm, particularly as seen on a standard PA chest film.

Councilman chisel An autopsy instrument used for splitting bone.

count Any enumeration of discrete objects in a specimen, such as cells of a certain type in blood.

crenated Having a shriveled or pitted surface.

crepitation, crepitus Crackling.

cribriform Perforated like a sieve.

cut A tomogram or CT section or image; a scan.

cyanotic Showing an abnormal bluish discoloration.

cyst Any fluid-filled abnormal structure.

debris Amorphous material resulting from injury, degeneration, or necrosis of tissue.

demineralization Reduction in the amount of calcium present in bone, due to disease or immobilization.

denuded Uncovered, deprived of a normal surface.

depth The deepest portion of a surgically excised specimen, as in "The margins and depths of the specimen are free of malignant cells."

DIC Disseminated intravascular coagulation, a condition in which widespread clotting of blood in vessels consumes clotting factors and leads to hemorrhage.

dilated Enlarged.

dosimeter A device worn continuously by a person whose occupation involves exposure to x-rays or other radiation, to monitor cumulative exposure. Also called a *film badge*.

double contrast technique A modification of a barium contrast procedure for radiographic examination of the digestive system. After the standard barium enema examination has been performed and the barium has passed out of the area under study, air or gas is injected. The coating of barium remaining on the surface may outline masses or defects nor seen during the standard examination.

ectasia Expansion or dilatation of a duct or vessel.

ectopia Abnormal location of a tissue or structure.

effacement Abnormal flattening of the contour of a structure.

efferent Conducting away from a structure.

effusion An oozing or outpouring of fluid.

electrode A component of an electrical device that conducts or detects electricity.

emphysema Abnormal presence of air within tissues.

end point The point in an analysis at which the chemical reaction is complete, or at which the reading or interpretation of test results is feasible.

endosteum The connective-tissue lining of the marrow cavity of a bone.

enterotome An autopsy instrument used for opening the intestine.

eosinophilia (1) Affinity for eosin and other acidic stains. (2) An abnormal increase of eosinophils in the circulating blood or in tissue.

epistaxis Nosebleed.

erythema Abnormal redness.

erythroderma Redness of the skin.

eschar A crust or scab of exudate or devitalized tissue forming at the site of a burn or other injury.

etiology The study of the causes of disease; often used in the sense of "cause."

excrescence An abnormal nodule or mass growing away from a surface.

exophytic Growing away from a surface.

extension Straightening of a joint so that both bones form a straight line.

extravasate To leak or ooze from vessels.

extravasation of contrast medium Leakage of contrast medium from the structure into which it is injected through a perforation or other abnormal orifice.

fascia A general term for a binding or enveloping sheet of connective tissue such as that which lies under the skin surface and those that surround muscles or muscle groups.

fascicle A small bundle.

fibrofatty Consisting of fibrous and fatty connective tissue.

fibrovascular Consisting of fibrous connective tissue and blood vessels.

filiform Threadlike.

filling defect A zone within a tubular structure that is not filled by injected contrast medium (usually a neoplasm or abnormal mass).

film badge A device worn continuously by a person whose occupation involves exposure to x-rays or other radiation, to monitor cumulative exposure. Also called a *personal dosimeter*.

first pass view An image or set of images obtained immediately after the injection of radionuclide into the circulation, when its concentration in the blood pool is at its highest.

fixation device Any appliance placed surgically in or on a bone to stabilize a fracture during healing.

flaccid Limp, not spastic or rigid.

flagellum A whiplike process characteristic of certain protozoans.

flexion Bending of a joint to a more acute angle.

florid Fully developed, as in "florid cirrhosis."

flush method An angiographic technique in which contrast medium is injected into a relatively large vessel so as to visualize all the organs or tissues supplied by it.

focal Confined to one or several distinct sites or foci.

frank Fully developed, obvious, unequivocal, as in "frank pus."

Franseen needle A needle used for aspiration biopsy as well as for removal of a solid core of tissue.

free air Air or gas in a body cavity where it does not belong, usually after escape from the gastrointestinal tract.

friable Crumbly, readily broken up.

frogleg view A radiographic study of one or both hip joints for which the subject lies supine (face up) with thighs maximally abducted and externally rotated and knees flexed so as to bring the soles of the feet together.

full-bladder technique An ultrasonographic examination of the pelvic organs performed while the subject's bladder is distended with urine. This is done to improve the recognition of the bladder outline, which cannot be distinguished adequately when the bladder is empty.

fungating Growing rapidly and irregularly, like a fungus, usually said of a neoplasm.

fusiform Spindle-shaped; an elongated structure that is thicker in the middle than at either end.

galvanometer A device for measuring electrical potential (voltage).

gas density line A linear band of maximal radiolucency, representing or appearing to represent a narrow zone of air or gas.

gastroesophageal reflux Abnormal backflow of material from the stomach into the lower esophagus.

gated view An image obtained by a technique synchronized with motions of the heart to eliminate blurring.

gemistocyte A swollen astrocyte with an eccentric nucleus.

genupectoral position (knee-chest position) A position for examination or therapeutic procedures in which the subject kneels on the examining table and bends forward so that the weight of the upper body rests on the chest.

Gluck rib shears An autopsy instrument used to cut through the costosternal joints.

granular Speckled or grainy in appearance or texture.

great vessels The major vascular trunks entering and leaving the heart: the superior and inferior venae cavae, the pulmonary arteries and veins, and the aorta.

Greene needle A biopsy needle used for aspiration and also for removal of solid tissue specimens.

grumous Lumpy; said of a liquid or semisolid material with small, denser masses or bodies suspended in it.

gumma A rubbery nodule of inflammation and necrosis, characteristic of tertiary syphilis.

hematemesis Vomiting blood.

hemoglobinuria The presence of hemoglobin, as distinct from whole blood, in the urine.

hemoptysis Coughing up blood from the respiratory tract.

hepatomegaly Enlargement of the liver.

hepatosplenomegaly Enlargement of the liver and spleen.

hereditary Inherited; affecting the genetic makeup of an organism.

hertz (Hz) A unit corresponding to a frequency or wave motion of 1 cycle per second (cps).

high normal A quantitative test result that is near the upper limit of normal, though within the normal range.

Holter monitor A portable ECG machine worn by the subject for 24-48 hours to record intermittent abnormalities in cardiac rate, rhythm, or conduction.

host The person or animal in whom an infection or infestation occurs.

Howship lacuna A pit or cavity resulting from resorption of calcium from bone.

Hutchinson teeth Notched incisor teeth in congenital syphilis.

hypercapnia Excess of carbon dioxide in the blood.

hypermetropia Far-sightedness.

hyperventilation Breathing that is deeper and more rapid than required for normal oxygen and carbon dioxide exchange.

hypoaeration Abnormal reduction in the amount of air in lung tissue.

hypokinesis Abnormal reduction of mobility or motility; reduced contractile force in one or both cardiac ventricles.

hypoxia Deficiency of oxygen.

iatrogenic Referring to a condition, abnormality, disease, or injury that results from medical or surgical treatment or from a diagnostic procedure.

idiopathic Arising as if spontaneously; said of a disease or abnormality whose cause is unknown.

ileus Small-bowel obstruction due to failure of peristalsis.

impingement Contact or pressure, generally abnormal, between two structures.

in situ (Latin, 'in position') In its original or normal position; said of a malignancy that has not begun to extend or invade beyond its tissue of origin.

in vitro (Latin, 'in glass') Referring to a condition, change, or reaction existing or occurring in a test tube or other laboratory vessel.

in vivo (Latin, 'in the living') Referring to a condition, change, or reaction existing or occurring in the living body.

indicator A chemical substance that changes color in the presence of certain other substances or in response to variations in acidity or alkalinity.

indifferent electrode An ECG or EEG electrode whose input is used to bal-

ance the input of the recording electrode.

induration Abnormal hardening of tissue.

injection Hyperemia; dilatation of blood vessels causing redness of a surface or tissue.

inoculation Introduction of infectious material into a living host or culture medium.

inspissated Dried out, thickened; said of fluid or semisolid materials.

interstitial markings The radiographic appearance of lung tissue, as opposed to the appearance of air contained in the lung.

interval change Change in the radiographic appearance of a structure or lesion in the interval between two examinations.

invasive Said of diagnostic procedures that require the introduction of instruments such as vascular catheters into the body.

isometric Without change of length, said of a measurement of force in which no motion takes place between the thing measured and the recording instrument.

isotonic Without change of force, said of a measurement of force in which movement takes place between the thing measured and the recording instrument.

Jamshidi needle A biopsy needle.

karyorrhexis Fragmentation of cell nuclei.

K-complex A brief series of slower waves of higher voltage noted on the EEG during sleep.

keratic precipitates Inflammatory deposits of cells and protein on the posterior surface of the cornea, as seen with a slit lamp.

keratoacanthoma A benign epidermal tumor resembling squamous cell carcinoma.

koilocytosis A hollow appearance of cells.

label To render a substance radioactive by incorporating a radionuclide in it.

lamellated Layered.

laminated Layered.

lead A wire conducting electrical information from the subject to a recording instrument (e.g., ECG or EEG). Also, the tracing that reflects data obtained by a particular lead.

Lee needle A cutting biopsy needle.

lesion Any local, objectively perceptible abnormality in tissues resulting from injury or disease.

leukocytosis Abnormal increase in circulating leukocytes.

leukoderma Abnormal whiteness of skin.

leukopenia Abnormal decrease in circulating leukocytes.

level A numerical (quantitative) test result showing the amount or (more often) concentration of a substance in a specimen.

ligneous Woody.

lipidosis Any abnormal condition characterized by an increased amount of lipid.

lipophage A macrophage that has ingested lipid material.

lithotomy position A position for examination or therapeutic procedures in which the subject lies supine (face up) with the feet supported in stirrups, the hips and knees flexed, and the knees spread apart.

loculated effusion A collection of fluid whose distribution is limited by adjacent normal or abnormal structures.

low normal A quantitative test result that is near the lower limit of normal, though within the normal range.

lucent defect An abnormal zone of decreased resistance to x-rays, appearing darker on the x-ray film.

lumen The interior of a hollow body passage (blood vessel, intestine) or of a tubular instrument (catheter, endoscope).

lytic (osteolytic) lesion A disease or abnormality resulting from or consisting of focal breakdown of bone, with reduction in density.

macrometastasis A grossly evident metastasis.

macrophage A blood or tissue cell that phagocytizes invading microorganisms, foreign material, or debris from degenerating cells or tissues.

macula The central, most light-sensitive part of the retina; in full, macula lutea.

Madayag needle A biopsy needle used for aspiration and also for removal of solid tissue specimens.

malar Pertaining to the cheeks.

manometer A device for measuring pressure.

marantic Pertaining to cachexia or wasting.

marasmus Wasting, cachexia, particularly when due to protein and caloric deficiency in children.

mass effect Anything that occupies space within the body and is not normal tissue.

meaty Having the appearance or texture of raw meat.

mediastinum That part of the thoracic cavity lying between the lungs.

melena Tarry black stools, generally due to bleeding within the digestive tract.

mesangial Pertaining to the mesangium, a membrane that supports the capillary loops of a glomerulus.

metabolic equivalent (MET) The oxygen consumption of a subject at complete rest, defined as 3.5 mL of oxygen per kilogram of body weight per minute.

metabolism A general term referring to the sum of biochemical processes taking place in a living organism, or to specific groups of such processes, as in "carbohydrate metabolism."

microcalcification A very small deposit of calcium in breast tissue, as seen in a mammogram. Clustered microcalcifications are highly suggestive of malignancy.

micrometastasis A microscopic metastasis.

midline shift Displacement of a structure that is normally seen at or near the midline of the body, such as the pineal gland or the trachea.

mmHg Millimeter of mercury, a unit of pressure, also called *torr*.

mononucleosis Excessive numbers of mononuclear cells in circulating blood.

morphology The study of the shape or appearance of structures; often used as a synonym for "shape" or "appearance."

mottled Irregularly covered with darker or lighter spots.

mucopus A mixture of mucus and pus.

multi-echo images (MRI) A series of spin echo images obtained with various pulse sequences.

mummification Necrosis of tissue (as in gangrene) or of a dead body accompanied by extreme drying and shriveling, with only slight evidence of putrefaction.

myalgia Muscular pain.

mycosis Any fungal infection.

mycotic aneurysm An aneurysm due to local infection with a fungus. Although this is the literal meaning of the term, in practice it usually refers to local infection caused by bacteria carried in the circulation from another site.

mydriatic A medicine that dilates the pupil.

myopia Nearsightedness.

negative control A specimen that is known to be normal, or that should yield a negative test.

nephrocalcinosis Deposition of calcium salts in the tissue of the kidney.

normocephalic Having a normal head.

nosocomial Pertaining to a hospital, and particularly to an infection contracted by a hospitalized person.

nuclear dust Fragments of a nucleus that has undergone karyorrhexis.

obliteration Complete removal of a structure, or complete filling of a cavity or passage.

obturator A solid plug placed temporarily inside a hollow instrument such as an anoscope to facilitate insertion.

occult Hidden, not evident; said of abnormalities or diseases that are not readily apparent but may be revealed by diagnostic investigation.

oliguria Abnormal reduction in the volume of urine.

opacification An increase in the density of a tissue or region, with increased resistance to x-rays and lighter appearance on the x-ray film.

opportunistic Said of microorganisms that seldom invade healthy persons but often cause infections in persons with diminished immunity or in tissues already damaged by injury or disease.

organogenesis Formation of organs during embryonic development.

orthochromatic Showing normal or expected staining properties.

osteoblastic Referring to development or overdevelopment of bone tissue.

osteolytic Referring to absorption or destruction of bone tissue.

osteophyte An abnormal growth of calcified, bonelike material from the surface of a bone.

ostium A small orifice.

palisade A configuration created by structures lined up like the palings of a fence.

palpation Feeling a structure or tissue for diagnostic purposes.

panic level An abnormal test result level that may indicate a severe or life-threatening condition.

papillary Showing nipplelike projections.

paracentesis Removal of fluid from a cavity, especially the abdominal cavity, with a hollow needle.

parameter Although this term has a specific meaning in mathematics, in medical jargon it means any variable that can be measured.

parenchyma The distinctive and functioning cells and tissues of any organ, as opposed to the connective tissue stroma. See *stroma*.

patchy Occurring in irregularly shaped and irregularly distributed areas.

patent Open, unobstructed.

pedunculated Attached to a surface by a stalk.

percutaneous Through the skin.

perforation Creation of an abnormal opening, usually in a hollow structure.

perfusion The flow of fluid through the vessels of a structure, generally referring to blood circulation.

peribronchial cuffing Thickening of bronchial walls by edema or fibrosis, as seen on chest x-ray in asthma, emphysema, cardiac failure, and other acute and chronic respiratory and circulatory disorders.

perichondrium The connective-tissue covering of cartilage.

peristalsis The coordinated wave of muscular contractions in a tubular organ such as the intestine by which its contents are propelled forward.

peritoneum The serous membrane that lines the abdominopelvic cavity and covers the abdominal viscera.

phagocytosis The process whereby a blood or tissue cell surrounds, engulfs, and removes or destroys microorganisms, foreign materials, or tissue debris.

phlebolith A calcified thrombus inside a vein.

phlegmon An indurated zone of inflammation and necrosis caused by pyogenic bacteria.

photic Pertaining to light.

pinna The shell-like, sound-collecting part of the external ear.

plain film A radiographic study performed without contrast medium.

plantar Pertaining to the sole of the foot.

plasmacytic Pertaining to plasma cells.

pleocytosis An increase in the number of cells, particularly in the cerebrospinal fluid.

pleomorphic Occurring in various forms.

pleura The serous membrane that lines the thoracic cavity and covers the lungs.

pleural effusion An abnormal accumulation of fluid in the pleural cavity.

polarity Orientation of elongated structures, particularly with respect to an axis.

polygonal Many-sided.

polyhedral Many-sided.

porencephaly The presence of cysts or cavities in the cerebral cortex.

portable film An x-ray picture taken with movable equipment at the bedside or in an emergency department or operating room when it is not feasible to more the patient to the radiology department.

positive control A specimen that is known to be abnormal, or that should yield a positive test.

posterior sulcus The groove formed by the intersection of the diaphragm and the posterior thoracic wall, as seen in a lateral chest x-ray.

prenatal Before birth.

primary Said of a disease or condition not known to result from some other disease or abnormal condition; cf. *secondary*.

primordium The earliest discernible rudiment of a structure during embryonic development; anlage.

probe patent Allowing the passage of a probe; said of an orifice or hollow or tubular structure.

proliferation Reproduction, growth through increase in number of components.

protuberant Bulging, protruding.

proud flesh Granulation tissue of skin or mucous membrane.

pruritus Itching.

psammoma body A small, concentrically laminated mass of calcareous material found in certain neoplasms.

pseudomembrane A film of exudate or tissue debris resembling a membrane.

punctate Forming or resembling a spot or dot.

pyrexia Fever.

pyriform Pear-shaped.

QNS Quantity not sufficient; usually indicating that the specimen submitted is inadequate for the performance of the test requested.

radiolucent Offering relatively little resistance to x-rays, and hence appearing darker on an x-ray film (by analogy with *translucent*).

radionuclide A radioactive isotope; a species of atom that spontaneously emits radioactivity.

radiopaque Resisting penetration by x-rays, and hence appearing light or white on an x-ray film.

rate A laboratory determination involving time; usually a measure of change occurring in a specimen or reagent during a fixed interval of time.

reagent A chemical substance that is made to react with one or more other substances, usually in an analytic procedure.

real-time examination Ultrasonographic examination performed by sweeping the ultrasound beam through the scan plane at a rapid rate, generating up to 30 images per second. This display of images at this frequency is in effect a motion picture, providing visualization of movement of internal structures as it actually occurs.

reconstitution Maintenance of flow in an artery beyond an area of narrowing or obstruction by establishment of collateral circulation.

reconstruction Generation of an image by computer processing of scan data.

recording electrode That one of an array of ECG or EEG electrodes whose input is balanced against the input of one or more indifferent electrodes.

refractile Transmitting light rays in the manner of glass or water, with deviation of rays as they pass into the surrounding air.

Rein rib-cutting knife Autopsy instrument for severing the costosternal joints.

REM sleep The phase of sleep characterized by rapid eye movement, during which most dreaming occurs.

resolution The ability of an optical, radiographic, or other image-forming device to distinguish or separate two closely adjacent points in the subject. In CT, resolution is measured in lines per millimeter. The higher the resolution, the sharper and more faithful the image.

rest (1) A mass of surviving embryonic cells. (2) A mass of cells misplaced during embryonic development (e.g., adrenal tissue in the kidney).

retroperitoneal Behind the peritoneal cavity.

rhythm strip A long, continuous tracing made from lead II of the standard ECG in order to record intermittent disturbances of rhythm.

rosette A ring-shaped cluster.

Rotex needle A cutting biopsy needle.

rouleau (plural, **rouleaux**) A roll of erythrocytes like a stack of coins.

runoff The flow of blood (and contrast medium) through the branches of an artery into which the medium has been injected.

saddle embolus An embolus consisting of a thrombus that comes to rest at the bifurcation of an artery, blocking both branches.

sand, brain Gritty material found in the pineal body, the choroid plexus, and other structures within the brain.

saponification Formation of soap or soaplike material.

sarcoplasm The cytoplasm of striated muscle fibers.

satellite A cell, structure, or lesion found in association with a larger one.

scaphoid Boatlike; said of an abdomen that appears concave when the subject is supine.

sclerosis Hardening.

scout film A plain x-ray study that is performed before the introduction of contrast medium, to assess the general anatomy of the region under study and ensure proper positioning of the patient.

secondary Due to some other condition or disease; as in "secondary hypertension" and "ischemia secondary to vascular occlusion." Cf. primary.

sensitize To introduce material into a fluid, tissue, or space for purposes of performing a radioactive scan; essentially the same as label.

septum A dividing wall or membrane.

serial scans A series of scans made at regular intervals along one dimension of a body region.

siderophage A macrophage that has ingested hemosiderin, a product of broken-down erythrocytes.

signal intensity (MRI) The strength of the signal or stream of radiofrequency energy emitted by tissue after an excitation pulse.

Sims position A position for examination or therapeutic procedures in which the subject lies on the left side with the hips and knees flexed, the right hip and knee more than the left.

skin slip Abnormal mobility of the skin over subcutaneous structures due to early putrefactive changes in a dead body.

sleep spindle A spindle-shaped complex of waves with a frequency of 14/sec, noted on the EEG during sleep.

slide test A test, usually qualitative, performed on a glass, plastic, or cardboard plate, strip, disc, or microscope slide; especially a test designed to be performed simply and rapidly by persons without technical training.

slough Complete separation of inflamed or devitalized tissue.

small-bowel transit time The time required for swallowed contrast medium to pass through the small bowel and appear in the colon.

sonolucent Offering relatively little resistance to ultrasound waves and hence generating few or no echoes (by analogy with *translucent* and *radiolucent*).

specimen Any material or object that is subjected to scientific examination, measurement, or analysis; generally a sample whose composition is assumed to be representative of the whole from which it is derived.

sphincter A ringlike muscle that acts as a valve around a natural body passage or orifice.

sphygmomanometer A device for measuring blood pressure.

spin echo image A magnetic resonance image obtained by the spin echo technique. With this technique, T2 is determined indirectly, as a function of TE, the echo time.

spondylitis Inflammation of one or more vertebrae.

spurring Formation of one or more jagged osteophytes, as in osteoarthritis.

stable Firm, displaying no abnormal mobility or looseness.

stacked scans Same as *contiguous images*.

standard A material of known properties that is used to calibrate an instrument or test system or to verify its correctness.

stat Immediately; refers to medical procedures performed on an urgent basis, including laboratory testing.

stellate Star-shaped.

stenosis Abnormal narrowing of an orifice or tubular structure.

stippling Speckling with fine dots.

storage disease A metabolic disorder that causes excessive accumulation of a substance such as glycogen in cells or tissues.

strandy infiltrate A pulmonic infiltrate that appears as strands or streaks of increased density (lighter on the x-ray film).

stress cystogram A radiographic study of the bladder intended to demonstrate stress incontinence. Contrast medium is instilled into the bladder and films are taken while the subject coughs and bears down.

stroma The supporting framework of an organ, made up of connective tissue rather than actively functioning cells. See also *parenchyma*.

subcutaneous emphysema Air or gas in subcutaneous tissues.

subcutaneous fat line The edges or borders of the subcutaneous fat layer as seen on an x-ray film.

suboptimal Not as good as might have been expected; usually referring to technical factors in an x-ray study, such as positioning, film quality, and patient cooperation.

substrate The material on which an enzyme acts. The substrate of a phosphatase is phosphate.

surface coil (MRI) A simple flat coil placed on the surface of the body and used as a receiver.

suture, cranial A joint between two of the bones of the cranial vault.

syndrome A combination of symptoms or abnormal signs having a common cause.

T1 (MRI) The time it takes for protons to return to their orientation to a static magnetic field after an excitation pulse.

T1 weighted image (MRI) A spin echo image generated by a pulse sequence using a short TR (0.6 seconds or less).

T2 (MRI) The time it takes for protons to go out of phase after having been shifted in their orientation by an excitation pulse.

T2 weighted image (MRI) A spin echo image generated by a pulse sequence using a long TR (2.0 seconds or more).

tachypnea Abnormally rapid respiratory rate.

takeoff of a vessel The origin of a branch from a larger vessel, as demonstrated radiographically with injected contrast medium.

TE (MRI) Echo time; the interval between the first pulse in a spin echo examination and the appearance of the resulting echo.

tenting of hemidiaphragm A distortion of the diaphragm by scarring, in which an upward-pointing angular configuration (like a tent) replaces all or part of the normal curved contour of a hemidiaphragm OR A tent-shaped distortion of the diaphragm due to scarring.

teratology The study of congenital and developmental abnormalities.

thermistor A device that measures temperature by converting heat to an electronic signal.

thermocoagulation Coagulation of tissue by excessive heat.

thora(co)centesis Removal of fluid from the thoracic cavity.

tinnitus A ringing or other abnormal noise in one or both ears.

titration A measurement or analysis in which an end point is reached after a series of small additions of reagent.

torr A unit of pressure corresponding to 1 millimeter of mercury (mmHg).

tortuous Twisted, winding.

toxicology The study of poisons and their effects on living organisms.

TR (MRI) Repetition time; the interval between one spin echo pulse sequence and the next.

trabecula A sheet or band of connective tissue that incompletely divides the parenchyma of an organ into segments.

traction artifact Abnormal appearances created in tissue by suction or stretching during the obtaining of a biopsy specimen.

transducer A device that converts one form of energy into another—for example, sound waves to electrical signals.

transect To cut across.

transudate A fluid low in fibrin and cells that has passed through a membrane.

trocar A sharp-pointed rod that is placed inside a cannula to facilitate its insertion by puncturing the skin or mucous membrane. See *cannula*.

Tru-Cut needle A cutting biopsy needle.

turnaround time The time that elapses between the ordering of a test (or the obtaining of a specimen) and the reporting of the test results by the laboratory.

Turner needle A biopsy needle for aspiration and cutting of solid tissue specimens.

umbilicated Having a central pit or dimple.

unattended death Death of a person not under medical care.

unremarkable Displaying no abnormal or unusual features.

uptake The absorption or concentration of a substance, particularly a radionuclide, by an organ or tissue.

urticaria Hives; a transitory eruption of itchy white papules (wheals) usually due to allergy.

vasoconstriction Constriction of blood vessels, principally arterioles.

vasodilatation Dilatation of blood vessels, principally arterioles.

ventricular ejection fraction That portion of the total volume of blood present in a ventricle at the end of filling (diastole) that is ejected during ventricular contraction (systole); usually expressed as a percent rather than a fraction.

vesicular Resembling a bladder; said of a cell nucleus whose chromatin has been displaced to the margin of the nucleus, creating a hollow or open appearance.

Virchow chisel An autopsy instrument used for splitting bone.

viremia The presence of a virus in the blood.

washout phase Scintiscanning of the lungs at the conclusion of the inhalation phase of a ventilation scan, after an interval during which all inhaled radionuclide would be expected to have been exhaled.

Westcott needle A cutting biopsy needle.

whorl A circular swirl or vortex.

WNL Within normal limits.

xeroderma Abnormal dryness of the skin.

zymogen granules Secretory granules in the cytoplasm of glandular epithelium, representing precursors of enzymes.

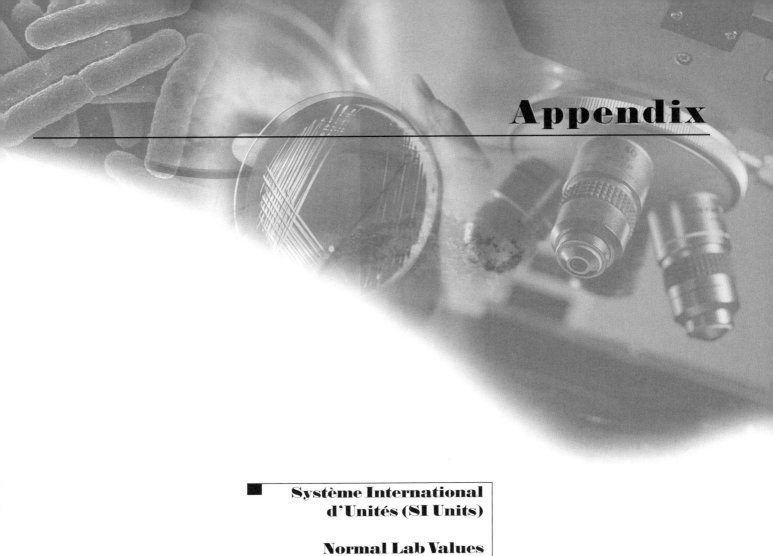

Appendix

- **Système International d'Unités (SI Units)**

  **Normal Lab Values
  Tests Performed on Whole
  Blood, Plasma, or Serum**

Système International d'Unités (SI Units)

This appendix shows only those SI units that are currently used in reporting clinical laboratory results.

The following conventions, some of them applicable also to the metric system, are observed with SI units.

1. A symbol is not followed by a period (except at the end of a sentence) and is not pluralized with final *s*. Thus, 21.3 mg (not 21.3 mg. or 21.3 mgs).

2. A numeral is followed by the abbreviation for the unit, not the full name of the unit. Thus, 10 mg (not 10 milligrams or ten mg).

3. Decimals are preferred to fractions. Thus, 1.75 cm (not 1³/₄ cm).

4. A zero is placed before a decimal less than 1. Thus, 0.25 U/L (not .25 U/L).

5. In a drug dosage, whether handwritten or keystroked, a whole number is not followed by a decimal point and a zero (2.0), nor is the last whole number to the right of the decimal point followed by a zero (2.50), because of the risk of misreading. Thus, 2 mg four times daily (not 2.0 mg four times daily, which might be misread as 20 mg four times daily); 5 mg/kg (not 5.0 mg/kg, which might be misread as 50 mg/kg). In physics and chemistry, however, the number of figures to the right of the decimal point in a numerical value indicates the degree of precision of the procedure that yielded the value. For that reason, a final zero to the right of the decimal point in a laboratory report should not be dropped. Thus, digoxin, 2.0 ng/mL (not 2 ng/mL); pH 7.40, not 7.4.

6. For numerals of five or more digits, spaces are preferred to commas to separate digits into groups of 3 starting from the decimal point. Thus, 2500 (not 2,500); 42 650 (not 42,650); 300 000 (not 300,000); 0.000 75 (not 0.000,75).

Prefixes and Their Abbreviations and Meanings

Multiples of Ten

kilo-	k	1000 (10^3)
hecto-	h	100 (10^2)
deca-	da	10 (10^1)

Submultiples of Ten

deci-	d	0.1 (10^{-1}) (one tenth)
centi-	c	0.01 (10^{-2}) (one hundredth)
milli-	m	0.001 (10^{-3}) (one thousandth)
micro-	µ (or mc)	0.000 001 (10^{-6}) (one millionth)
nano-	n	0.000 000 001 (10^{-9}) (one billionth)
pico-	p	0.000 000 000 001 (10^{-12}) (one trillionth)
femto-	f	0.000 000 000 000 001 (10^{-15}) (one quadrillionth)

Units of Length

Basic unit: meter (m)

1 kilometer	km	1000 m (10^3 m)
1 hectometer	hm	100 m (10^2 m)
1 decameter	dam	10 m (10^1 m)

Units of Length *(cont.)*

1 decimeter	dm	0.1 m (10^{-1} m)
1 centimeter	cm	0.01 m (10^{-2} m)
1 millimeter	mm	0.001 m (10^{-3} m)
1 micrometer	μm, mcm	0.000 001 m (10^{-6} m)
1 nanometer	nm	0.000 000 001 m (10^{-9} m)
1 picometer	pm	0.000 000 000 001 m (10^{-12} m)
1 femtometer	fm	0.000 000 000 000 001 m (10^{-5} m)

Units of Mass

Basic unit: gram (g)

1 kilogram	kg	1000 g (10^{3} g)
1 hectogram	hg	100 g (10^{2} g)
1 decagram	dag	10 g (10^{1} g)
1 decigram	dg	0.1 g (10^{-1} g)
1 centigram	cg	0.01 g (10^{-2} g)
1 milligram	mg	0.001 g (10^{-3} g)
1 microgram	μg, mcg	0.000 001 g (10^{-6} g)
1 nanogram	ng	0.000 000 001 g (10^{-9} g)
1 picogram	pg	0.000 000 000 001 g (10^{-12} g)
1 femtogram	fg	0.000 000 000 000 001 g (10^{-15} g)

Units of Amount of Matter

Basic unit: mole (mol)

1 kilomole	kmol	1000 mol (10^{3} mol)
1 hectomole	hmol	100 mol (10^{2} mol)
1 decamole	damol	10 mol (10^{1} mol)
1 decimole	dmol	0.1 mol (10^{-1} mol)
1 centimole	cmol	0.01 mol (10^{-2} mol)
1 millimole	mmol	0.001 mol (10^{-3} mol)
1 micromole	μmol, mcmol	0.000 001 mol (10^{-6} mol)
1 nanomole	nmol	0.000 000 001 mol (10^{-9} mol)
1 picomole	pmol	0.000 000 000 001 mol (10^{-12} mol)
1 femtomole	fmol	0.000 000 000 000 001 mol (10^{-15} mol)

Units of Volume

Basic unit: liter (L) = 1 cu dm

1 kiloliter	kL	1000 L (10^3 L)
1 hectoliter	hL	100 L (10^2 L)
1 decaliter	daL	10 L (10^1 L)
1 deciliter	dL	0.1 L (10^{-1} L)
1 centiliter	cL	0.01 L (10^{-2} L)
1 milliliter	mL	0.001 L (10^{-3} L)
1 microliter	μL, mcL	0.000 001 L (10^{-6} L)
1 nanoliter	nL	0.000 000 001 L (10^{-9} L)
1 picoliter	pL	0.000 000 000 001 L (10^{-12} L)
1 femtomole	fL	0.000 000 000 000 001 L (10^{-15} L)

Normal Lab Values
Tests Performed on Whole Blood, Plasma, or Serum

Note: Test results depend on methods used. Normal ranges and other interpretive data given in this book are intended solely for purposes of orientation and should not be applied to actual test results.

Analyte or Procedure	Normal Range (Metric)	Normal Range (SI)
A/G (albumin/globulin) ratio	1.5-3.0	1.5-3.0
AAT (alpha₁ antitrypsin)	100-300 mg/mL	20-60 mmol/L
acid phosphatase	<0.6 U/L	<0.6 U/L
ACTH (adrenocorticotropic hormone)	10-50 pg/mL	2.2-11.1 pmol/L
adrenocorticotropic hormone (ACTH)	10-50 pg/mL	2.2-11.1 pmol/L
AFP (alpha-fetoprotein)	<15 ng/mL	<15 mcg/L
albumin	3.5-5.0 g/dL	35-50 g/L
albumin/globulin (A/G) ratio	1.5-3.0	1.5-3.0
aldolase	2.5 U/L	2.5 U/L
aldosterone, recumbent	3-16 ng/dL	0.08-0.44 nmol/L
aldosterone, upright	7-30 ng/dL	0.19-0.83 nmol/L
alkaline phosphatase	20-120 U/L	20-120 U/L
alpha₁ antitrypsin (AAT)	100-300 mg/mL	20-60 mmol/L
alpha-fetoprotein (AFP)	<15 ng/mL	<15 mcg/L
ALT (alanine aminotransferase) (formerly SGPT)	8-45 U/L	8-45 U/L
ammonia, serum	15-45 mcg/dL	11-32 mcmol/L
amylase	<125 U/L	<125 U/L
anion gap	12-20 mEq/L	12-20 mmol/L
AST (aspartate aminotransferase) (formerly SGOT)	<35 U/L	<35 U/L
B cells	5-15%	5-15%
bands (banded neutrophils)	4-8%	4-8%
basophils	0-1%	0-1%
bicarbonate	24-30 mEq/L	24-30 mmol/L
bilirubin, direct	0.1-0.4 mg/dL	1.7-6.8 mcmol/L
bilirubin, indirect	0.1-0.9 mg/dL	1.7-15.3 mcmol/L
bilirubin, total	0.2-1.3 mg/dL	3.4-22.1 mcmol/L
bleeding time	< 4 minutes	< 4 minutes
blood urea nitrogen (BUN)	5-20 mg/dL	1.8-7.1 mcmol/L
BNP (brain natriuretic peptide)	<50 pg/mL	<50 ng/L
brain natriuretic peptide (BNP)	<50 pg/mL	<50 ng/L

Normal Lab Values

Analyte or Procedure	Normal Range (Metric)	Normal Range (SI)
BUN (blood urea nitrogen)	5-20 mg/dL	1.8-7.1 mcmol/L
calcitonin, male	0-15 pg/mL	0-4.20 pmol/L
calcium	8.2-10.2 mg/dL	2-2.5 mmol/L
carcinoembryonic antigen (CEA)	<2.5 ng/mL	<2.5 mcg/L
CD4 cell count	500-1500 cells/mm^3	0.5-1.5 x 10^9 cells/L
chloride	100-106 mEq/L	100-106 mmol/L
cholesterol	<200 mg/dL	<520 mmol/L
cholinesterase (pseudocholinesterase)	8-18 U/L	8-18 U/L
clotting time, Lee-White	6-17 minutes	6-17 minutes
copper	0.7-1.5 mcg/mL	11-24 mmol/L
cortisol, 8 a.m.	5-23 mcg/dL	138-635 nmol/L
cortisol, 4 p.m.	3-16 mcg/dL	83-441 nmol/L
creatinine	0.6-1.2 mg/dL	50-100 mcmol/L
electrolytes: see individual values for sodium, potassium, chloride, and bicarbonate		
eosinophils	2-4%	2-4%
EPO (erythropoietin)	5-30 mU/mL	5-30 U/L
erythrocyte sedimentation rate, Westergren	0-20 mm/hr	0-20 mm/hr
erythrocyte sedimentation rate, Wintrobe	0-15 mm/hr	0-15 mm/hr
erythropoietin (EPO)	5-30 mU/mL	5-30 mU/mL
estradiol	24-149 pg/mL	90-550 pmol/L
ferritin	20-200 ng/mL	20-200 mcg/L
fibrin degradation products (fibrin split products)	<3 mcg/mL	<3 mg/L
5´-nucleotidase	<12.5 U/L	<12.5 U/L
follicle-stimulating hormone (FSH), female	1.1-24 ng/mL	5.0-108 U/L
follicle-stimulating hormone (FSH), male	0.5-4.5 ng/mL	2.2-20.0 U/L
free fatty acids (FFA)	8-20 mg/dL	0.2-0.7 mmol/L
free T$_4$ index	0.9-2.1 ng/dL	12-27 pmol/L
FSH (follicle-stimulating hormone), female	1.1-24 ng/mL	5.0-108 U/L
FSH (follicle-stimulating hormone), male	0.5-4.5 ng/mL	2.2-20.0 U/L
FSP (fibrin split products)	<3 mcg/mL	<3 mg/L

Normal Lab Values

Analyte or Procedure	Normal Range (Metric)	Normal Range (SI)
gamma-glutamyl transpeptidase (GGT)	< 65 U/L	< 65 U/L
gastrin	21-125 pg/mL	10-59.3 pmol/L
GFR (glomerular filtration rate)	90-135 mL/min/1.73 m^2	0.86-1.3 mL/sec/m^2
GGT (gamma-glutamyl transpeptidase)	< 65 U/L	< 65 U/L
globulin, total	1.5-3.0 g/dL	15-30 g/L
glomerular filtration rate (GFR)	90-135 mL/min/1.73 m^2	0.86-1.3 mL/sec/m^2
glucagon	50-200 pg/mL	14-57 pmol/L
glucose	60-115 mg/dL	3.3-6.4 mmol/L
glycosylated hemoglobin (hemoglobin A_{1C}), normal	4-7%	4-7%
acceptable diabetic control	<8%	<8%
haptoglobin	40-180 mg/dL	0.4-1.8 g/L
HDL (high density lipoprotein) cholesterol	35-80 mg/dL	1-2 mmol/L
hematocrit	40-48%	40-48%
hemoglobin	12-16 g/dL	(7.5-10 mmol/L)
hemoglobin A_{1C} (see glycosylated hemoglobin)	4-7%	4-7%
hexosaminidase A	2.5-9 U/L	2.5-9 U/L
high density lipoprotein (HDL) cholesterol	35-80 mg/dL	1-2 mmol/L
homocysteine	<1.6 mg/L	<12 mcmol/L
insulin	5-25 mcU/mL	34-172 pmol/L
iron, males	50-160 mcg/dL	9.0-28.8 mcmol/L
iron, females	45-144 mcg/dL	8.1-26 mcmol/L
iron-binding capacity	250-350 mcg/dL	45-63 mcmol/L
lactate dehydrogenase (LDH)	<110 U/L	<110 U/L
lactic acid	4.5-19.8 mg/dL	0.5-2.2 mmol/L
LDH (lactate dehydrogenase)	<110 U/L	<110 U/L
LDL (low density lipoprotein) cholesterol	40-130 mg/dL	1-3 mmol/L
leucine aminopeptidase, serum (SLAP)	< 40 U/L	< 40 U/L
LH (luteinizing hormone), females	0.5-2.7 mcg/mL	4.5-24.3 U/L
LH (luteinizing hormone), males	0.4-1.9 mcg/mL	3.6-17.1 U/L
lipase	<1.5 U/L	<1.5 U/L
low density lipoprotein (LDL) cholesterol	40-130 mg/dL	1-3 mmol/L

Normal Lab Values

Analyte or Procedure	Normal Range (Metric)	Normal Range (SI)
luteinizing hormone (LH), females	0.5-2.7 mcg/mL	0.4-1.9 mcg/mL
luteinizing hormone (LH), males	4.5-24.3 U/L	3.6-17.1 U/L
lymphocytes	25-40%	25-40%
magnesium	1.5-2.3 mg/dL	0.6-1.0 mmol/L
MCH (mean corpuscular hemoglobin)	27-31 pg/cell	27-31 pg/cell
MCHC (mean corpuscular hemoglobin concentration)	32-36 g/dL	320-360 g/L
MCV (mean corpuscular volume)	82-92 mcm3	82-92 fL
mean corpuscular hemoglobin (MCH)	27-31 pg/cell	27-31 pg/cell
mean corpuscular hemoglobin concentration (MCHC)	32-36 g/dL	320-360 g/L
mean corpuscular volume (MCV)	82-92 mcm3	82-92 fL
melatonin, 8 a.m.	0.8-7.7 pg/mL	3.5-33 pmol/L
melatonin, midnight	3.7-23.3 pg/mL	16-100 pmol/L
methemoglobin	<3%	<3%
monocytes	4-6%	4-6%
myeloid/erythroid ratio	2.0-4.0	2.0-4.0
myoglobin	14-51 mcg/L	0.8-2.9 mol/L
osmolality, serum	280-295 mOsm/kg	280-295 mOsm/kg
oxygen saturation	95-100%	95-100%
parathyroid hormone	11-54 pg/mL	1.2-5.6 pmol/L
partial pressure of carbon dioxide (pCO_2)	35-45 torr	35-45 torr
partial pressure of oxygen (pO_2)	75-100 torr	75-100 torr
partial thromboplastin time (PTT)	22-37 seconds	22-37 seconds
pCO_2 (partial pressure of carbon dioxide)	35-45 torr	35-45 torr
pepsinogen	124-142 ng/mL	124-142 mcg/L
pH	7.35-7.45	7.35-7.45
phenylalanine	2-4 mg/dL	121-242 mcmol/L
phosphorus	2.5-4.5 mg/dL	0.8-1.5 mmol/L
platelets	150 000-400 000/mm^3	150-400 x 10^9/L
pO_2 (partial pressure of oxygen)	75-100 torr	75-100 torr

Normal Lab Values

Analyte or Procedure	Normal Range (Metric)	Normal Range (SI)
potassium	3.5-5.0 mEq/L	3.5-5.0 mmol/L
progesterone	0.1-28 ng/mL	0.3-89 nmol/L
prolactin (nonpregnant)	2.5-19 ng/mL	1.1-8.6 nmol/L
prostate specific antigen (PSA)	<4 ng/mL	<4 mcg/L
prothrombin time (PT)	12-14 seconds	12-14 seconds
PSA (prostate specific antigen)	< 4 ng/mL	<4 mcg/L
pseudocholinesterase (cholinesterase)	8-18 U/L	8-18 U/L
PT (prothrombin time)	12-14 seconds	12-14 seconds
PTT (partial thromboplastin time)	22-37 seconds	22-37 seconds
RDW (red cell distribution width)	< 15%	< 15%
red blood cells	4 800 000-5 600 000/mm^3	4.8-5.6 x 10^{12}/L
red cell distribution width (RDW)	< 15%	< 15%
renin, reclining	0.2-2.3 ng/mL	4.7-54.5 pmol/L
renin, upright	1.6-4.3 ng/mL	38-102 pmol/L
reticulocytes	0.5-1.5%	0.5-1.5%
sedimentation rate (erythrocyte sedimentation rate)		
segmented neutrophils	40-70%	40-70%
SGGT (see GGT)		
SGOT (serum glutamic oxalo-acetic transaminase) (now AST)	<35 U/L	<35 U/L
SGPT (serum glutamic pyruvic transaminase) (now ALT)	8-45 U/L	8-45 U/L
SLAP (serum leucine aminopeptidase)	< 40 U/L	< 40 U/L
sodium	136-145 mEq/L	136-145 mmol/L
somatotropin, child	5-10 ng/mL	232-465 pmol/L
somatotropin, adult	< 2.5 ng/mL	<116 pmol/L
T cells	55-65%	55-65%
T$_3$	70-190 ng/dL	1.1-2.9 nmol/L
T$_3$ uptake	25-38%	0.25-0.38
T$_4$ (thyroxine)	4.5-12.0 mcg/dL	58-154 nmol/L
testosterone, male	300-1200 ng/d	10.5-42 nmol/L
thyroid stimulating hormone (TSH)	0.4-4.2 mcU/mL	0.4-4.2 mU/L

Normal Lab Values

Analyte or Procedure	Normal Range (Metric)	Normal Range (SI)
thyroxine (T_4)	4.5-12.0 mcg/dL	58-154 nmol/L
transferrin	250-430 mg/dL	2.5-4.3 g/L
triglycerides	<160 mg/dL	<1.80 mmol/L
tropinin I	<1.5 ng/mL	<1.5 mcg/L
tropinin T	<0.029 ng/mL	<0.029 mcg/L
TSH (thyroid stimulating hormone)	0.4-4.2 mcU/mL	0.4-4.2 mU/L
two-hour (2-hour) postprandial glucose	<140 mg/dL	<7.7 mmol/L
uric acid	3.4-7 mg/dL	202-416 mcmol/L
vasopressin	2-12 pg/mL	1.85-11.1 pmol/L
white blood cells	5-10 x 10^9/L	5000-10 000/mm^3
zinc	0.75-1.4 mcg/mL	11.5-21.6 mcmol/L

Index

Answers to Exercises

Responses to the Short Answers questions are representative and are not necessarily the only correct answers. Answers to Activities for Application and Further Study are subjective and are not included.

Chapter 1. General Introduction

FILL IN THE BLANKS
1. supplemental diagnostic tests that lie outside the scope of the physical examination
2. screening test
3. evaluate disease and response to treatment, screen for hidden conditions, biomedical research
4. quantitative
5. (1) a unit of measure, (2) standard or yardstick, (3) a basis of interpretation
6. validity, usefulness
7. dimensionless measurements
8. accuracy, precision
9. comparison to known ranges of expected or normal values and to values obtained previously on the same patient
10. median, average, mean

MULTIPLE CHOICE
1. A
2. E
3. C
4. A
5. E
6. E
7. B
8. C
9. A
10. A

SHORT ANSWERS
1. Define or explain.
   a. action level—levels above or below which a situation may exist that requires immediate treatment or further assessment.
   b. CLIA—Clinical Laboratory Improvement Amendments, uniform standards of quality, passed by Congress in 1988 for all clinical laboratories in the U.S., as well as registration, surveillance, and enforcement procedures.
   c. CPT—*Physicians' Current Procedural Terminology*, a system that assigns a unique five-digit code number to each type of service rendered to a patient by a health care provider to establish each service as a discrete, standardized entity to which a dollar value can be assigned for health insurance claim processing.
   d. percentile—1/100 of the total range of values. A value falling on the 50th percentile is thus halfway between the highest and the lowest number in the distribution. Widely used in comparing the heights and weights of children to other children of the same gender and age.
   e. screening test— performed on a person who is thought to be well or in whom this particular test has a low statistical probability of proving abnormal and also for social, legal, or occupational reasons.
   f. SI—Système International d'Unités. A metric system revision with the addition of ampere (a unit of electrical current), the candela (a unit of luminous intensity), the kelvin (a unit of temperature), and the mole (a unit of amount of matter), a fully coherent system and its units are defined with the greatest possible precision.
   g. torr—the unit of pressure corresponding to 1 mmHg, in honor of Evangelista Torricelli, inventor of the mercury barometer.
2. Examples of tests performed directly on the patient
   a. cardiac catheterization
   b. endoscopy
   c. electrodiagnostic (EKG, EMG, EEG)
3. Examples of tests performed on specimens
   a. blood tests (CBC)
   b. urine tests
   c. genetic tests
4. How is range of normal established? Data from a sufficiently large population of subjects is necessary to provide a meaningful basis for comparison. Some factors used to determine normal include the median (the middle value in a distribution), the mode (the value occurring most frequently), the average, or arithmetic mean, (the sum of all the values divided by the number of values), and the standard deviation (how far a given value varies from the average or expected value, usually 2 SD).
5. Distinguish between sensitivity and specificity of a test.
   sensitivity—the ability to yield abnormal results consistently when performed on abnormal material usually expressed as a percent. A 90% sensitivity reflects 90 abnormal or positive results and 10 false negative results out of 100 abnormal specimens.
   specificity—refers to ability to reflect only a specific abnormality, not to be influenced by other factors. An 84% specificity means that 84 normal or negative results and 16 false positives would result from 100 normal specimens.
6. Four possible reasons for a false negative result.
   a. improper securing or preservation of the specimen
   b. malfunction or improper calibration of equipment
   c. mistakes in reading or recording results
   d. faulty identification of the source of the specimen
7. Which of these could also cause a false positive result?
   All of the above.

Chapter 2. Anthropometry, Musculoskeletal Measurements, and Clinical Pelvimetry

FILL IN THE BLANKS

1. low birth weight, failure to thrive.
2. obesity
3. between 25 and 30 kg/m2, 30 kg/m2 or more
4. skinfold measurement, underwater weighing
5. cardiovascular disease, type 2 diabetes mellitus
6. body surface area (BSA)
7. achondroplastic dwarfism, Marfan syndrome
8. emphysema
9. goniometry
10. quantitative muscle strength
11. isometric
12. dystocia
13. pelvimetry
14. diagonal conjugate

MULTIPLE COICE

1. D	7. B
2. B	8. E
3. D	9. C
4. A	10. A
5. C	11. B
6. D	

SHORT ANSWERS

1. Define or explain.
   a. anthropometry—a science pertaining to basic body measurements such as height, weight, girth, and arm span, and more complex values derived from them such as body mass index or waist-hip ratio.
   b. dystocia—difficult or protracted labor.
   c. goniometry—measures the passive range of motion.
   d. isometric testing—the subject exerts full force against a resistance that does not move appreciably, and the force is converted by a strain gauge (pressure transducer) into a measurable electronic signal.

   e. passive range of motion—the extent to which an examiner can move a joint in various standard directions, the limit of motion being the point at which the examiner feels resistance to further movement.
   f. skinfold caliper—a spring-loaded device that provides constant tension and yields mechanical or digital (electronic) readings of skinfold thickness.
   g. waist-to-hip ratio—calculated by dividing the circumference of the waist by the circumference of the hip; the distribution of fat as indicated by these measurements is a significant predictor of cardiovascular disease and type 2 diabetes.

2. Why does a pediatrician measure the circumference of a child's head? To detect hydrocephalus (increase in the pressure and volume of cerebrospinal fluid, causing enlargement of the head and compression of the brain).

3. Give three reasons for performing goniometry.
   a. Useful in determining mobility of a joint
   b. Adjunct in the diagnosis, treatment, and rehabilitation of injuries or diseases that affect joints and the structures around them
   c. Useful in establishing job restrictions for disabled workers, in planning physical therapy and assessing its effects, and in designing braces and adaptive equipment.

4. Give three reasons for measuring BSA?
   a. to compute the ideal dosages of certain drugs
   b. to determine fluid and electrolyte needs of children
   c. to determine caloric needs of infants and small children

5. What is the weight in kilograms of a person who weighs 186 pounds? 84.37 kg.

6. Is the person in question 5 obese? Explain.
   Not necessarily. Subcutaneous fat, height, and body mass index have to be taken into account.

Chapter 3. Measurement of Vision and Hearing

FILL IN THE BLANKS

1. Snellen
2. Jaeger
3. refraction
4. myopia
5. hypermetropia
6. astigmatism
7. diopter
8. higher
9. visual field testing, Amsler grid
10. perimetry
11. color-blindness
12. audiometry
13. tinnitus
14. audiometry
15. conductive hearing loss, sensorineural hearing loss
16. lower range (250-2000 Hz)
17. higher pitches
18. eighth cranial nerve
19. dysequilibrium, vertigo
20. nystagmus

MULTIPLE CHOICE

1. D	6. B
2. A	7. B
3. C	8. A
4. E	9. E
5. C	10. E

SHORT ANSWERS

1. Define or explain:
   a. decibel—1/10 of a bel, or the smallest difference in intensity between two sounds that can be appreciated by the human ear.
   b. diopter—One diopter is the reciprocal of the focal length of the lens in meters. The stronger the lens, the shorter its radius of curvature and its focal length. Hence a higher diopter indicates a stronger lens.

c. myopia—nearsightedness, the ability to see things that are close but not those farther away.

d. nystagmus—involuntary cyclical back-and-forth movement of the eyes).

e. refraction—the use of an instrument containing lenses of various powers to measure deficiencies of near and distant vision more precisely than is possible with vision charts alone.

2. How is it possible to test the vision of a person who cannot read?
Charts with pictures or symbols are used.

3. List two tests mentioned in this chapter that are often used to screen persons without symptoms of abnormality or disease.
a. Vision testing
b. Audiometry

4. What test described in this chapter does not depend on the patient's report of what is perceived or experienced?
caloric stimulation

5. What two functions are served by the eighth cranial nerve?
a. hearing
b. balance

6. Discuss the advantages and disadvantages of automated audiometry as compared to that performed by a technician.
Technician-performed audiometry is more time-consuming and less precise than automatic audiometry, and requires a skilled technician. It may, however, be preferable with an examinee whose intelligence or ability to concentrate is limited, or who is unable to use the automatic equipment. Manual testing may also be of use to check questionable results of automatic testing and to detect malingerers.

The automatic audiometer produces a written result of test results. This record may be either a graph or a digital printout. The graphic record requires slightly more skill to interpret but is more

precise and conveys more information. Digital records are highly reproducible and can be evaluated and compared by nonprofessional persons, but they round off decibel readings to the nearest multiple of 5, and give no information about the configuration of the response curves. They record no threshold when responses at any pitch are erratic.

7. Define and explain the acronym COWS (cold to the opposite, warm to the same).
The normal response to unilateral caloric stimulation of the vestibule is a transitory nystagmus (involuntary back-and-forth movements of the eyes). Nystagmus consists of alternating quick lateral movements in one direction (fast component or phase) followed by slower return movements (slow phase) in the opposite direction. A nystagmus is said to beat in the direction of the fast component. Nystagmus induced by cool water beats in the direction opposite to the ear being stimulated, while nystagmus induced by warm water beats in the same direction as the ear being stimulated.

Chapter 4. Measurement of Temperature, Rates, Pressures, and Volumes

FILL IN THE BLANKS

1. vital signs
2. pyrexia
3. tertian, quartan
4. crisis, lysis
5. intraocular pressure
6. Schiøtz tonometer
7. applanation tonometry
8. pneumotonometry
9. peristalsis
10. sphincter
11. manometry
12. systole, diastole
13. pulse deficit
14. bounding, thready
15. pulsus alternans
16. pulsus paradoxus, constrictive pericarditis, pericardial tamponade

17. shock
18. ambulatory blood pressure
19. invasive
20. cardiac catheterization
21. spirometry
22. incentive spirometry
23. plethysmography
24. tracer gas studies

MULTIPLE CHOICE

1.	D	13.	E
2.	E	14.	A
3.	B	15.	E
4.	A	16.	B
5.	C	17.	C
6.	C	18.	A
7.	D	19.	D
8.	A	20.	B
9.	B	21.	B
10.	D	22.	E
11.	C	23.	C
12.	B	24.	A

(angioplasty is interventional, not diagnostic)

SHORT ANSWERS

1. Define or explain:
a. apical pulse—the actual heart rate gained by auscultation over the cardiac apex.

b. central venous pressure—the pressure in the superior or inferior vena cava. It closely reflects the volume of circulating blood and is therefore a useful index of the degree of shock and the response to its treatment.

c. fever of unknown origin—a documented fever (temperature of 101°F [38.3°C] or higher) lasting more than three weeks and not explainable by history or findings on physical examination and laboratory studies.

d. forced vital capacity—the maximum volume of air that can be forcefully exhaled after a maximal inspiration, in liters.

e. peristalsis—the coordinated action of the muscles of the GI tract, consisting of waves of alternating contraction and relaxation, by which the contents of the digestive tract are moved forward.

f. sphincter—a ring of muscle surrounding a normal bodily opening or passage and serving as a valve to control the release of material.

g. tilt table test—The patient lies horizontal on a motorized tilting table while baseline readings of pulse and blood pressure are obtained. Continuous electrocardiographic monitoring may also be performed. The table is then gradually tilted to a nearly vertical position, with the patient supported by a strap and a foot rest. Changes in cardiovascular measures are noted and recorded. Used to evaluate incipient shock or orthostatic hypotension.

h. Swan-Ganz catheter—a type of catheter with a balloon near its tip, which can be inflated by injection of 1-2 mL of air through one of its lumens. Once the balloon is inflated, the forward flow of blood causes the catheter to become wedged in one of the smaller branches of the pulmonary artery.

i. carbon monoxide diffusion capacity (DL_{CO}) test—The patient takes a maximum inhalation of a mixture of air, helium, and carbon monoxide and holds it for ten seconds. The exhaled breath is then analyzed, and from the concentrations of gases present the diffusing capacity is calculated as the volume of gas transferred per minute per millimeter of mercury of difference between the gas pressure of alveolar air and capillary blood.

j. nitrogen washout test—The subject breathes 100% oxygen and the nitrogen composition of exhaled air is determined serially. The finding of a nitrogen concentration greater than 2.5% after 7 minutes indicates erratic pulmonary gas diffusion.

2. List three methods of measuring intraocular pressure.

a. Indentation tonometry measures the depth to which a weighted plunger indents the cornea.

b. Applanation tonometry measures the amount of force necessary to flatten a fixed area of the cornea.

c. Pneumotonometry uses a puff of air to flatten the cornea.

3. Which heart chamber is not readily accessible by cardiac catheterization? How are pressure readings for that chamber determined indirectly?

For mechanical reasons it is seldom feasible to pass an arterial catheter through the aorta and left ventricle into the left atrium. A close estimate of left atrial pressure can, however, be obtained by measuring pulmonary wedge pressure (Ppw), also called pulmonary capillary wedge pressure (PCWP), with a Swan-Ganz catheter inserted through a peripheral vein.

4. List five types of observation besides pressure recordings that may be performed during cardiac catheterization.

a. detection of septal defects and abnormal shunts

b. sampling of blood for determination of oxygen concentration

c. assessment of valve function

d. identify and localize coronary artery disease and assess its severity

e. measure left ventricular dysfunction (congestive heart failure, myocarditis), and diagnose or assess congenital or acquired abnormalities of cardiac anatomy

5. Give two examples of vascular catheterization procedures that may be performed without fluoroscopic guidance.

a. pulmonary wedge pressure (Ppw), also called pulmonary capillary wedge pressure (PCWP)

b. the placement of a central venous pressure line, often with access through an internal jugular or subclavian vein

6. Give two examples of restrictive lung disease.

a. pulmonary diseases causing scarring of the lungs or filling of air spaces with fluid or exudate

b. diseases of the chest wall (pleura, ribs) impairing respiratory effort

7. Give two examples of obstructive lung disease.

a. emphysema

b. chronic bronchitis

8. Measurements of lung volumes and flow rates do not assess the function of the lungs, which is to exchange oxygen and carbon dioxide between the atmosphere and the blood. Carbon monoxide diffusion capacity and the nitrogen washout test are two types of pulmonary function tests.

Chapter 5. Electroencephalography, Electromyography, and Related Studies

FILL IN THE BLANKS

1. electroencephalography (EEG)
2. monopolar
3. bipolar
4. hyperventilation, photic stimulation
5. sleep spindles
6. K-complex
7. spike
8. polysomnography
9. ganzfeld
10. electromyography (EMG)

MULTIPLE CHOICE

1.	D	4.	D
2.	E	5.	C
3.	A	6.	B

SHORT ANSWERS

1. Define or explain.
   a. alpha rhythm—waves characteristic of the resting state in the normal waking adult that have a frequency of 8-13 Hz.
   b. coaxial needle electrodea—has an insulated tip and uses the barrel through which it passes as the indifferent electrode.
   c. photic stimulation—a provocation measure to elicit a significant response by exposing the patient to a rapidly flashing light.
   d. polysomnography—the simultaneous performance of several monitoring activities during sleep.
   e. REM sleep—a period of sleep in which the sleeper's body lies immobile and inert and the eyes undergo spells of rapid, irregular movement.
   f. electromyogram—The EMG procedure consists of inserting one or several needle electrodes into voluntary muscles in the area under study. The usual indication for the procedure is unexplained local or general muscle weakness.
   g. nerve conduction study—often performed in conjunction with an EMG, a small electrical stimulus is delivered by a surface electrode placed over a nerve trunk in an extremity, and the rate and amplitude of transmission of the electrical impulse through the nerve are detected by other surface electrodes placed along the course of the nerve.
2. What are some reasons for performing an electroencephalogram?
   a. seizure disorders
   b. sleep disorders
   c. toxic encephalopathies
   d. certain dementias
3. What measures may be used to evoke particular responses during the performance of an electroencephalogram?

Standard provocative measures are hyperventilation (deep and rapid breathing, which lowers the subject's plasma carbon dioxide concentration) and photic stimulation by exposure to a rapidly flashing light.

4. Describe the findings of an EEG positive for petit male and grand mal seizures.
   Series of spike-and-wave (spike-and-dome) complexes occurring at a rate of 3/second are highly characteristic of petit mal epilepsy but are noted only during seizure activity. Spike-and-wave complexes with a frequency of 10/second are seen during a grand mal seizure. Between seizures, the EEG of a person with grand mal epilepsy may show widespread paroxysmal bursts of irregular spikes and spike-wave complexes.
5. List the indications for a polysomnogram.
   a. chronic insomnia
   b. obstructive sleep apnea
   c. narcolepsy
   d. sleep pattern disorders.
   e. parasomnias such as sleep walking
6. Distinguish between an electrooculogram and an electroretinogram.
   a. Electrooculogram is sometimes performed in conjunction with electroretinogram and evaluates the ability of the retinal pigment layer to adapt to changes in light intensity.
   b. Electroretinogram records electrical activity in the retina after photic stimulation, useful in the diagnosis of retinitis pigmentosa, cone dystrophy, diabetic retinopathy, and central retinal vein occlusion.
7. Distinguish between the two meanings of electrooculogram.
   One type of electrooculography evaluates the ability of the retinal pigment layer to adapt to changes in light intensity. The term is also applied to a diagnostic study of eye movements, performed with electrical recording equipment while

the subject reads and watches a swinging pendulum.
8. List five disorders in which an electromyogram might yield abnormal results.
   a. muscular dystrophy
   b. myositis
   c. myasthenia gravis
   d. amyotrophic lateral sclerosis
   e. nerve entrapment

Chapter 6. Electrocardiography

FILL IN THE BLANKS

1. electrocardiography
2. electrodes, waves, deflections
3. heart rate, rhythm, conduction, ischemia
4. tissue death, ischemia
5. sinoatrial (SA) node
6. atrioventricular (AV) node, bundle of His
7. Purkinje fibers
8. sinoatrial (SA) node
9. depolarization, repolarization
10. bipolar
11. recording electrode
12. depolarization, repolarization
13. deflection
14. unipolar
15. augmented
16. precordial, V1 through V6
17. frontal plane, cross-section
18. rhythm strip
19. atrial
20. amplitude, polarity
21. Bruce
22. metabolic equivalent (MET)
23. dobutamine

MULTIPLE CHOICE

1. B	8. D	15. B
2. C	9. E	16. E
3. B	10. C	17. D
4. D	11. B	18. A
5. A	12. C	19. C
6. E	13. A	20. E
7. A	14. D	21. B

SHORT ANSWERS

1. Define or explain.
   a. Holter monitor—a compact ECG machine worn by a patient for 24-48 hours to pro-

vide continuous recording of cardiac electrical activity. Stored on tape, the data are analyzed by a computer at the end of the testing period.

b. PR interval—the time elapsed between the beginning of the P wave and the beginning of the R wave, representing the interval between the beginning of atrial depolarization and the beginning of ventricular depolarization.

c. precordial leads—six leads, labeled V_1 through V_6, placed on the chest.

d. pulse oximeter—a method of monitoring the oxygen saturation of circulating hemoglobin, as detected by a probe attached to the patient's finger or earlobe. It also detects pulse rate.

e. SA node—sinoatrial node, a small nubbin of tissue in the upper part of the right atrium known as the pacemaker of the heart,

f. stress testing—any standardized diagnostic measure designed to assess the effects of stress on the function of the heart. Stress may be induced by physical exercise on a motorized treadmill or bicycle ergometer, or by injection of a drug.

g. AV node—atrioventricular node, a mass of specialized tissue located low in the right atrium that picks up and transmits the depolarization wave from the SA node to the bundle of His.

h. bundle of His—a bundle of fibers that carries the depolarization wave to the interventricular septum.

i. Purkinje fibers—tissues that penetrate the walls of the ventricles, transmitting the depolarization wave causing the ventricles to contract.

j. QRS interval—the time duration of a typical QRS complex, which represents the whole process of ventricular depolarization.

2. List three reasons for performing electrocardiography.
   a. identifying and analyzing abnormalities in heart rate and rhythm
   b. identifying abnormalities in the size or shape of the heart or one or more of its chambers
   c. identifying transitory or permanent effects of impairment of the coronary circulation
   Additional answers might include: Diagnosis of pericarditis, in verifying the function of an artificial pacemaker, and in assessing various systemic and metabolic disorders that affect heart function.

3. List three reasons for performing stress testing.
   a. to identify and grade coronary artery disease in patients with angina pectoris or a history of myocardial infarction
   b. to predict future cardiac events
   c. to monitor rehabilitation after myocardial infarction.
   Also: to judge the need for coronary artery bypass surgery or balloon angioplasty

4. What kind of information about heart function can be learned from any ECG lead?
   Any given recording electrode can supply information about the rate and rhythm of ventricular contractions, and may also show abnormalities of impulse formation or conduction or evidence of ischemia or infarction.

5. What kind of information may require examination or comparison of several leads?
   Standard locations provide precise information not only about heart rate and rhythm but also about the shape and size of the heart chambers and the state of health of the heart muscle or any sign of disease affecting parts of the heart other than those facing the recording electrode.

6. What is the significance of deep, wide Q waves in an ECG lead?

It is evidence of myocardial infarction.

7. Explain the mnemonic for remembering the limb leads I, II, and III. The Roman numeral gives the number of L's.
   Lead I: Right Arm, Left Arm
   Lead II: Right Arm, Left Leg
   Lead III: Left Arm, Left Leg

8. In the leads denoted by the letters aVR, aVL, aVF, what do the letters "a" and "V" stand for?
   The "a" stands for augmented (the unipolar lead deflections are smaller, so recording sensitivity is increased); the "V" stands for vector (the recording electrode of a unipolar lead registers a quantity having both magnitude and direction). The third letter stands for the site of the electrode, right arm (R), left arm (L), left leg (F for foot).

9. What is the axis of the heart? How is it determined on an ECG? What does deviation of the axis indicate?
   The electrical axis, or still more simply the axis, is an imaginary line representing the direction along which the mean or maximum electrical activity passes down through the heart during each cardiac cycle. The axis as projected in the frontal plane is determined by a comparison of the heights of the R waves in the first six leads of the ECG. Axis deviation to right or left can indicate asymmetric enlargement of a heart chamber, aberrant conduction of cardiac impulses, or other abnormality.

Chapter 7. Visual Examinations of the Eyes, Ears, Nose, and Respiratory Tract

FILL IN THE BLANKS

1. slit lamp
2. "flare and cells"
3. keratic precipitates (KPs)
4. funduscopy
5. ophthalmoscopy
6. retina
7. optic disk
8. neovascularization
9. "choked disk"

10. naris, nares
11. epistaxis
12. anterior rhinoscopy
13. posterior rhinoscopy
14. otoscopy
15. pinna
16. light reflex
17. operating otoscopes
18. direct laryngoscopy, indirect laryngoscopy
19. epiglottis
20. indirect laryngoscopy
21. bronchoscopy

MULTIPLE CHOICE

1. E (Glaucoma is evaluated with applanation tonometry; a slit-lamp examines the anterior portion of the eye; the uvea is in the posterior eye.)
2. D (Not E; the macula is part of the retina.)
3. B
4. A
5. E
6. C
7. D
8. A
9. E
10. B

SHORT ANSWERS

1. Define or explain.
   a. cerumen—earwax.
   b. choana—posterior naris.
   c. fiberscope—A fiberoptic endoscope (fiberscope) contains a compact bundle of 25-50,000 flexible rods of fibrous glass that direct a beam of light to the tip of the instrument and convey images back to the examiner.
   d. mydriatic—drops instilled before an examination to dilate the pupil so as to provide maximal visualization of structures behind the iris.
   e. ocular fundus—the curving inner surface of the posterior portion of the eyeball.
   f. speculum—device that dilates the opening of a body passage or cavity and may also direct or reflect light into it. Specula

in routine use in modern medicine include the nasal speculum, the otoscope, the vaginal speculum, and the anoscope.

2. Compare advantages and disadvantages of rigid and flexible laryngoscopy.
   Rigid laryngoscopy is used in emergency situations and does not require anesthesia. It allows the examiner to observe down to the larynx but does not store images. Flexible laryngoscopy is elective but requires the nostril and pharynx be sprayed with anesthetic. It also is equipped with video cameras to provide immediate display and digital storage of findings.

3. What kind of information about a patient's general health can be learned from funduscopy?
   The effects of systemic diseases such as arteriosclerosis, hypertension, and diabetes mellitus may be reflected more clearly in the retina than elsewhere.

4. What type of examination mentioned in this chapter requires the cooperation and participation of the patient?
   Posterior rhinoscopy; patients sometimes have difficulty holding still enough for the insertion of the mirror that reflects light into the nasopharynx and gagging occurs. Ophthalmoscopy and slit-lamp examinations also require the patient's cooperation.

5. Which examinations described in this chapter might be performed as emergency procedures?
   Laryngoscopy, bronchoscopy

6. Describe the features and purpose of the ophthalmoscope.
   It is a handheld instrument with a light source and a set of lenses mounted on a wheel-like diaphragm that compensate for any visual in the patient. The strength of the lens in use, measured in diopters gives a rough measure of how far the patient's vision varies from normal. The ophthalmoscope also includes red and green filters to emphasize certain features of the

fundus, a grid for estimating distances, and a means of adjusting the intensity of the light and the size of the aperture through which it is projected into the eye.

7. What is meant by a "2-diopter choke"?
   In evaluation of the optic disk with an ophthalmoscope, the difference between the strength of the lens needed to examine the retina and the strength of the lens needed to examine the optic disk is 2 diopters.

8. What are the limitations and advantages of nasal speculum examination, anterior rhinoscopy, and posterior rhinoscopy?
   The nasal speculum allows only minimal examination of the nose but is sufficient for evaluation of epistaxis (nosebleed), local inflammation, ulceration, polyps (lumpy swellings of mucous membrane, usually due to nasal allergy) or other tumors, foreign bodies, trauma, or septal deviation or perforation. Anterior rhinoscopy allows examination of the middle meatus, into which the frontal, maxillary, and anterior ethmoidal sinuses and the nasolacrimal duct all drain and may require topical anesthesia. Posterior rhinoscopy is indirect and more difficult, requiring patient cooperation, but is undertaken to investigate nasal obstruction, bleeding sites, tumors, and foreign bodies.

9. Compare and contrast rigid and flexible bronchoscopy.
   The indications are the same for both procedures. Rigid bronchoscopy requires general anesthesia as well as topical anesthetic of the throat to prevent gagging, and the scope is inserted through the mouth into the throat. Flexible bronchoscopy can usually be performed with local anesthesia, and the scope is inserted through the nostril.

Chapter 8. Endoscopy of the Digestive Tract and Genitourinary System

FILL IN THE BLANKS

1. visualization, discomfort, perforation
2. esophagogastroduodenoscope
3. of the coiling, irregular course of the sigmoid colon
4. hemorrhoid
5. fissure
6. fistula in ano
7. allows gravity to expand and unfold the rectum
8. colonoscopy
9. cecum
10. resectoscope
11. speculum examination of the vagina and cervix
12. acetic acid, Lugol

MULTIPLE CHOICE

1. A
2. E
3. C
4. C
5. D
6. B
7. D
8. E
9. B
10. A
11. C
12. D
13. E
14. B
15. D

SHORT ANSWERS

1. Define or explain.
   a. colposcopy—performed in conjunction with a vaginal speculum to provide a magnified view of the cervix and the vaginal mucosa to evaluate lesions or abnormal zones of the cervix, in identifying areas of cervical dysplasia in a patient with an abnormal Pap smear, and as an aid in biopsy or minor surgical procedures.
   b. hematemesis—vomiting of blood.
   c. lithotomy position—position in which the patient lies supine, with the hips flexed, the thighs abducted, and the feet supported in stirrups, used for endoscopic examinations of the female GU tract and reproductive system.
   d. meatotomy—one or more slits to enlarge the external urethral meatus.
   e. obturator—a metal plug with a rounded, cone-shaped tip used to facilitate the insertion of a rigid endoscope into the anus or rectum.
   f. sigmoid colon—the zig-zag portion of the colon just above the rectum, the limits of the colon that can be reached with a rigid endoscope.

2. List three indications for each of the following procedures:
   a. cystoscopy—to evaluate hematuria, acute or chronic cystitis, vesical calculi, and ulcerative lesions or tumors of the bladder. It is also used for placement of ureteral catheters in the investigation of ureteral obstruction and to instill contrast medium for retrograde pyelography.
   b. gastroduodenoscopy—peptic ulcer, stenosis due to scarring, diverticulum, or tumor of the duodenum, as well as indications for esophagogastroscopy. It may also be performed in conjunction with ERCP.
   c. hysteroscopy—indicated in the study of abnormal uterine bleeding, uterine masses (fibroids, polyps), infertility, habitual abortion (repeated miscarriage), and congenital malformations of the reproductive system. It can also be used to direct chorionic villus biopsy.
   d. proctoscopy—the same as for anoscopy (to evaluate pain, bleeding, swelling, hemorrhoids, fissures, fistula in ano), and also include masses or swellings felt on digital examination of the rectum and rectal foreign body.

3. List four examination positions mentioned in this chapter and indicate some types of examination for which each is appropriate.
   a. Sims position: anoscopy, colonoscopy
   b. Genupectoral: proctoscopy
   c. Left lateral position: sigmoidoscopy (but the knee-chest position allows better visualization); colonoscopy
   d. Lithotomy position: cystoscopy, urethroscopy on the female, speculum exam of the vagina, colposcopy, and hysteroscopy

4. Which examinations discussed in this chapter might be done to discover a source of bleeding?
   All of them.

5. Which examinations discussed in this chapter might be part of a routine health examination for certain patients?
   Sigmoidoscopy as surveillance for colorectal cancer in persons at heightened risk because of age or personal or family history.
   Speculum examination of the vagina and cervix is part of the routine health evaluation of women.

Chapter 9. Endoscopic Examinations Requiring Incisions

FILL IN THE BLANKS

1. minimal-access, keyhole, buttonhole, or Band-Aid surgery
2. cannula
3. trocar
4. pleural effusion
5. empyema
6. thoracoscope
7. mediastinum
8. pleural surface
9. mediastinoscopy
10. thoracoscope
11. laparoscopy
12. pneumoperitoneum
13. culdocentesis
14. arthroscopy

MULTIPLE CHOICE

1. B
2. D
3. E
4. A
5. E
6. B
7. C
8. C

SHORT ANSWERS

1. Define or explain.
   a. cul-de-sac—the rectouterine pouch of Douglas, a pocket of peritoneum lying between the rectum and the uterus.
   b. empyema—pus in the pleural cavity.
   c. insufflation—carbon dioxide gas is introduced into the peritoneal cavity under pressure.
   d. mediastinum—the middle portion of the chest cavity, the anatomic region between the lungs that contains the heart and great vessels, the trachea, and the esophagus. Lymph nodes and the thymus gland also occupy this region.
   e. trocar—a sharp-pointed obturator that fits inside the cannula and is used to pierce the skin and introduce the cannula into the resulting opening, after which the trocar is removed.
   f. Veress needle—a needle inserted through a skin puncture, usually just below the umbilicus used for insufflation of CO_2 gas into the peritoneal cavity.

2. Mention some circumstances in which an open surgical procedure might be preferred to endoscopic surgery.
   Answers may vary (not discussed in text) but include obesity, excessive adhesions, excessive bleeding or inaccessibility of organ during endoscopic procedure.

3. List five reasons for performing mediastinoscopy.
   a. examination and biopsy of mediastinal lymph nodes
   b. investigation of disorders of the trachea
   c. investigation of disorders of the esophagus
   d. investigation of disorders of the pericardium
   e. diagnosing and staging of lung cancer

4. What procedures discussed in this chapter might be performed in emergency situations?
   Thoracoscopy, which may be used to diagnose fluid or pus in the pleural space; laparoscopy for abdominal trauma, and arthroscopy for joint trauma.

5. What two procedures discussed in this chapter provide access to the same bodily region by different anatomic approaches?
   Thoracoscopy (in which a small-caliber endoscope is inserted through a skin incision between two ribs to provide a view of the interior of the pleural cavity) and mediastinoscopy (in which an endoscope is inserted through an incision in the midline just above the sternum) are both examinations of the chest regions.

Chapter 10. Plain Radiography

FILL IN THE BLANKS

1. computed tomography
2. ultrasonic waves
3. nuclear imaging
4. radiologist
5. clinical correlation
6. fluoroscopy
7. negative
8. radiolucent
9. radiopaque
10. posteroanterior or PA
11. anteroposterior or AP
12. Bucky grid
13. plain film
14. atelectasis
15. lordotic
16. pneumothorax
17. air bronchogram
18. scout film
19. KUB (kidneys, ureters, bladder)
20. flat plate
21. flat, upright, and left lateral decubitus
22. all structures are superimposed in one composite 2-D image
23. anteroposterior (AP), lateral, and oblique
24. stress film
25. mammography
26. permit a lower dose of radiation, reduce the risk of movement during the exposure.
27. mediolateral oblique, craniocaudal
28. irregularly clustered or spiculated
29. because mineral density must be decreased by about one-third before any reduction is apparent in an x-ray image
30. bone densitometry

MULTIPLE CHOICE

1. D
2. E
3. E
4. B
5. A
6. C
7. C
8. D
9. A
10. E
11. B
12. A
13. D
14. E
15. B

SHORT ANSWERS

1. Define or explain.
   a. cardiothoracic ratio—on a standard PA chest film, comparison of the width of the cardiac shadow at its widest to the width of the thorax at its widest (heart width divided by thoracic width).
   b. contrast medium—liquid that block x-rays and therefore create an image in an x-ray picture
   c. fluoroscopy—a continuous stream of x-rays passing through a part of the body is made to create an image on a television screen.
   d. osteoporosis—characterized by decreased mass and decreased mineral density of bone, with increased susceptibility to fractures.
   e. radiopaque—a structure or object that blocks x-rays, resulting in less exposure of the film and a lighter or white area.
   f. tomography—also called laminography; a technique for focusing on a particular site or level within the subject. The x-ray source and the film-holder, both mounted on a rigid frame that maintains an exact distance between them, rotate simultaneously in an

arc, in opposite directions, with the subject between them. The point within the subject about which this rotation occurs will produce an image of maximum clarity on the film, while tissues closer to and further away from that point will be blurred or invisible. Individual images in the series of tomograms are called slices or cuts.

2. What might be some emergency indications for performing a chest x-ray?

Chest trauma, complications' of surgery, exposure to toxic airborne substances, infiltrates, atelectasis, pneumothorax.

3. List three radiographic studies mentioned in this chapter that have been supplanted by safer or more informative methods.
   a. X-ray pelvimetry replaced by clinical pelvimetry.
   b. CT, MRI, angiography have largely supplanted plain skull films in the assessment of brain disorders and in evaluating injury or disease of the vertebrae.
   c. Computed tomography (CT) is more accurate in the diagnosis of acute and chronic sinusitis, and shows nasal polyps better.

4. List several factors that might interfere with the quality or usefulness of an x-ray examination.

Improper patient positioning, faulty developing technique, poor patient preparation (necklace left in place for chest x-ray, stool in the colon during barium enema examination), poor patient cooperation or movement during exposure of films. (Section IV Introduction)

5. What procedures are followed to reduce unnecessary exposure of patients and technicians to radiation during radiographic examinations?

X-ray machines are regularly recalibrated and their shielding checked; minimum voltage and exposure time are used; the radiation beam is restricted to the area of clinical interest; settings are carefully checked to avoid need for repeated exposures; gonadal shielding may be used on some patients; lead aprons, lead gloves, stationary or movable shields are used to protect radiologists and technicians; and anyone exposed occupationally to radiation must wear a radiation dosimeter. (Section IV Introduction)

6. Explain how the use of contrast material has helped to overcome the limitations of plain radiography. Contrast media can outline a hollow structure such as the stomach or the colon, or a tubular system such as the circulation, the bile ducts, or the urinary tract. Contrast media can be swallowed, injected, or introduced through a tube, catheter, or enema apparatus. Air or gas can be introduced into a hollow structure to serve as a negative contrast medium.

7. List the radiographic views of the chest discussed in the text and the advantages of each.

The PA view, the most common, can reveal a variety of abnormal conditions: tumors, fluid collections, infiltrates, abnormalities in cardiac silhouette.

The lateral view shows substantially more of the lung bases than a PA view, and may reveal abnormalities concealed by the heart shadow in the PA view.

A left lateral film (with the left side of the chest nearest to the film holder) is usually preferred because it provides a sharper image of the heart.

Right and left oblique views of the chest may be obtained to clarify the diagnosis.

A lordotic view is an anteroposterior chest film in which the x-ray beam is aimed slightly upward to improve visibility of the apices of the lungs, which are partly concealed by the clavicles in a PA film.

Recumbent may show pleural fluid better than upright films.

8. Discuss the strengths and weaknesses of plain films of the abdomen.

They are less valuable than chest films because most of the abdominal organs are of the same (water) density. Abdominal films are useful, however, in identifying disorders characterized by abnormal distribution of air or gas (distention of bowel due to obstruction, gas in the peritoneal cavity from a ruptured bowel), in confirming the presence and location of kidney stones and swallowed foreign bodies, and in identifying certain other disorders.

Chapter 11. Contrast Radiography

FILL IN THE BLANKS

1. most of the structures represented in the image are of the same (water) density
2. contrast medium
3. myelogram
4. arthritic osteophytes
5. spinal stenosis
6. headache
7. air or gas
8. barium sulfate
9. filling defects
10. ulcerations
11. stricture
12. swelling, tumors, or hemorrhage
13. motility
14. air contrast, double contrast
15. esophagram
16. perforation
17. esophageal varices
18. hiatal hernia
19. gastroesophageal reflux
20. stomach
21. duodenum
22. pylorus
23. volvulus
24. intussusception
25. hematochezia
26. distention of the colon with barium or injected air may rupture it
27. diverticulosis
28. ulcerative colitis, Crohn's disease
29. cholangiography

30. percutaneous cholangiography
31. cholecystokinin
32. vesicoureteral reflux
33. stress incontinence
34. hysterosalpingography
35. angiography
36. right or left femoral artery
37. guidewire
38. atheromatous disease
39. left anterior descending (LAD)
40. deep venous thrombosis (DVT)
41. venography, phlebography
42. sialography, ptyalography
43. dacryocystography
44. galactography (ductogalactography)
45. fistulography (sinography)

MULTIPLE CHOICE

1.	C	14.	A
2.	D	15.	A
3.	B	16.	D
4.	B	17.	B
5.	E	18.	C
6.	A	19.	D
7.	D	20.	A
8.	B	21.	C
9.	E	22.	A
10.	B	23.	D
11.	C	24.	E
12.	A	25.	B
13.	D		

SHORT ANSWERS

1. Define or explain.
   a. barium sulfate—the standard contrast for gastrointestinal studies for many decades. Pure barium sulfate forms white or yellowish crystals and is odorless, tasteless, virtually insoluble, chemically inert, and nontoxic when consumed orally. Concentration used depends on examination performed.
   b. biplane imaging—particularly in angiography of the central nervous system and abdominal aorta, two images at right angles to each other (an AP and a lateral view) may be obtained and recorded in rapid sequence during a single injection of medium; this biplane imaging lends a 3-D element to the interpretation of the study.
   c. cholecystokinin—a natural polypeptide hormone produced by the small intestinal mucosa, affects motility of the upper GI tract and on its supply of digestive juices. IV administration during biliary tract imaging studies stimulates contraction of the gallbladder and increases bile flow as well as secretion of pancreatic and intestinal digestive juices.
   d. double contrast study—air or gas is introduced into the digestive tract to distend its walls after most of the barium has passed through or, in the case of a barium enema, has been expelled from the colon. Also, air contrast study.
   e. embolus—a clot (thrombus) that has formed in a systemic vein and broken loose from its site of origin
   f. IVP—intravenous pyelogram, the delineation of the urinary tract (renal pelves, ureters, bladder, and urethra) by means of a contrast agent administered intravenously.
   g. scout film—a preliminary plain film performed prior to a contrast study or surgery.
   h. sialography—or ptyalography, a contrast study of a parotid gland duct performed to diagnose obstruction of the duct by calculus or tumor.
   i. T-tube cholangiogram—contrast medium is injected into the biliary tract through a T-tube, a temporary drain placed in the biliary tract after cholecystectomy

2. Why is a scout film routinely made before the injection of contrast medium?
   The scout film gives basic structural information, confirms that the patient and the x-ray equipment are properly positioned for the desired examination, and may alert the radiologist or the technician to potential problems.

3. List some examinations discussed in this chapter that might be done as emergency procedures.
   Esophagram, gastroscopy, and colonoscopy may be done for foreign body or bleeding; percutaneous cholangiography for rapid detection of biliary tract obstruction; pulmonary angiography for embolus.

4. List some examinations discussed in this chapter that have been largely supplanted by safer or more informative examinations.
   Encephalography (ventriculography, pneumoencephalography) has been rendered obsolete by the superior sensitivity and greater safety of MRI and CT. Contrast bronchography with iodine media has been largely supplanted by CT studies with inhaled xenon as a contrast medium. Oral and intravenous cholangiography have largely been replaced by ultrasound because of its superior definition of the biliary tract and gallstones and because in oral cholangiography, it takes 12-15 hours for the contrast to appear in the gallbladder (if it does), and reactions to injected medium are frequent. Because venography is an invasive procedure which may aggravate existing inflammation or thrombosis, other diagnostic measures such as Doppler ultrasonography and MRI may be preferred.

5. What are some possible adverse consequences or complications of angiography?
   The injection of iodide solution causes a local sensation of burning or flushing and often dizziness or nausea. In some patients, particularly those with pre-existing renal disease, dehydration, or congestive heart failure, iodide contrast media can cause transitory or permanent kidney damage. Angiographic examinations are therefore contraindicated in patients with these conditions.

6. Describe the limitations of contrast studies of the gastrointestinal tract.
Anatomic variations due to tumors, ulceration, scarring, or external factors are visible only when they affect the outer margin of the image as seen in any given projection.

7. What are the advantages of cholangiography over plain radiography in diagnosing disorders of the biliary tract and gallbladder?
Plain radiography can show gallstones that contain calcium salts (not all of them do), but it cannot clearly indicate their position in the biliary tract. The tract itself cannot be seen in a plain x-ray study unless it contains air or gas.

8. What advantage does the retrograde pyelogram have over an intravenous pyelogram? What disadvantage?
Contrast medium appears immediately in full concentration in the ureter under examination, regardless of impairment in renal function. However, unlike an IVP this examination must usually be done under spinal or general anesthesia and requires placement of catheters by a urologist.

9. Angiography differs from most other contrast studies in two important respects. What are they?
The structures that are to be outlined (blood vessels) are already full of fluid, and that fluid is in motion. Because injected contrast medium immediately becomes diluted by the blood, it must be highly concentrated in order to retain its potency as an opacifying agent. And because the medium is immediately swept along through the vessels by the flow of blood, an x-ray exposure must be made at the same instant as the injection.

10. Distinguish among arteriography, venography, and lymphangiography.
Arteriography, which records the flow of contrast medium through some part of the arterial system, is by far the most important and widely used form of angiography. A major application of arteriography is in the evaluation of the chambers and valves of the heart, the coronary arteries, and the aorta and pulmonary arterial circulation. Arteriography is also extensively used to assess the circulation of the brain, the abdominal viscera, and the extremities. Venography (phlebography), the angiographic study of veins, and lymphography (lymphangiography), the study of lymphatic vessels, are less widely used but can yield information of crucial importance in certain settings.

Chapter 12. Computed Tomography

FILL IN THE BLANKS
1. acquisition, reconstruction
2. multiplanar reconstructions
3. xenon
4. supine (face up), from the subject's feet
5. Housfield unit

MULTIPLE CHOICE
1. B   3. C
2. A   4. E

SHORT ANSWERS
1. Define or explain.
   a. scintillation counter—device that detects and measures radiation.
   b. virtual endoscopy—3-dimensional imaging, so-called because the images generated are similar to what could be seen by actual inspection with an endoscope.
   c. xenon— a colorless, odorless, and chemically inert elemental gas that when inhaled can aid in the CT examination of the respiratory tract, circulation, abdominal viscera, and cerebral blood flow.
2. List some types of examination for which CT scanning is superior to conventional radiography.
CT provides superior visualization of enlarged or displaced organs and of soft-tissue masses (cysts, neoplasms, hemorrhage), and is particularly valuable in diagnostic screening of the head, thorax, abdomen, and pelvis. It is more sensitive in detecting variations in calcification and bone density and in identifying subtle fractures. CT examinations of the head are useful in identifying and localizing epidural or subdural hematoma and, in stroke, to rule out hemorrhage before administration of a thrombolytic agent. In the diagnosis of pulmonary embolism, CT is approximately as accurate as a ventilation-perfusion scan. Helical CT and multiplanar imaging have application in the diagnosis of bronchial disease and asthma and in screening high-risk populations (e.g., smokers over 60) for lung cancer. CT is valuable in diagnosing ureteral calculus, bowel obstruction, and appendicitis, deep vein thrombosis.

3. What are some advantages of CT angiography over conventional angiography? Iodide contrast medium is infused intravenously rather than being introduced into an artery by catheter.

4. In what ways does helical CT differ from the more conventional procedure?
In helical (or spiral) CT, the x-ray tube emits radiation continuously as it rotates through a predetermined arc while the table supporting the subject moves at a constant speed at a right angle to this arc to yield a series of cuts as opposed to the x-ray source moving from one position to another in stepwise fashion around the patient while exposures are made individually. Breathing movements and random shifts in the patient's position between slices can introduce artifacts during conventional CT.

5. What might be the advantage of producing contiguous CT images of a body area?
Helical CT allows an entire organ or body region (for example, the

liver or the thorax) to be scanned during a single session.

6. Why would a radiographer choose to limit the range of densities to be displayed? Give examples.

The data from a single scan can be processed repeatedly with different windows to accentuate different features of the part examined. A window ranging from -200 to 300 might be chosen to emphasize subtle contrasts in the densities of mediastinal soft tissues in a CT examination of the thorax.

Chapter 13. Ultrasonography

FILL IN THE BLANKS

1. ultrasonography (or sonography)
2. sound waves, frequency (pitch)
3. the treatment of acute or chronic soft-tissue pain and to shatter urinary calculi (lithotripsy)
4. transducer
5. acoustical impedance
6. echo time
7. intensity
8. high echogenicity
9. hypoechoic
10. real time scanning
11. beating heart
12. open wounds or dressings
13. it displaces bowel and creates a readily observable reference point
14. sonohysterography
15. crown-rump length
16. transverse width of skull, age
17. estimating fetal size and weight
18. ventricular ejection fraction
19. hypokinesis
20. asyneresis
21. ejection fraction

MULTIPLE CHOICE

1.	B	10.	A
2.	E	11.	B
3.	C	12.	A
4.	A	13.	D
5.	E	14.	E
6.	C	15.	D
7.	B	16.	B
8.	A	17.	A
9.	E	18.	C

SHORT ANSWERS

1. Define or explain.
   a. acoustic shadowing—a phenomenon in which a highly echogenic structure, such as a bone, prevents sound waves from generating images of tissues behind it.
   b. Doppler effect—refers to the change in the observed frequency of sound waves (or other waves) when the distance between the source of the waves and the observer is changing.
   c. pixel—"picture element," smallest discrete component of an image.
   d. polyhydramnios—excessive amniotic fluid
   e. sonolucent—anechoic, that is not reflecting sound waves at all. Water and other fluids are said to be anechoic or sonolucent (by analogy with translucent and radiolucent).

2. List some body areas for which ultrasonography is superior to conventional x-ray.
   Because no harmful radiation is involved, it is particularly useful during pregnancy and in the examination of children. It is a standard procedure in evaluating masses or swellings in the thyroid gland, liver, pancreas, spleen, kidney, and prostate because it can determine the size of masses and distinguish between cysts and solid tumors. It is particularly useful in obstructive disease of the biliary and urinary tracts because it can show gallstones and urinary calculi clearly. It can also be used to guide the performance of a biopsy, particularly of the prostate, or (during surgery) the placement of a needle in a cyst or other lesion.

3. Ultrasonography is used in neurosurgery to aid the placement of instruments or localization of structures in the brain. It is not used, however, for routine examinations of the brain or spinal cord. Why not?

The skull blocks sound waves from penetrating the brain and the vertebrae block sound waves from reaching the spinal cord.

4. What are some indications for performing obstetric ultrasonography before 18 weeks' gestation?
   To confirm the presence of pregnancy or, in cases of vaginal bleeding, to assess fetal viability and rule out ectopic pregnancy.

5. What types of ultrasound examination might be performed in an emergency situation?
   Obstetrical ultrasonography may be performed to assess fetal viability or rule out ectopic pregnancy in cases of vaginal bleeding.

6. Describe how ultrasound works.
   Ultrasound waves pass through air, gas, and fluid without being reflected. However, they bounce back from rigid structures such as bone and gallstones, creating an echo that can be detected by a receiver. Solid organs such as the liver and kidney partially reflect ultrasound waves in predictable patterns. Waves are also reflected from the interface between two structures having different acoustic properties, such as fluid and the structure that contains it (e.g., cyst, urinary bladder).

Chapter 14. Magnetic Resonance Imaging

FILL IN THE BLANKS

1. yields similar cuts or cross-sectional images
2. an unequal number of protons
3. spin
4. shorter
5. gradient magnetic field
6. pulse sequences
7. hyperintense
8. hypointense
9. STIR (short T1 inversion recovery) sequence
10. FLAIR (fluid-attenuated inversion-recovery) sequence
11. gadolinium

MULTIPLE CHOICE

1.	B	6.	A
2.	A	7.	D
3.	C	8.	B
4.	E	9.	D
5.	C		

SHORT ANSWERS

1. Define or explain.

    a. gadolinium—a biologically inert metallic element used as an imaging agent in MRI; it enhances the MRI signal of any tissue or area in which it accumulates by shortening the T1 of adjacent protons.

    b. pulse sequence—a number of different pulses and time intervals used in predetermined series.

2. List some types of examination for which MRI is preferred to conventional radiography, applications in which it provides superior discrimination among tissue densities.

    In the examination of the central nervous system, MRI shows the plaques of demyelination characteristic of multiple sclerosis. MRI is a more sensitive indicator (than CT) of early ischemia and infarction, and of lesions in the posterior cranial fossa (brain stem and cerebellum). It is valuable in determining the location, size, and shape of tumors, particularly in the brain and liver, and in the diagnosis of bone and joint disorders (internal derangements, ligamentous tears, spinal cord compression due to disk herniation or spinal stenosis). MRI may detect tumors at an earlier stage than mammography, and has been recommended by some authorities for annual surveillance of women at high risk.

3. In what circumstances might MRI examination not be feasible?

    MRI is contraindicated for patients with ferrous metal prostheses or implanted cardiac pacemakers. Patients with claustrophobia may have problems due to the length of time they must spend inside the magnet. MRI examination is often not feasible in the critically ill or injured patient who may require supportive care and frequent assessment.

4. What types of examination mentioned in this chapter might be performed in an emergency situation? Diagnosing of early ischemia and infarction in the brain or spinal cord and internal derangements or ligamentous tears of the bones or joints as well as spinal cord compression due to disk herniation or spinal stenosis.

5. List some differences between a T1 weighted image and a T2 weighted image.

    In a T1 weighted image, water and watery fluids (urine, cerebrospinal fluid) appear dark; fat, fresh hemorrhage, slowly moving blood, and fluids with high protein content such as mucus appear bright. Water is hyperintense in a T2 weighted image and soft tissues including muscle and fat appear dark. Regardless of weighting, bone, calcifications, and air or gas are always hypointense, appearing dark in an MR image. The ACOG and the NRPB have advised against the use of MRI during the first trimester of pregnancy.

6. How does MRI differ from standard x-rays and ultrasonography?

    An x-ray examination detects varying resistance of tissues to penetration by x-rays, and ultrasonography detects varying resistance to penetration by sound waves, MRI detects varying concentrations or densities of hydrogen atoms (protons) in tissues.

7. Summarize how MRI images are made.

    The patient is placed inside a static magnetic field. A pulse of radio waves (excitation pulse) is then used to create briefly a second magnetic field at a right angle to the static field. This causes the hydrogen ions (protons) change their orientation, which go back to their previous orientation to the static magnetic field when the second field is turned off giving off a stream of radiofrequency energy or "signal," which can be detected by a receiving coil. The signal intensity given off by any tissue is proportional to the hydrogen ion concentration (or proton density) of that tissue. Muscle emits a very high signal, bone a very low one, air or gas almost none. These signals are converted to images by a computer.

Chapter 15. Nuclear Imaging

FILL IN THE BLANKS

1. radioactivity
2. half-life, one-half
3. radiopharmaceutical
4. radioactive tracer
5. technetium
6. millicuries (mCi)
7. geiger counter
8. curie
9. multiple-gated acquisition (MUGA)
10. positron emission tomography (PET)
11. positron emission tomography
12. single-photon emission computed tomography
13. ventilation
14. perfusion
15. pulmonary embolism
16. apatite
17. osteoblastic
18. osteomyelitis

MULTIPLE CHOICE

1.	B	6.	B
2.	C	7.	A
3.	E	8.	E
4.	D	9.	E

SHORT ANSWERS

1. Define or explain.

    a. HIDA scan—hepatobiliary iminodiacetic acid scan; outlines the biliary tract, showing obstruction by stones or tumor.

    b. isotope—atoms of a given element that vary in the number of neutrons in their nuclei, and hence in their mass numbers, are called isotopes of that element.

c. photon—In the context of a particle theory of radiation, a photon is a quantum of electromagnetic energy, assumed to have zero mass and no electrical charge.

d. ventilation-perfusion scan—a procedure done when acute pulmonary embolism is suspected; two scans of the lungs are performed in succession with different radionuclides administered by different routes. First a ventilation scan with inhaled radioactive xenon gas is done to show which parts of the lungs are filled with inspired gas and which, if any, are not. After all of the xenon has been washed out of the respiratory tract with ordinary air, technetium Tc 99m macroaggregated albumin is administered intravenously. A second lung scan is then performed to assess the perfusion (circulatory distribution) of radionuclide through lung tissue.

2. What is the essential difference between nuclear imaging and all other standard imaging techniques? Unlike other imaging techniques, nuclear imaging appraises the function of the structures under study rather than their anatomy (size, shape, position). The significance of increased or decreased uptake of a radiotracer depends on the tissue under study and the biochemical nature of the substance into which the radioisotope has been incorporated.

3. List some situations in which nuclear imaging is standard.
MUGA scan permits calculation of the ejection fraction.
HIDA scan outlines the biliary tract, showing obstruction by stones or tumor.
PET scan provides valuable information about brain function in Alzheimer and other dementias, parkinsonism, epilepsy, brain tumors, and stroke. This technique

is also used to assess coronary blood flow and to study solitary pulmonary nodules and other masses. SPECT scan provides information about regional blood flow, in assessing disorders of the heart and lungs, and in the evaluation of head injuries, seizure disorders, stroke, brain tumors, and dementia. Ventilation-perfusion scan is used to detect acute pulmonary embolus. Bone scintigraphy is useful in detecting osteomyelitis, primary and metastatic tumors of bone, and subtle fractures missed by x-ray studies.

4. List some circumstances in which nuclear imaging would not be feasible.
Nuclear imaging is contraindicated in women who are or may be pregnant, because of the sensitivity of the fetus to even small amounts of radiation, after recent administration of a radiopharmaceutical, such as radioactive iodine, and after recent performance of another nuclear diagnostic procedure.

5. List some nuclear imaging procedures that might be performed in emergency situations.
SPECT and ventilation-perfusion scans may be performed in emergency situations. See question 3 above for indications.

6. How is the mass number of an isotope represented?
By convention, the mass number is shown as a superscript number before the symbol of the element (^{32}P, an isotope of phosphorus with a mass number of 32; ^{14}C, an isotope of carbon with a mass number of 14). Alternatively the mass number may follow the symbol of the element, without a hyphen: P 32, C 14.

7. Why is a simple perfusion scan often not adequate to diagnosed acute pulmonary embolism?
Although pulmonary embolism may be evident on a simple perfusion scan, an abnormal scan can also result if a zone of lung tissue has poor circulation because of

pre-existing disease. Hence a ventilation scan is also done, so that any areas of lung tissue with chronic impairment of circulation can be identified. A ventilation-perfusion mismatch—an area with normal ventilation but blocked perfusion—probably represents a zone of acute pulmonary artery blockage due to embolism.

Chapter 16. Normal Anatomy and Histology

FILL IN THE BLANKS

1. pathology
2. pathologists
3. anatomic pathology, clinical pathology, forensic pathology
4. medical technologists
5. systems, organs, tissue, cells
6. viscus, viscera
7. septa, trabeculae
8. outer cortex, medulla
9. mucosa, tunica mucosa
10. fibrosa, tunica fibrosa
11. serosa, tunica serosa
12. pericardium
13. mature cartilage, central nervous system
14. arterioles, capillaries
15. epithelial, endothelium
16. venule, vein
17. spermatozoa, oocytes
18. mitosis
19. neutrophils
20. artifact
21. staining properties
22. squamous
23. stratified
24. basement membrane
25. acinus, alveolus
26. exocrine
27. endocrine, hormones
28. mesothelium, endothelium
29. fibroblast, fibrocyte
30. collagenous, elastic, reticular
31. smooth muscle
32. skeletal, striped, voluntary
33. cardiac
34. dendrites, axons
35. neuron
36. glial cells
37. plasma
38. lymphoid tissue

MULTIPLE CHOICE

1. C	12. A	23. D
2. E	13. B	24. E
3. A	14. E	25. D
4. D	15. C	26. A
5. B	16. D	27. C
6. B	17. C	28. A
7. C	18. E	29. D
8. E	19. A	30. C
9. B	20. B	31. B
10. D	21. B	32. C
11. A	22. A	33. E

SHORT ANSWERS

1. Define pathology. Name and define its three principal branches.

   Pathology is the branch of medicine that studies the structural and functional changes produced in the living body by injury or disease. Anatomic pathology is concerned with the gross and microscopic changes brought about in living human tissues by disease. Clinical pathology refers to the laboratory examination of bodily fluids and waste products such as blood, spinal fluid, urine, and feces. Forensic pathology involves the application of knowledge comprised by the other two branches to certain issues in both civil and criminal law.

2. Define or explain.
   a. cortex—the outer surface of some organs, such as the kidney and the adrenal gland,
   b. medulla—the inner surface of some organs, such as the kidney and the adrenal gland,
   c. organ—an anatomically differentiated and isolated structure with a specific function.
   d. parenchyma—the specialized cells that are unique to solid organs, such as the liver or kidney, and that enable the organ to perform its function,
   e. stroma—the supporting framework of connective tissue of a solid organ. The stroma is also called interstitial tissue.
   f. system—a division of the human body, each having a general biological function. Each system is composed of

organs, each organ having a specialized function.
   g. tissue—the material of which organs are made, A tissue is made up of cells. The cell is the smallest and simplest independent unit of living matter.

3. Describe the basic structural features of a cell. Each cell is isolated from its surroundings by an enclosing membrane. Within each cell is a fluid called cytoplasm, which is a colloidal suspension of proteins, amino acids, carbohydrates, and electrolytes in water. The cell membrane is neither an impermeable barrier nor a biologically inert one. The most conspicuous internal feature of a cell is generally its nucleus, a dense and roughly spherical mass of protein, DNA, and RNA, which controls such cellular functions as energy metabolism and protein synthesis. The nucleolus is a sharply defined body containing RNA that is often visible within the nucleus. Structural elements besides the nucleus can be seen in the cytoplasm of some cells. These, collectively known as organelles or organoids, include mitochondria, microsomes, the central body or centrosome, and the Golgi apparatus. Standard histologic preparations often show cytoplasmic granules that are characteristic of certain cells. In addition, the cytoplasm of some cells may contain pigment, fat globules, or minute bubbles of air or gas called vacuoles.

4. What are mitotic figures?
   Clearly distinguishable bands of DNA called chromosomes that result from the splitting of the normally tangled chromatin (genetic) material of a cell nucleus.

5. What is the general term for the type of tissue that forms coverings and lining membranes?
   Most of the surfaces in the body, including skin and mucous membranes, the linings of hollow and tubular organs in the digestive, respiratory, and urogenital systems, and the linings of the chest and

abdominal cavities, consist of a tissue called epithelium.

6. In what kind of structure is endothelium found?
   Endothelium is the type of epithelium lining blood vessels.

7. What basic type of tissue contains the highest proportion of noncellular material?
   Connective tissues contain a higher proportion of noncellular material than other tissues, chiefly because bundles and networks of fibers provide more strength, cohesion, and durability than aggregations of living cells.

8. What is the function of fibroblasts?
   The function of the fibroblast is to produce fibers. In mature, healthy connective tissue, the fibroblasts are few and not especially active. In tissue that is growing or undergoing repair, fibroblasts are more numerous and more active.

9. In what type of tissue are haversian systems found?
   The microscopic structural unit of bone is the osteon or haversian system, consisting of ten or more thin layers called lamellae arranged concentrically around a haversian canal. These haversian canals branch and intersect to serve as passages for blood vessels and nerves.

10. State two important differences between smooth and skeletal muscle.
    a. Smooth muscle consists of long, spindle-shaped cells usually found tightly packed together in sheets. Skeletal, striped, or voluntary muscle consists of long cylindrical strands or fibers, which are bunched into groups called fasciculi.
    b. Smooth muscle is also called involuntary muscle because it responds only to stimuli from the autonomic nervous system and is not under voluntary control. Skeletal muscle is found in the large muscle masses of the trunk and extremities, which hold the

body erect and serve for loco-motion and other voluntary activities.

11. What type of cell has processes called axons and dendrites?
Nerve cells.

12. What English words are synonymous with Latin *tunica* and *lamina*?
Coat and layer.

13. What is the difference between visceral and parietal peritoneum?
The parietal membrane covers the walls of the abdominal cavity; the visceral peritoneum covers the organs.

14. What structures are typically found in a neurovascular bundle?
An artery, one or more veins, and a nerve.

15. Connective tissue can be divided on the basis of its structural organization into six distinct types. List and give examples of each type.
Loose connective tissue is found in the subcutaneous fascia and in the stroma or structural framework of solid organs such as the liver, kidney, and pancreas.
Dense connective tissue occurs in ligaments, tendons, and the dermis.
Reticular connective tissue forms the framework of lymphoid organs (spleen and lymph nodes) and of bone marrow.
Adipose tissue is distributed in variable amounts in the subcutaneous tissue and forms cushioning layers around certain organs such as the kidney and the eye.
Cartilage: Hyaline cartilage is found in the nose, larynx, trachea, and bronchi, and as a covering for the joint surfaces of bones; elastic cartilage occurs in the external ear and the epiglottis; fibrous cartilage (or fibrocartilage) is found in the intervertebral disks.
Bone forms the skeletal structure of the human body—skull, extremities, ribs are examples.

16. List and give a brief, one-sentence definition for each of the five tissue types discussed in this chapter.
a. epithelial—comprises most of the surfaces in the body, including skin and mucous membranes, the linings of hollow and tubular organs in the digestive, respiratory, and urogenital systems, and the linings of the chest and abdominal cavities.
b. connective—includes bone, cartilage, tendons, ligaments, the dermis or true skin, subcutaneous fat, and many other supporting and investing structures.
c. muscle-consists of bundles or sheets of long, narrow cells arranged in parallel and having the capacity to shorten under appropriate electrochemical stimulation.
d. nerve—the most highly specialized type of tissue in the body, nerve cells show the most extreme differentiation of structure and have the unique property of conducting electrochemical impulses.
e. hemolymphatic—which can be addressed as
blood—consists of a fluid called plasma in which various cells or "formed elements" (red blood cells, white blood cells, and platelets) are suspended.
lymphoid—not really a separate tissue type, it consists of large numbers of lymphocytes (small white blood cells with relatively large nuclei, essential components of the immune system) in a meshwork of reticular connective tissue. More highly organized masses of lymphoid tissue occur in the spleen, thymus, lymph nodes, and tonsils.

Chapter 17. Procedures and Practices in Anatomic Pathology

FILL IN THE BLANKS
1. specimens taken from living patients, autopsy specimens
2. tissues or organs, biopsy specimens
3. fixative
4. formalin is made by bubbling formaldehyde gas through water
5. immediate gross examination
6. to allow penetration of processing chemicals
7. serial number or accession number
8. three planes
9. histopathology
10. paraffin, cellulose
11. microtome
12. all of the tissue spaces are filled with the infiltrating medium
13. stains
14. mordant
15. polychrome stain
16. counterstain
17. metachromatic stain
18. hematoxylin and eosin (H&E)
19. blue and purple
20. pink to red
21. mounting medium (balsam)
22. more the detail, smaller the zone of tissue
23. incisional biopsy
24. excisional biopsy
25. to determine whether all abnormal tissue has in fact been excised
26. smear
27. fine-needle aspiration
28. to determine as precisely as possible the cause of death
29. objective anatomic evidence
30. body, cadaver, deceased or decedent, patient, remains, or subject
31. prosector, dissector, operator, autopsy surgeon, pathologist
32. diener
33. livor mortis (postmortem lividity, hypostasis)
34. rigor mortis
35. lividity
36. pathology conference

MULTIPLE CHOICE
1.	D	13.	E
2.	B	14.	B
3.	C	15.	C
4.	E	16.	B
5.	E	17.	D
6.	A	18.	A
7.	E	19.	D
8.	B	20.	C
9.	C	21.	E
10.	D	22.	B
11.	B	23.	D
12.	A		

SHORT ANSWERS

1. Define or explain.
   a. Bethesda system—a method for categorizing the findings on a Pap smear.
   b. biopsy—the removal of tissue from a living patient for pathologic examination.
   c. counterstain—a contrasting color stain applied to a slide after the slide has been washed to remove the color that has not chemically bonded to the tissue.
   d. cytology—the study of cells, often used in the narrow sense of a study of cells that have been detached from a surface for microscopic study.
   e. fixative—a fluid into which specimens are placed in order to arrest the process of decomposition that begins almost at once in devitalized tissue, to kill bacteria and fungi in or on the specimen, and to begin hardening the tissue to facilitate preparation for microscopic study.
   f. mordant—a substance applied to a tissue section to render it chemically more receptive to staining.
   g. Pap smear—Papanicolaou smear, the most frequently performed cytologic test for detection of abnormal cells from the uterine cervix.
   h. polychrome stain—a mixture of two or more coloring agents in one solution.
2. What is the most widely used fixative?
   The most commonly used fixative is a 10% aqueous solution of formalin.
3. What does the pathologist do with a surgical specimen after completing the gross examination?
   The trimmed pieces of tissue are placed in small, flat, round or oblong cassettes of perforated metal or plastic with lids of the same material, in which they will remain during the first stages of processing.

4. What are some ways by which a surgeon might indicate the origin or anatomic orientation of a specimen taken for pathologic study?
   The surgeon may cut the specimen to a certain shape to indicate its origin or its orientation in the patient's body or place a suture at a certain place in the specimen, such as at the uppermost point of a tumor excised from the skin.
5. Name some kinds of surgical specimens that are not routinely sectioned for microscopic study.
   Hernia sacs, blood clots, varicose veins, healthy bone (e.g., a section of rib removed for access to thoracic organs), and teeth.
6. Why must embedding of tissue in paraffin be preceded by dehydration and clearing?
   It is dehydrated by replacing the water with a series of organic solvents to make it harder and cleared with xylene (xylol), benzene, cedarwood oil, or chloroform to replace the dehydrating agent and make it transparent.
7. What is meant by making serial sections of a specimen?
   Every tenth or twentieth slice of a paraffin block, to provide the pathologist with a three-dimensional concept of a tissue or lesion.
8. What two methods can be used to obtain cells for study from fluids with low cell counts?
   a. The cells may be concentrated by centrifugation.
   b. The cells may be or separated by filtration.
9. What is the principal advantage of the frozen section technique?
   It makes it possible for a pathologist to perform a histologic examination of tissue within minutes after it is removed from the patient.
10. List several reasons for performing an autopsy.
    In certain cases (homicide, suicide, fatal accident, death due to poison or drug overdose, and others), the law requires that an autopsy be performed by or under the auspices of a coroner or medical examiner. In

addition, an autopsy may be ordered by legal authorities when a person dies during the first 24 hours after hospital admission or after surgery, or when a person with no known health problems dies suddenly.
11. What two points must always be verified by the pathologist before an autopsy is begun, except in a forensic setting?
    a. identification of the body
    b. that a consent form has been signed
12. What is postmortem lividity?
    Livor mortis (postmortem lividity, hypostasis) is a purplish discoloration of the skin due to engorgement of capillaries that occurs shortly after death. Lividity affects whatever parts of the body are lowermost, but does not appear in areas of the skin that have been in firm contact with a supporting surface.
13. Which major organ is sometimes removed but not opened at the time of autopsy? Why?
    Because brain tissue is extremely soft in its natural state, it is usually allowed to harden in fixative for several days before being cut for gross and microscopic study.
14. List two reasons why a frozen section might be requested during surgery?
    a. The histologic character of a tumor may determine whether the surgeon can be content with simple excision or whether a more radical procedure must be performed at once.
    b. When the resection of a malignancy involves extensive, mutilating surgery, the surgeon may choose to remove tissue in stages, submitting a specimen from each stage for pathologic study before deciding whether to close the incision or remove more tissue.
15. What are the three components of the Bethesda system of reporting Pap smear findings?

a. a statement of the adequacy of the specimen

b. general categorization (negative for intraepithelial lesion or malignancy; epithelial cell abnormality; or other)

c. descriptive diagnosis, elaborating on the general categorization and including mention of all significant abnormalities (e.g., evidence of inflammation or infection with *Candida* or *Trichomonas*) as well as of the patient's hormonal status (when vaginal cells are present in the smear)

Chapter 18. Pathologic Change and Pathologic Diagnosis

FILL IN THE BLANKS

1. hereditary
2. congenital
3. hereditary
4. may not be
5. dysplasia
6. inborn errors of metabolism
7. ectopic, heterotopic
8. hamartoma
9. teratogen
10. increase, differentiation
11. malabsorption syndromes
12. dystrophy
13. metaplasia
14. chemotaxis
15. lymphocytes
16. chronic
17. infiltrate
18. exudate
19. suppuration
20. proliferation of microscopic organisms
21. they can be transmitted in one way or another from one person to another
22. opportunistic
23. very small segment of genetic material (DNA or RNA)
24. hyperemia, edema
25. active hyperemia
26. passive hyperemia
27. atherosclerosis
28. identification of the poison by chemical analysis of blood, tissue, secretions, or waste products

29. neoplasia
30. cancerous, malignant, benign

MULTIPLE CHOICE

1. B	13. E	25. A
2. C	14. D	26. C
3. D	15. B	27. E
4. A	16. E	28. E
5. D	17. C	29. D
6. C	18. A	30. B
7. E	19. B	31. A
8. B	20. D	32. A
9. D	21. C	33. B
10. D	22. B	34. E
11. C	23. A	35. C
12. A	24. B	

SHORT ANSWERS

1. Define pathology. Name and define its three principal branches.
   Pathology is the branch of medicine that studies the structural and functional changes produced in the living body by injury or disease. Anatomic pathology is concerned with the gross and microscopic changes brought about in living human tissues by disease. Clinical pathology refers to the laboratory examination of bodily fluids and waste products such as blood, spinal fluid, urine, and feces. Forensic pathology involves the application of knowledge comprised by the other two branches to certain issues in both civil and criminal law.

2. Define or explain.
   a. anaplasia—the presence of primitive cells, or more undifferentiated cells than are normally present in the affected tissue, a possible characteristic of a malignant tumor.
   b. ascites—the presence of edema fluid in the abdominal (peritoneal) cavity.
   c. desmoplasia—exuberant production of connective tissue fibers appearing as a dense, woody or stony consistency, such as is present in a scirrhous tumor.
   d. embolism—the process of formation or release of anything other than fluid blood (embolus) into the circulation

   e. thrombosis—the process of formation of a clot (thrombus) within the circulatory system.
   f. hyperchromasia—the characteristic of nuclei to stain more darkly.
   g. infarction—necrosis or death of tissue due to severe acute interruption of blood supply to a tissue.
   h. ischemia—a reduction in the supply of blood to a tissue or organ as a result of obstruction of a single major artery by a clot or external compression, or from generalized narrowing of arterioles by vascular disease.
   i. necrosis— death of tissue (see infarction).
   j. pleomorphism—a variation from normal of shape of malignant cells.
   k. putrefaction—the decomposition of the body as a whole after death, due in part to the action of bacteria normally resident in the intestine and in part due to the breakdown of cells and tissues by the action of their own chemical components.
   l. shock—an acute, life-threatening state of hypotension (subnormal blood pressure) with inadequate blood flow through vital organs.

3. What information does a pathologist's report contain besides a record of abnormalities found in the specimen?
   The dictation always begins with basic identifying data: the patient's name as shown on the label of the container and on the laboratory requisition accompanying the specimen, and a general indication of what material has been submitted. Alternatively, a serial number or accession number may be assigned to the specimen container and the pertinent data kept in a register. If only one specimen is taken during an operation, as in an appendectomy, it may be unnecessary to

identify it other than by the patient's name.

4. What kinds of change in the gross and microscopic features of a tissue specimen are taken into account by the pathologist in arriving at a diagnosis?

In performing a gross examination of a tissue specimen, the anatomic pathologist looks for departures from expected color, size, shape, surface texture, internal consistency, and homogeneity, as well as for any tumors, cysts, hemorrhage, exudate, tissue death, scarring, or abnormal deposition of materials such as fat or calcium. In examining microscopic sections of tissue the pathologist observes the type, size, shape, number, and distribution of cells present, the configuration and staining properties of their nuclei, cytoplasmic granules, vacuoles, or deposits, the type and distribution of intercellular material such as connective-tissue fibers, extravasated blood, fibrinous or other exudates, and any variations from expected tissue architecture.

5. Distinguish the following:
   a. hypoplasia—refers to underdevelopment of a structure.
   b. aplasia—extreme underdevelopment of a structure.
   c. agenesis—complete failure of formation (congenital absence).

6. What are the three germ layers?
   a. The ectoderm, or outer layer, forms the epidermis, the nervous system including the specialized sensory structures of the eye and ear, and the enamel of the teeth.
   b. The mesoderm, or middle layer, forms connective tissue (including cartilage and bone), muscle (all types), the circulatory and genitourinary systems, and the spleen.
   c. The endoderm, or inner layer, forms the epithelial linings of the respiratory, digestive, and excretory systems, the liver, and the pancreas.

7. How does hypertrophy differ from hyperplasia?

Hyperplasia is an increase in the number of cells or other structural elements, hypertrophy an increase in the size of cells or fibers.

8. List various causes of inflammation.

Causes of inflammation can be divided into two broad categories: pathogenic (disease-causing) microorganisms, and physical or chemical injury. The latter category includes cutting, crushing, burning, freezing, electrical shock, radiation, various types of foreign body, and irritation or poisoning by chemical agents. In addition, certain processes originating inside the body —tissue death due to circulatory impairment, the formation and spread of a malignant tumor, the production of abnormal antibodies that attack normal tissue—can set off an inflammatory response.

9. What is responsible for the redness and heat in inflamed tissue?

The capillaries in a zone of inflamed tissue dilate. At the same time, capillary walls thicken, so that the net effect is congestion or engorgement of tissues with blood rather than an increased flow of blood through the tissues. This increased amount of blood in the tissues, or hyperemia, accounts for the familiar observation of redness and heat in an inflamed part.

10. What is phagocytosis?

A reaction to inflammation or invasion of foreign bodies in which histiocytes (macrophages), neutrophils and monocytes collectively assemble with remarkable speed, engulfing, breaking down, and removing dead tissue, foreign material, or invading microorganisms.

11. Distinguish beneficial from harmful types of antibody formation.

Antibodies are a normal reaction against foreign substances (antigens) introduced into the body, but sometimes antibodies react with the body's own tissues to induce local inflammation and destruction resulting in autoimmune disorders known as collagen diseases.

12. Name some autoimmune or collagen diseases.

Rheumatoid arthritis, lupus erythematosus, periarteritis nodosa

13. In what important ways do viruses differ from bacteria and fungi?

Viruses are not living organisms but pieces of DNA or RNA that take over a cell's function. Virus particles are much too small to be seen by light microscopy, but cells infected with virus show characteristic changes that may enable the pathologist not only to recognize that infection is present but even to identify the specific virus involved.

14. What are some ways in which a parasite may affect the health of the host?

Parasites cause varying degrees of disease by depriving the host of nutrients, invading or disrupting tissues, and eliciting allergic and inflammatory reactions.

15. Mention some types of atrophy that are normal or expected.

The thymus gland usually undergoes atrophy during infancy, the tonsils after puberty. Atrophy of the ovaries and breasts normally follows menopause.

16. What is the name of the pigment normally found in the skin and the iris?

Melanin.

17. List four major differences between benign and malignant neoplasms.
   a. A malignant tumor is more likely to display anaplasia— the presence of primitive cells, or more undifferentiated cells than are normally present in the affected tissue—than a benign one.
   b. A malignant tumor typically enlarges by infiltration and invasion of surrounding tissues, whereas a benign tumor expands while remaining sharply localized and readily distinguishable from surrounding normal tissue. Often a benign tumor has a definite capsule.
   c. A malignant tumor tends to grow faster than a benign one.

d. A malignant tumor is capable of metastasis—establishing secondary foci of malignant cells at sites remote from the primary tumor.

18. Distinguish between grading and staging of malignant neoplasms.

The grade of a malignant neoplasm is a quantitative estimate of its malignant potential, generally based on the percentage of anaplastic (undifferentiated) cells it contains. Grading correlates generally with the expected future behavior of a tumor. Staging of a malignancy is a formulation of its current extent, an attempt to describe its behavior up to the present.

19. In what ways do the following substances normally found in the body cause problems?

a. Cholesterol is deposited as atherosclerosis in the lining of arteries which, accompanied by fibrosis, is a major cause of stroke and heart attack, it may form deposits in the wall of the gallbladder, especially when the gallbladder is chronically inflamed. In addition, cholesterol is an important constituent of gallstones.

b. Calcium is deposited in chronically inflamed, fibrotic, or degenerating tissue, as in tendinitis, osteoarthritis, pulmonary tuberculosis, and in aging blood vessels; metastatic calcium is deposition of calcium in normal tissues as a result of an excessive level of calcium in the blood.

c. glycogen deposited in cells occurs in diabetes mellitus and in hereditary abnormalities of glycogen storage.

d. uric acid salts, a normal breakdown product of certain foods, accumulate in the blood and tissues in gout and other metabolic disorders. Formation of urate crystals in joints causes the pain and swelling of acute gouty arthritis. Urates may also contribute to the formation of urinary calculi.

e. bilirubin, when elevated, causes jaundice.

f. melanin may be increased in certain abnormal conditions, including melanoma, chronic inflammation or trauma in the skin and in the cartilage and urine (ochronosis) of persons with alkaptonuria, an uncommon inborn error of metabolism.

20. List three types of trauma that can cause changes in tissues detectable by gross and microscopic examination.

a. fractures
b. burns
c. radiation

Chapter 19. Hematology, Coagulation, and Blood Typing

FILL IN THE BLANKS

1. biochemistry
2. immunology
3. molecular biology
4. smears, cultures
5. antibiotics
6. panel, profile
7. alkaline phosphatase
8. antibodies
9. albumin, total protein
10. venipuncture, phlebotomy
11. arterial
12. pricking a finger (pinprick)
13. erythrocytes
14. rouleaux
15. leukocytes
16. polymorphonuclear leukocytes
17. monocyte
18. unsegmented neutrophils, stab cells, band cells, bands
19. B cells
20. T cells
21. cytotoxic (killer) T cells
22. null cells
23. CD4 protein, CD8 protein
24. CD4+ cells, T4 cells
25. hemogram
26. anemia, erythrocytopenia
27. extramedullary hematopoiesis
28. differential count (or white blood cell differential)
29. shift to the left or a left shift

30. CD4 count, 20%
31. Downey cells or virocytes
32. collagen diseases and some malignancies, particularly those of the bone marrow
33. idiopathic thrombocytopenic purpura, thrombotic thrombocytopenic purpura, and disease or toxic states associated with damage to the bone marrow
34. platelet aggregation
35. activated partial thromboplastin time (PTT)
36. aspiration, biopsy
37. blood typing
38. hemolytic disease of the newborn, erythroblastosis fetalis
39. attempts to disprove paternity
40. incompatibility, contraindication

MULTIPLE CHOICE

1.	D	25.	C
2.	C	26.	D
3.	E	27.	A
4.	A	28.	E
5.	B	29.	D
6.	D	30.	B
7.	C	31.	C
8.	A	32.	A
9.	C	33.	B
10.	B	34.	E
11.	E	35.	D
12.	B	36.	C
13.	D	37.	B
14.	C	38.	A
15.	E	39.	C
16.	E	40.	B
17.	A	41.	A
18.	C	42.	E
19.	B	43.	B
20.	D	44.	D
21.	B	45.	C
22.	E	46.	A
23.	B	47.	C
24.	A		

SHORT ANSWERS

1. Briefly explain the scope of the following branches of clinical pathology (Introduction)

a. Hematology refers both to a subspecialty of internal medicine concerned with abnormalities in the formation and function of blood cells (such as anemia and leukemia) and to a branch of laboratory technology concerned with the performance of quantitative and qualitative assessments of blood cells.

b. Clinical chemistry the application of biochemistry to diagnostic medicine. In practice, clinical chemistry refers almost exclusively to quantitative chemical analysis of blood specimens.

c. Urinology is a branch of medical technology that involves basic microscopic and chemical examination of urine specimens.

d. Microbiology is concerned with the study of microscopic living things. Medical microbiology concentrates on bacteria, fungi, and other microorganisms capable of causing human disease. Bacteriology, parasitology, mycology (the study of fungi), and virology are divisions of medical microbiology.

e. Serology is a branch of immunology that studies antigen-antibody reactions, particularly with respect to the diagnosis of infectious diseases.

2. What is meant by quantitative data? Give examples of the difference between qualitative and quantitative data. (Introduction)
They count discrete components or measure concentrations, rates, or other features of a specimen that are capable of being expressed numerically. The shape, grouping, and staining characteristics of cells in a fluid such as blood or urine are examples of purely qualitative observations. The size and relative or absolute numbers of various cells present are quantitative measurements.

3. How is "normal" defined in practice? (Introduction)
For most tests, a range of results called a normal range or reference range has been established as being compatible with normal function or absence of disease or impairment. This range is ordinarily based on a statistical analysis of large numbers of results obtained by testing apparently healthy persons. Test results above or below this range are considered abnormal. For some tests, one set of normals is appropriate for women and another for men. Various sets of normal values may be applied depending on the patient's age.

4. What factors govern the physician's choice of a laboratory procedure when several similar methods are available?
The choice of method for performing a given test may be governed by such considerations as cost, speed of performance, availability of special equipment or reagents or of appropriately trained technicians, as well as the comparative sensitivity and specificity of the various methods available.

5. What examinations make up the complete blood count?
Red blood cell count, hemoglobin, hematocrit with red cell indices consisting of mean corpuscular volume (hematocrit ÷ red blood cell count), mean corpuscular hemoglobin (hemoglobin ÷ red blood cell count), and mean corpuscular hemoglobin concentration (hemoglobin ÷ hematocrit); white blood cells with a differential count of white blood cells; and platelets.

6. What is the significance of the reticulocyte count?
The normal reticulocyte count is 0.5 to 1.5% of all red blood cells. Increase in this count (reticulocytosis) suggests heightened erythropoiesis in response to blood loss or hemolysis.

7. List some basic tests that are included in a coagulation panel.
Platelet count, bleeding time, clotting time, prothrombin time, partial thromboplastin time, and clot retraction. In addition, plasma assay for specific coagulation factors is possible.

8. List blood groups and explain their clinical significance.
A, B, AB, O. The most important antigen-antibody relationships of the red blood cell are those involved in the ABO system, which makes blood type A incompatible with blood type B. A hemolytic reaction due to transfusion of incompatible blood is manifested by fever, chills, shock, and renal failure. The mortality rate is high. The Rh antibody is another factor in incompatibility. A person who is Rh negative may receive a first transfusion of Rh positive blood with impunity. After forming antibody to the Rh antigen in this blood, however, such a person may not receive further transfusions of Rh positive blood without risk of hemolytic reaction.

9. Sickle cell disease differs from sickle cell trait in what ways?
a. Persons with sickle cell trait (the heterozygous form) produce some red blood cells containing hemoglobin S, and persons with sickle cell disease (the homozygous form) produce more.

b. Sickle cell trait is often asymptomatic, sickle cell disease commonly causes developmental abnormalities, splenomegaly, recurrent bouts of abdominal and extremity pain, and susceptibility to aseptic necrosis of long bones and to infections with *Salmonella* organisms.

10. Describe the procedure performed to test for erythrocyte survival time.
A specimen of the patient's blood is labeled with chromium Cr 51 sodium chromate and reinjected into the patient. Specimens of blood obtained at intervals during the next several weeks are tested to determine what percent of the cells in the specimen remain in the circulation. Nuclear imaging may also be performed to detect any sites of high concentration of radioisotope.

11. List the six different types of white cells and the significance of each.

    a. neutrophils, segmented—increased in acute bacterial infections, toxemia, uremia, acidosis, burns, leukemia, and lymphoma. Reduced in toxic states, chemical poisoning, typhoid fever, measles, influenza, overwhelming bacterial infection, miliary tuberculosis, and after irradiation.

    b. neutrophils, bands—The more acute and intense the neutrophilic response, the greater the number of immature cells (bands) that are likely to be present.

    c. eosinophils—increased in various allergic states (asthma, urticaria), parasitism (trichinosis, echinococcosis), polyarteritis nodosa, sarcoidosis, Hodgkin disease, chronic myelogenous leukemia, and after splenectomy. Decreased after chemotherapy, irradiation, or treatment with adrenocortical steroid.

    d. basophils—increased in chronic myelogenous leukemia, polycythemia, Hodgkin disease, and after splenectomy. Decreased in hyperthyroidism and after chemotherapy, irradiation, or administration of adrenocortical steroid.

    e. monocytes—increased in some bacterial (tuberculosis, infective endocarditis), rickettsial (typhus, Rocky Mountain spotted fever), or protozoal (malaria, trypanosomiasis) infections, and in some collagen diseases, sarcoidosis, Hodgkin disease, polycythemia vera, and monocytic leukemia. Reduction in the number of monocytes (monocytopenia) is not often recognized but may accompany conditions involving destruction or suppression of bone marrow.

    f. lymphocytes—increased in many viral infections (mumps, infectious hepatitis, infectious mononucleosis), tuberculosis, brucellosis, thyrotoxicosis, and lymphatic leukemia. Relative lymphocytosis accompanies marked neutropenia. Reduced in autoimmune disorders, particularly systemic lupus erythematosus, and in some congenital and acquired immune deficiencies including AIDS. Relative lymphopenia occurs with absolute neutrophilia.

12. The myeloid/erythroid ratio, that is, the ratio of leukocyte to erythrocyte precursors in the marrow is useful for evaluating what kinds of conditions?

    The ratio is increased in chronic myelogenous leukemia and in disorders resulting in loss of erythroid elements. The ratio is decreased in agranulocytosis and in disorders resulting in overgrowth of erythroid elements.

Chapter 20. Blood Chemistry

FILL IN THE BLANKS

1. centrifuge, plasma
2. hemolysis
3. serum
4. gravimetric, volumetric, quantitative
5. electrolyte, ionizes
6. sodium and potassium, chloride and bicarbonate
7. sodium (Na)
8. hypernatremia, hyponatremia
9. diuresis
10. hyperkalemia, hyperpotassemia
11. hypokalemia, hypopotassemia
12. hyperchloremia
13. hypochloremia
14. bicarbonate
15. alkaline
16. alkalosis, acidosis
17. respiratory alkalosis
18. phosphorus
19. hypoparathyroidism
20. iron-binding capacity
21. calcium, phosphorus
22. arterial blood gases
23. enzyme
24. indicate disease in its tissue of origin
25. serum glutamic-oxaloacetic transaminase (SGOT)
26. serum glutamic-pyruvate transaminase (SGPT)
27. creatine phosphokinase (CPK)
28. storage disease
29. hormone
30. hormones
31. radioimmunoassay (RIA)
32. hypophysis
33. antidiuretic hormone (ADH)
34. gonadotropins
35. pineal gland
36. albumin, globulin, fibrinogen.
37. amino acids
38. troponin I (TnI), myocardial necrosis
39. congestive failure
40. acute phase reactants
41. therapeutic range

MULTIPLE CHOICE

1.	C	24.	A
2,	A	25.	D
3.	D	26.	E
4.	E	27.	B
5.	B	28.	B
6.	D	29.	C
7.	A	30.	B
8.	B	31.	A
9.	C	32.	D
10.	E	33.	E
11.	C	34.	C
12.	B	35.	B
13.	A	36.	A
14.	D	37.	E
15.	E	38.	A
16.	B	39.	D
17.	C	40.	C
18.	D	41.	B
19.	A	42.	E
20.	E	43.	C
21.	B	44.	A
22.	A	45.	D
23.	C		

SHORT ANSWERS

1. Define or explain.
    a. A/G ratio—the quotient obtained by dividing albumin level by globulin level.

b. anion—an ion that has a negative charge because it has gained one or more electrons

c. buffer—a substance that resists changes in pH by combining with or releasing hydrogen ions so as to keep their concentration constant in a solution. The principal buffer of the serum is bicarbonate ion. Phosphate ion and the serum proteins (albumin and globulin) also act as buffers, but to a much lesser extent.

d. cation—an ion that has a positive charge because it has lost one or more electrons.

e. hypercapnia—increase in carbon dioxide tension.

f. hypokalemia—decrease in potassium.

g. isoenzyme—a group of two or more enzymes having the same action but differing in chemical structure.

h. pH—The acidity or alkalinity of a solution depends on its hydrogen ion concentration. This is measured in pH units derived from the logarithm of the hydrogen ion concentration.

i. trace elements—elements that occur in only small concentrations in body fluids and tissues, such as copper, zinc, and certain other metallic elements.

2. List some reasons why several tests are often done together in a group or "panel."

Automation makes performing multiple tests on a single specimen faster, easier, cheaper. Several constituents of a specimen may be inter-related, such as CBC, liver function tests, lipid tests, renal function tests. A group or panel of enzyme tests are done and diagnostic inferences drawn from a consideration of all the information thus gained.

3. Give an example of a laboratory value derived by calculation from other laboratory values.

A/G ratio, LDL, bicarbonate, oxygen saturation.

4. Why is it usually important to separate red blood cells from plasma promptly and completely in a blood specimen intended for chemical testing?

Keeping cells and plasma completely segregated is important because otherwise some red blood cells may leak or burst (hemolyze) and release their contents into the plasma while the specimen is awaiting analysis.

5. What are some advantages of automated chemical testing of blood?

Automated analytic devices can perform 20 or more tests on blood samples at a rate of one sample or more a minute. Despite their great expense, these analyzers reduce the cost of chemical testing because they are capable of processing a much higher volume of material than a human technician. In addition, they permit better standardization of results and eliminate many potential sources of human error.

6. What are the principal serum electrolytes?

Sodium and potassium, chloride and bicarbonate.

7. What is the point of determining the cholesterol level in an apparently healthy person?

Persons with elevated cholesterol are at increased risk of atherosclerosis, an inflammatory and degenerative disorder of arteries in which plaques of lipid material reduce caliber and obstruct blood flow.

8. What important class of substances is included in the gamma globulin fraction of plasma?

All known circulating antibodies, including IgG (more than 75% of the total globulin fraction), IgA (15%), IgM (10%), IgD (less than 1%), and IgE (less than 0.1%).

9. What is the principal nitrogenous waste product excreted in urine?

Urea, a form of nitrogen which in turn is a breakdown product of protein.

10. List three factors affecting the glomerular filtration rate.

a. systemic blood pressure.

b. the resistance of glomerular capillaries to blood flow.

c. the integrity of the glomerular basement membrane, which is subject to damage by a variety of inflammatory, degenerative, and toxic factors.

11. List the three distinct operations performed on the glomerular filtrate by the tubules of the kidney that determine the eventual volume and composition of urine.

a. They passively reabsorb most of the water and dissolved electrolytes.

b. They actively reabsorb certain substances (sodium, chloride).

c. They actively secrete other substances (potassium, hydrogen ions, urea).

12. List two ways in which aldosterone affects tubular function.

a. It promotes the renal tubular retention (that is, the reabsorption from glomerular filtrate) of sodium, the principal cation (positively charged ion) of the blood and extracellular fluid, and of chloride, the principal anion (negatively charged ion).

b. It also promotes the tubular excretion of potassium, the principal cation of intracellular fluid.

13. Hyponatremia may be a reflection of what two factors?

a. an increase in serum water content (dilutional hyponatremia), as in congestive heart failure or hepatic or renal disease

b. true depletion of sodium, as by vomiting, sweating, or excessive renal excretion of sodium in renal disease, adrenal cortical deficiency (Addison disease), or as an effect of certain diuretics.

14. List the components of an arterial blood gas study and the importance of each.

a. The partial pressure of oxygen (PO_2) normally declines with age, may be increased in hyperventilation, or reduced in any condition that depresses or inhibits respiratory movements, any condition that prevents normal oxygen exchange in lung tissue, or reduction of available oxygen in the atmosphere.

b. Oxygen saturation can also be calculated from the PO_2 and the concentration of hemoglobin; a reduction below 95-100% has essentially the same significance as a reduction in the partial pressure of oxygen.

c. The partial pressure of carbon dioxide (PCO_2) may be increased by most of the same conditions that reduce oxygen (except reduction in available oxygen) and in response to metabolic alkalosis, reduced in hyperventilation and in response to metabolic acidosis.

d. The pH and bicarbonate concentration of the specimen is also determined to identify acidosis or alkalosis and to permit indirect calculation of the bicarbonate ion concentration.

15. List the serum enzymes often found elevated to varying degrees in hepatic disease and in injury or infarction of muscle, particularly cardiac muscle.

    a. alanine aminotransferase (ALT)
    b. aspartate aminotransferase (AST)
    c. creatine phosphokinase (CPK)
    d. lactic dehydrogenase (LDH)
    e. gamma-glutamyl transpeptidase (GGT)

16. If the serum leucine aminopeptidase (SLAP) and the 5′-nucleotidase are elevated in conjunction with an elevated alkaline phosphatase, what is the most likely diagnosis? If they are normal in the presence of an elevated alkaline

phosphatase, what is the most likely diagnosis?
These typically rise in hepatic disease but not in bone disease and so help interpret a rise in alkaline phosphatase.

17. Numerous congenital disorders consist in the lack of genes that encode specific enzymes. List number of these enzymes and the diseases associated with their deficiency.

    a. Deficiency of beta-glucosidase (also called glucocerebrosidase and glucosylceramidase) results in Gaucher disease.
    b. Congenital deficiency of hexosaminidase A results in Tay-Sachs disease.
    c. People with a deficiency of acetylcholinesterase (actually detected by blood tests for pseudocholinesterase [serum cholinesterase]) are abnormalities sensitive to succinylcholine, a muscle relaxant used in general anesthesia.
    d. Hereditary deficiency of glucose-6-phosphate dehydrogenase (G-6-PD) in red blood cells was is a cause of hemolytic anemia after exposure to certain drugs, chemicals, and foods.

18. List the five anatomically discrete endocrine (ductless) glands and the hormones they produce.

    a. pituitary—follicle-stimulating hormone, luteinizing hormone, prolactin, thyroid-stimulating hormone, adrenocorticotropic hormone, and somatostatin are produced in the anterior pituitary; oxytocin and vasopressin (antidiuretic hormone, ADH) in the posterior pituitary.
    b. thyroid gland—thyroxine or T_4, triiodothyronine or T_3, calcitonin
    c. parathyroids—parathormone
    d. adrenals—cortisol, deoxycortisol, aldosterone
    e. pineal—melatonin

19. List the areas, other than the endocrine glands, where zones of specialized tissue contain secretory cells and the chemical products they send directly into the blood.
Pancreas (insulin, glucagon), ovary (estradiol, estriol, progesterone), testicle (testosterone), liver, lung, kidney (renin and the product of its action, angiotensin II), digestive tract (gastrin), the placenta (chorionic gonadotropin, human placental lactogen, estriol), and nervous system.

20. List the fractions of cholesterol and their significance.
high density lipoproteins (HDL), low density lipoproteins (LDL), and very low density lipoproteins (VLDL). Lipoprotein assay provides additional diagnostic information in cases of hypercholesterolemia. The normal level of HDL cholesterol is 35-80 mg/dL [1-2 mmol/L], and the normal level of LDL cholesterol is 40-130 mg/dL [1-3 mmol/L]. A relative preponderance of HDL, which carry cholesterol away from tissues, is associated with lower risk of atherosclerosis, while a preponderance of LDL, which deposit cholesterol in tissues, implies increased risk of atherosclerosis.

21. List six tumor markers and their significance.

    a. Carcinoembryonic antigen (CEA) is not of much use in screening or diagnosis but is valuable in testing treated cancer patients for recurrence or metastases.
    b. Alpha-fetoprotein (AFP) is elevated in hepatocellular carcinoma, viral hepatitis, hepatic cirrhosis, and various teratocarcinomas and embryonal carcinomas of gonadal origin and also in pregnancy but extremely high levels in maternal serum may indicate fetal neural tube defects (anencephaly, spina bifida) or fetal death.

c. A prostate specific antigen (PSA) above 10 usually is indicative of prostate carcinoma.

d. CA (cancer antigen) 19-9 is elevated in some patients with malignant tumors of the stomach, bowel, liver and pancreas.

e. CA 125 elevations occur in a majority of ovarian cancers, but also in digestive tract neoplasms, in some benign tumors of the reproductive tract, and in normal pregnancy.

f. CA 27.29 is elevated in one-third of early breast cancers and in two-thirds of later-stage breast cancers.

g. HER-2 protein is expressed in many breast cancers

22. Discuss the importance of monitoring drug levels.

Monitoring of drug levels is particularly important with drugs having narrow margins between therapeutic and toxic effects (gentamicin, lithium, theophylline, tobramycin), drugs used to control cardiac arrhythmias (digitoxin, digoxin, procainamide, quinidine), and drugs used to prevent seizures (carbamazepine, phenobarbital, phenytoin, valproic acid). For some drugs, determination of both peak (maximum) and trough (minimum) levels in the serum is necessary to monitor drug metabolism so as to avoid levels above or below the therapeutic range.

Chapter 21. Microbiology

FILL IN THE BLANKS
1. source of a specimen
2. bacteriology
3. smear
4. gram-positive
5. urinary tract infection
6. human papillomavirus, rotavirus, hepatitis

MULTIPLE CHOICE
1. B
2. C
3. E
4. A
5. A
6. D
7. B
8. C
9. E
10. D

SHORT ANSWERS
1. Define or explain.
   a. agar—a vegetable gum which gives them a stiff gel-like consistency below 45°C. Organisms grown on agar present more distinctive cultural characteristics than those grown in broth, and individual colonies can be observed and sampled.
   b. Gram stain— In this technique, crystal violet is first applied, along with a mordant (an agent that causes the stain to react chemically with some components of the smear) that contains iodine. Certain bacteria, called gram-positive, take up this stain and resist decolorization with alcohol. Other organisms, called gram-negative, do not retain the stain after washing with alcohol. These are counterstained red with safranin in the final step of the technique.
   c. mycology— the study of pathogenic fungi.
   d. normal flora— nonpathogenic organisms normally found in the source material or bodily region in question.
   e. sensitivity test— disks impregnated with known concentrations of various antibiotics are incorporated in the culture medium. Zones of inhibition of bacterial growth around certain disks indicate sensitivity of the organism to those antibiotics.
2. What are the two basic laboratory procedures in bacteriology?
   a. microscopic examination of stained smears, in which a translucent layer of fluid or semisolid material thinly spread over a microscope slide.
   b. the culture of microorganisms under controlled artificial conditions in the laboratory, when only a few organisms are present and could be missed by a stain.
3. In what ways can culturing a pathogenic microorganism contribute to its identification?
   Culturing permits isolation of various organisms from a mixture for individual study. Observation of the growth characteristics of organisms in a culture supplies additional identifying data, and pure colonies from the culture can be studied in stained smears. By the addition of nutrients and inhibitors to a culture medium, certain types of organisms can be favored while others are suppressed. Reagents and indicators added to the culture medium allow prompt detection of distinctive products of bacterial growth through color change.
4. What is the standard medium for throat cultures?
   Throat cultures are performed on blood agar, a medium containing whole blood of animal origin, to facilitate identification of streptococci.
5. Mention two types of pathogenic microorganism that cannot be grown in cultures.
   a. viruses
   b. parasites
6. Mention two types of pathogenic microorganism that take several weeks to grow in cultures.
   a. Cultures for acid-fast organisms (mycobacteria) require 6-8 weeks of incubation
   b. Special culture media are required for fungi; incubation, usually at room temperature, must be continued for several weeks.
7. Explain the procedure to ensure that the urine specimen is representative of bladder urine and to reduce the risk of contamination by extraneous bacteria and other materials.

To obtain a midstream specimen the patient begins voiding into the toilet, catches 1-2 ounces (30-60 mL) of urine in a container, and then finishes voiding into the toilet. (In contrast, when the urine will be tested by DNA probe or other methods for microorganisms in urethral cells, the first portion of urine passed must be preserved.) Women patients are instructed to cleanse around the urethral meatus with cotton balls saturated with antiseptic to remove any vaginal secretions, including menstrual blood.

Chapter 22. Immunology

FILL IN THE BLANKS

1. immunology
2. serology
3. complement fixation (CF)
4. radioimmunoassay (RIA)
5. enzyme-linked immunosorbent assay (ELISA)
6. nonspecific antigens
7. VDRL, RPR (rapid plasma reagin)
8. cold agglutinins
9. LE cell
10. wheal, pseudopods

MULTIPLE CHOICE

1. B   6. E
2. D   7. E
3. C   8. D
4. A   9. A
5. B   10. C

SHORT ANSWERS

1. Define or explain.
   a. convalescent serum—a four-fold rise in the titer of antibody to the infecting organism from the acute phase specimen to a specimen drawn two weeks later in the convalescing phase.
   b. febrile agglutinins—sometimes performed in cases of fever of unknown origin, a typical panel includes agglutination titers for typhoid (Widal O and H), paratyphoid, brucellosis, tularemia, leptospirosis, and rickettsiae (Weil-Felix).
   c. STS—serologic test for syphilis; sometimes the term "serology" is used to refer to this test.
2. What basic type of reaction is studied in a serologic test?
   The identification of an antibody or an antigen by bringing about an antigen-antibody reaction under controlled conditions.
3. What are some reasons for preferring serologic testing to culture of pathogenic microorganisms?
   Serologic testing is often easier, less expensive, faster, and more specific than routine procedures for isolation and identification of infecting organisms, particularly viruses.
4. List three purposes for serologic testing.
   a. to identify acute infections due to certain bacteria, fungi, viruses, and parasites
   b. to detect immunity to certain pathogenic organisms resulting from prior infection or from administration of vaccine
   c. to diagnose some noninfectious diseases, particularly autoimmune disorders and neoplasms
5. Give an example of a diagnostic antibody test that uses a nonspecific antigen.
   Sheep or horse red blood cells that react with heterophile antibodies in infectious mononucleosis.
6. List some serologic tests that are used to diagnose diseases or conditions that are not infections.
   Radioallergosorbent test (RAST) is useful in diagnosing allergies; the lupus erythematosus cell test (LE cell prep), antinuclear antibody (ANA), and rheumatoid factor (RF) to diagnose autoimmune disorders, and serologic tests for AFP, CEA to diagnose neoplasms.
7. When several methods may be available to detect and measure a given antigen or antibody, including molecular biology methods, what then does the choice of method depend on?
   The cost, the availability of materials, equipment, and trained personnel, the volume of testing performed by the laboratory, turnaround time, relative sensitivity and specificity of procedures, and other factors.
8. What is the fluorescent antibody technique useful for? Describe the procedure.
   Fluorescent antibody technique is valuable in identifying intracellular organisms, such as *Chlamydia*, which stain poorly if at all by standard staining techniques. A smear is treated with a combination of monoclonal antibody to a suspected organism and a fluorescent dye such as rhodamine. If the anticipated antigen-antibody reaction occurs, sites of fixation of the fluorescent antibody can be observed by microscopic examination of the smear with fluorescent lighting.
9. Describe the method of using serial dilutions to determine antibody titer. Is this a qualitative or quantitative analysis?
   A row of test tubes are prepared in which each tube contains a higher dilution of serum or specimen material than the one before it. Test material is added to each tube, and the results of the test are reported as the highest dilution of serum in which antibody activity can still be detected. A report of 1:200 means that antibody activity occurred in all tubes up to and including the one containing the 1:200 dilution of serum, but not at 1:400 or higher dilutions. This is a quantitative analysis.
10. Which test gets its name based on a pun? Explain.
   A man named Southern gave his name to a method of locating specific DNA sequences by blotting the specimen to a membrane; later a similar method for identifying RNA was named the Northern blot. When a third blotting procedure was developed, it was called the Western blot.

Chapter 23. Molecular Biology

FILL IN THE BLANKS

1. molecular biology
2. heredity, DNA molecule
3. DNA probe
4. fluorescent in situ hybridization
5. genital warts
6. human papillomavirus (HPV)
7. atypical squamous cells of undetermined significance (ASC-US), low-grade squamous intraepithelial lesion (LGSIL)
8. chromosomes
9. two X, an X and a Y
10. mitosis
11. long arm (q), a short arm (p)
12. recessive
13. mutation
14. aneuploidy
15. tumor suppressor gene
16. BRCA1, BRCA2
17. amniocentesis.

MULTIPLE CHOICE

1. B	10. B
2. A	11. A
3. D	12. E
4. D	13. D
5. C	14. C
6. A	15. A
7. B	16. B
8. E	17. B
9. C	

SHORT ANSWERS

1. Define or explain.
   a. codon—a sequence of three bases (for example, AAG or CUG) that conveys a distinct piece of chemical information; most direct the incorporation of specific amino acids into a polypeptide chain, but a few direct chain initiation or chain termination.
   b. gene—a segment of a DNA molecule, the unit of heredity.
   c. karyotype—a form on which cut-outs of photographs of individual chromosomes are pasted in a standard order, autosomes 1 to 22 followed by

sex chromosomes (X and, if one is present, Y).
   d. oncogene—a gene whose possession confers an increased risk of cancer.
   e. polymerase chain reaction—a method for the repeated copying of DNA in a particular gene sequence, widely used to amplify very small quantities of biological material so as to provide adequate specimens for laboratory study.
   f. viral load—the number of copies of viral RNA per mL of plasma, it indicates the prognosis of persons infected with HIV and helps in deciding when to start antiretroviral therapy, and to assess the response to therapy.

2. List three nonmedical applications of molecular biology.
   a. determining paternity and maternity
   b. establishing the identity of an individual
   c. matching biological material left at a crime scene with that of a suspect

3. Explain the difference between a recessive gene and a dominant gene.
   A dominant gene expresses the trait for which it is coded even when paired with a gene that is not identical to it. Traits associated with recessive genes are expressed only when both genes at a given locus are be identical. If a recessive gene appears on only one chromosome of a pair, the trait for which it codes is not expressed.

4. How does polymerase chain reaction technology improve the sensitivity of laboratory testing?
   In PCR, very small quantities of biological material can be amplified by combining specimen DNA with specially designed primers which are then enzymatically induced to replicate many times. Replication can be triggered repeatedly by changing the temperature of the system, each cycle yielding many

copies of the DNA strands produced in the previous cycle. PCR technology is thus highly sensitive and highly specific, and does not require prior purification

5. What are some reasons for doing prenatal genetic testing?
   Advanced maternal age (which increases the risk of Down syndrome), genetic disease in either parent, a history of a birth defect with a previous pregnancy, and abnormal findings on prenatal ultrasound examination.

6. How does cell division in gametes differ from that of non-gamete cells?
   In nongamete cells, daughter cells are formed by a process called mitosis, splitting into two identical cells with identical nuclei and identical chromosomes. In sex cells, the chromosome pairs divide by a process called meiosis, so that each daughter cell has only 23 chromosomes instead of 23 pairs of chromosomes. When sperm and oocyte unite, the full complement of 23 pairs of chromosomes is restored, one of each pair having come from each parent.

7. List and explain three aberrations that can occur in the process by which chromosomes divide up during meiosis and then pair off after conception.
   a. Translocation is an interchange of fragments between two chromosomes.
   b. Inversion means that a fragment broken off from a chromosome has rotated end-for-end before reattaching.
   c. Deletion is the complete loss of part of a chromosome.

Chapter 24. Examination of Urine, Stool, and Other Fluids and Materials

FILL IN THE BLANKS

1. first-voided specimen
2. blood cells in urine rupture early, bacterial growth in a standing specimen may alter its chemical composition

3. smoky brown color, Coca-Cola
4. high-power field
5. squamous epithelial cells (squames), amorphous sediment
6. dipstick, reagent
7. albuminuria
8. glycosuria
9. bilirubinuria, hemolysis or liver disease
10. sodium, potassium, chloride
11. microalbuminuria (microproteinuria)
12. diabetic nephropathy
13. vitamin B12, pernicious anemia
14. antacids, vitamin C, red meat, horseradish
15. viral encephalitis, meningitis, tuberculous meningitis
16. pyogenic (bacterial) meningitis, encephalitis, brain abscess
17. intracranial hemorrhage, traumatic tap
18. increased, reduced
19. transudate, exudate
20. septic arthritis

MULTIPLE CHOICE

1.	B	12.	B
2.	C	13.	C
3.	E	14.	E
4.	E	15.	C
5.	A	16.	D
6.	D	17.	D
7.	A	18.	A
8.	C	19.	B
9.	B	20.	C
10.	D	21.	E
11.	A	22.	D

SHORT ANSWERS

1. Define or explain.
   a. choluria—the appearance of bilirubin in the urine, also called bilirubinuria.
   b. clean catch—a clean-voided specimen obtained after cleansing the area around the urethral meatus (usually with liquid soap and cotton balls) to prevent contamination of the specimen with material from outside the urinary tract.
   c. glycosuria—glucose in the urine, generally an indication of an abnormal elevation of plasma glucose, a cardinal finding in diabetes mellitus.
   d. lumbar puncture—spinal tap, a method of obtaining cerebrospinal fluid for cell count, chemical testing, and smear and culture.
   e. occult blood—blood present in insufficient quantity to alter the color of the urine.
   f. pyuria—pus in the urine.
   g. specific gravity—the weight of a liquid compared to distilled water, it varies in direct proportion to the concentration of dissolved materials.

2. What procedures can be used to limit contamination of a urine specimen by cells or secretions from outside the urinary tract?
   Obtaining a clean-voided specimen after cleansing the area around the urethral meatus (usually with liquid soap and cotton balls) to prevent contamination of the specimen with material from outside the urinary tract, obtaining a midstream specimen, or obtaining a catheterized specimen.

3. What examinations make up the standard urinalysis?
   Direct observation of the specimen for color, turbidity, and other obvious characteristics; determination of specific gravity; microscopic examination of sediment for cells, crystals, and other formed elements; determination of pH; and chemical testing for glucose, protein, occult blood, and perhaps bilirubin and acetone.

4. What is the origin of casts in the urine?
   Casts are microscopic cylindrical bodies that have been formed by concretion of cells or insoluble material within renal tubules and subsequently excreted in the urine. Casts are always abnormal.

5. What conditions other than diabetes mellitus may account for the appearance of glucose in the urine?
   It can occur after rapid absorption of dietary glucose (alimentary glycosuria) and in some persons with abnormally low renal thresholds for glucose (renal glycosuria).

6. List some constituents of urine for which analysis requires collection of a 24-hour specimen.
   Electrolytes (sodium, potassium, chloride), calcium and phosphorus, albumin (protein), amino acids, copper, acid mucopolysaccharides (AMP), amylase, coproporphyrin, delta-aminolevulinic acid.

7. What two factors might account for an alkaline pH in the urine?
   The pH might be as much as 8 for the person who is a vegetarian or has a *Proteus* urinary tract infection.

8. What constituent of the stool is likely to be increased in malabsorption syndromes?
   Fat (steatorrhea is malabsorption of fat).

9. Which tests are routinely performed on stool specimens?
   Qualitative analysis for occult blood and fat; quantitative determination of urobilinogen; smears for leukocytes, parasites, and parasite ova; Gram stain for pathogenic organisms; and culture in infectious diarrheas.

10. What routine examinations are performed on cerebrospinal fluid?
    White blood cell count, red blood cell count (if any), total protein concentration. Spinal fluid is examined by smear and culture for pathogenic microorganisms, and immunologic study for antigens or antibodies indicative of specific pathogens, autoimmune disorders, or certain neoplasms.

11. In what conditions are abnormalities of gastric acid secretion noted?
    Gastric acid secretion is increased in duodenal ulcer and greatly

increased in Zollinger-Ellison syndrome. It is decreased or absent in gastric carcinoma, achlorhydria, and pernicious anemia.

12. What diagnostic procedures can be performed on amniotic fluid?

Elevation of alpha-fetoprotein (AFP) occurs in neural tube defects (anencephaly, spina bifida). The lecithin/sphingomyelin ratio, determined by thin-layer chromatography, is less than 1.0 before fetal lungs mature, more than 1.0 when lung maturity has been attained.